Bite Back

The publisher and the University of California Press Foundation gratefully acknowledge the generous support of the Anne G. Lipow Endowment Fund in Social Justice and Human Rights.

Bite Back

PEOPLE TAKING ON CORPORATE FOOD
AND WINNING

*Edited by Saru Jayaraman and
Kathryn De Master*

Foreword by Marion Nestle

UNIVERSITY OF CALIFORNIA PRESS

University of California Press
Oakland, California

© 2020 by the Regents of the University of California

Library of Congress Cataloging-in-Publication Data

Names: Jayaraman, Sarumathi, 1975– editor. | De Master, Kathryn, 1966–
    editor. | Nestle, Marion, writer of foreword.
Title: Bite back : people taking on corporate food and winning / edited by
    Saru Jayaraman and Kathryn De Master ; foreword by Marion Nestle.
Description: Oakland, California : University of California Press, [2020] |
    Includes bibliographical references and index.
Identifiers: LCCN 2019041691 (print) | LCCN 2019041692 (ebook) |
    ISBN 9780520289352 (cloth) | ISBN 9780520289369 (paperback) |
    ISBN 9780520964051 (ebook)
Subjects: LCSH: Food security—United States. | Food industry and trade—
    United States.
Classification: LCC TX360.U6 B549 2020 (print) | LCC TX360.U6 (ebook) |
    DDC 338.4/76640973—dc23
LC record available at https://lccn.loc.gov/2019041691
LC ebook record available at https://lccn.loc.gov/2019041692

Manufactured in the United States of America

28 27 26 25 24 23 22 21 20
10 9 8 7 6 5 4 3 2 1

CONTENTS

FOREWORD

Our food system—how we produce, process, distribute, and consume food—is broken, and badly. We know this because roughly a billion people in the world go hungry every day for lack of a reliable food supply while, perversely, about two billion are overweight and at increased risk for chronic diseases. All of us bear the consequences of atmospheric warming due, in part, to greenhouse gases released from industrial production of the animals, plants, and products we eat.

It is true that a great many factors have contributed to the breakdown of our food system, but one in particular stands out as a cause: the companies that produce our food put profits above the health and well-being of the public. Capitalism demands that food corporations prioritize their fiduciary responsibilities to stockholders.

If we want to reverse this priority, we are going to have to get organized, mobilize, and act. *Bite Back* tells us how.

Bite Back is a manifesto. It is a call to action to reverse the many harms caused by the corporate takeover of our food system. It is an advocacy manual for, as Kathryn De Master and Saru Jayaraman put it, "disrupting corporate power through food democracy." It is a guidebook for empowering all of us to resist corporate power and to collectively make our own decisions about how to create a food system that best prevents hunger, improves health, and reverses climate change.

The operative phrase here is "food democracy." This book embeds democracy in its very structure. Each part of the book contains two chapters. The first chapter focuses on how Wall Street's requirement that corporations stress profit over the public good has harmed workers, undermined small farmers, imperiled health, damaged the environment, and imposed highly processed "junk" foods on world populations.

The second chapter in each part is about democracy in action. Each highlights the work of individuals or groups who have resisted corporate power—and succeeded in doing so. Here, we see how community organizing, grassroots advocacy, and genuine leadership can stop or reverse some of the more egregious corporate damage. These chapters make it clear that advocacy can succeed. They demonstrate that resistance to corporate power is not only necessary; it is also *possible*.

The food movement in the United States has been criticized for its focus on personal food access rather than on mobilizing individuals and groups to gain real political power. Why, for example, do we not see a grassroots political movement emerging among participants in federal food assistance programs to demand better-paying jobs, safer communities, and better schools? I'm guessing that the power imbalance of such efforts seems too discouraging. This book aims to redress that imbalance by providing accounts of real change.

Bite Back presents voices from the food movement, all deeply passionate about their causes. Read here about the importance of grassroots organizing, why advocates must stay eternally vigilant to maintain the gains they have won, and why uniting advocacy organizations into strong coalitions is essential for gaining political power.

A particular gift is the afterword, which is anything but an afterthought. Subtitled "Taking Action to Create Change," it is a superb summary of the principal elements of successful advocacy. It explains the basic tools of community organizing—setting goals, building organizations and coalitions, identifying the people who can make desired changes, developing strategies and tactics, and gaining real power—and how to obtain and use those tools.

Together, these elements make *Bite Back* essential reading for anyone who longs for a food system healthier for people and the environment. This book is an inspiration for food advocates and potential advocates. Join organizations! Vote! Run for office! Whatever you do, get busy and act. Our food system and the world will be better—much better—as a result.

Marion Nestle
New York City
December 2019

Introduction

Kathryn De Master and Saru Jayaraman

CORPORATE POWER. Taming its relentless influence in our political systems, markets, and communities has been described as the "key political issue of our age."[1] Corporate power has grown rapidly over the last seventy years, first sparked by market deregulation and privatization in the decades following World War II, and then accelerating with President Ronald Reagan's "trickle-down" economics in the 1980s.[2] Today, corporations wield unbalanced power over our democracy, winning the right to operate as legal persons,[3] spend enormous amounts of money on political campaigns to curry the favor of politicians,[4] and use revolving doors in which corporate leaders influence or even control the very agencies that are intended to regulate them.

The food system is no exception to the advance of corporate power. In the last seventy years, as we have witnessed the industrialization and globalization of the food system, agrofood corporations have progressively expanded their reach and solidified their influence. Today nearly every food sector from farm gate to dinner plate is dominated by a handful of corporations that have restructured food production, reshaped markets, and radically altered what we eat.[5]

Like other multinational corporations in the United States, agrofood firms enjoy the protected constitutional rights of legal persons: they can sue and be sued, enter into contracts, make donations to political action committees, and even exercise some of the same religious freedoms that are granted to individuals. These rights and freedoms have allowed food corporations to protect their own interests and those of their shareholders over public goods, such as protecting workers and the environment. Indeed, food firms have a fiduciary *responsibility* to benefit their shareholders first.

In decades past, a clear vision of the corporate takeover of our food system was sometimes obscured by efforts to hold corporate power in check, through the enforcement of antitrust legislation, labor laws, environmental regulation, and campaign finance rules. Claiming to be "good corporate citizens," food firms also trumpeted their contributions to economic growth and "corporate social responsibility." McDonald's touted its recycled packaging, Starbucks its green-friendly cups, and Monsanto its climate-smart agriculture. Debates among scholars and activist groups focused on whether such efforts represented meaningful reform or simply proverbial lipstick-on-a-pig rebranding.

Now, however, such debates appear pointless, even naive. Pro-corporate tax giveaways have made it abundantly transparent not only that corporate elites hold the reins of economic and political power in the US and globally, but also that they do so *unapologetically*. While the current US political administration epitomizes unapologetic corporate elitism, the political and economic power grab of the Trump administration represents only the latest of a longstanding series of onslaughts to our democracy and our food system that have been documented by analysts for decades. Indeed, when David Korten first published the seminal contribution *When Corporations Rule the World* in 1995, he was referencing a longstanding series of economic trends that had been set in motion by the Bretton Woods institutions fifty years earlier.

As scholars and activists have extensively documented, corporate control and consolidation in the agrofood system is the norm, not the exception.[6] How have corporations typically consolidated their power in the US agrofood system? Most scholarly analyses of corporate concentration and power have examined discrete sectors to attempt to answer that question. For example, William Heffernan and Mary Hendrickson's foundational studies revealed how the concentration and vertical integration in the poultry, hog, and beef sectors completely transformed the meat industry, gradually eroding the decision-making power and freedoms of individual farmers.[7] More recently, our coauthors in this book, Wenonah Hauter and Phil Howard, have expanded upon these analyses of agriculture and food systems consolidation into extensive studies of many components of the agrofood supply chain—from seeds to grocery retailers to soda to beer to wine to the organic sector to dairy consolidation and more.[8] One important contribution these studies have made is demonstrating the ways in which concentration and vertical integration create conditions that allow corporate power structures to thrive. If a corporation controls an entire supply chain, it effectively creates a powerful monopoly or an oligopoly.

New trends in financial speculation, as well as an unprecedented number of corporate mergers and acquisitions, mean that food corporations are also increasingly entangled with one another, and even across food sectors. The boundaries between, say, Smithfield Foods and Perdue, or between Tesco and Walmart, or between Monsanto and Syngenta and Bayer, are increasingly blurry. While such firms may ostensibly compete with one another, their control of markets through the horizontal and vertical integration of their respective supply chains fosters oligopolies in which actual competition is extremely limited.

The result is that a mere ten companies now control the products on our grocery store shelves.[9] Three firms control nearly two-thirds of the market share of seeds.[10] Four corporations control over 60 percent of all chicken consumed in the US, dictating the terms of production for hundreds of contract poultry producers who can no longer compete with larger firms.[11] Four packing firms control over 70 percent of the pork market, while the top four beef-packing firms control roughly 85 percent of the market.[12] Ten corporations control over 50 percent of the fertilizer market globally.[13] Four companies control around 80 percent of cereal sales, even though nearly 250 varieties can be found in a typical cereal aisle.[14] Indeed, the illusion of consumer choice is carefully crafted through nearly limitless product offerings. From restaurants to soybean fields, from lettuce warehouses to factory hog farms, and from seed companies to supermarkets, corporate power increasingly determines what happens throughout our food system.

Members of the corporate elite often make their decisions from arm's length. Most leaders of food corporations, for example, do not trudge through muddy cow pastures, but those investors today are nevertheless catalyzing a blizzard of rural land reorganization through new forms of farmland speculation. Leaders of the National Restaurant Association do not wait tables for a living, but they nevertheless benefited when the Trump administration in fall 2017 declared tips the property of restaurant owners, not workers. Policymakers who decided that certain cancer-causing pesticides are legal and safe—after being lobbied by the manufacturers of those same pesticides—do not apply those chemicals to vegetable crops with backpack sprayers. And unlike the farmworkers of Earlimart, California (whom Jill Harrison describes in this book), elites typically live safely distant from pesticide drift. Such decision-making dominance in the food system is an exercise in *sovereignty*—one that has been methodically wrested from farm-workers, wait staff, and eaters.

To quell any resistance to this system, corporate messaging pervades nearly all media, as companies work to create loyal consumer acolytes. Most people in America are lulled into acquiescence through exposure to over 350 advertisements and approximately five thousand corporate messages daily.[15] Sloganeering—"Have it your way," "Eat fresh," "Lovin' it!"—keeps us primed to consume. Objections to this messaging are met with reminders of what Jack Kloppenburg, an organizer for the Open Source Seed Initiative, has called the "planetary patriotism" of agribusiness firms: promises of grand solutions to global crises ranging from climate change to hunger.[16]

This process—one in which corporations now have widespread control over most aspects of human sustenance—has been presented as natural, desirable, and inevitable. We contend that it is not.

In this book, we present a vision for disrupting corporate power through food democracy—a vision in which people affected by decisions made about their food system have voice, power, and agency to collectively influence those decisions. This vision is not new. We share it with countless advocates for food system change: labor organizers battling for workplace equity, anti-hunger advocates disrupting corporate charity, farmers protesting petro-chemical regimes, public plant breeders combatting germplasm privatization, and nearly two hundred million smallholder peasants worldwide who are fighting for food sovereignty.

We argue that achieving a democratic food system—one characterized by justice and sovereignty for producers, workers, and consumers—is not a trickle-down proposition. Rather, it foments up. Impolitely. It is nothing short of a rebellion.

We contend that such a rebellion involves interrogating three prevailing narratives often perpetuated about corporate power in the agrofood system. The first is what we term the "inevitability" narrative. In this familiar canard, corporations figure prominently as modern-day economic Goliaths—giants that march throughout the globe, crushing all who stand in their path. While it is true that many corporate monoliths now dominate, to assume the *inevitability* of that power overlooks history. It fails to account for the hundreds of ways that social movements have organized to powerfully combat myriad injustices—from slavery to structural racism and sexism to environmental destruction to workplace abuses. It also treats corporations like forces of nature to which immutable laws of physics apply. But as Jane Collins has incisively reminded us, there is nothing natural or inevitable about globalized corporate economic power, and viewing it "as an abstract force lets real actors off the hook. Globalization is not a ghost, and it is not like gravity. It is made up of decisions and actions, struggles and negotiations carried out in a large number of specific places where people live and work."[17] This inevitability myth misleads through cynicism, ignoring the ways that the targeted organizing of social movements can achieve, and has achieved, social and environmental change.

The second prevailing food system narrative we interrogate with this book is the "vote with our fork" solution. This model for change suggests that corporate power can—and should—be addressed by simply opting out of the current morally bankrupt system. Eating differently. Scholars and activists have repeatedly offered impressively robust critiques of the inherent limitations of this approach, but this popular narrative is nevertheless remarkably persistent.[18] We see it in endorsements of the host of initiatives focused on producing and consuming locally sourced, healthy, and ecologically sustainable food, specifically when those endorsements fail to recognize the need for structural change. Celebrations of the "local food" or "good food" movement abound: in a spate of popular blogs, books, and articles; at farmers' markets; in restaurants showcasing local foods; and on cooking shows. In the last twenty years, local food, organics, CSAs, and farmers' markets have spread like wildfire, catalyzing enthusiastic popular support for an alternative food system. But while efforts to build alternatives are exciting and laudable, the cost of alternative foods remains out of reach for most Americans— including many of the workers who produce them. Many alternatives rely on a conscientious, well-heeled consumer culture. And in spite of enthusiasm for local, organic, and "good" food offerings, and the exciting growth of alternative food systems, thus far the impact of such alternatives remains relatively modest, with the market for alternative food still a small fraction of the overall food market in the United States. More importantly, those advocating for alternative food systems have little or no ability to regulate conventional food systems. In fact, conventional food system actors continue to wield so much power as to influence the legal definitions of concepts such as "organic" by lobbying standards-setting bodies such as the USDA. Also, in some cases—as we see, for example, with organic agriculture— alternatives can be frequently overtaken by the same corporate structures and systems they initially set out to oppose.[19] Absent meaningful structural change, well-intended alternatives can easily replicate wage inequities, reproduce environmentally extractive farming practices, perpetuate racism and sexism, and create market oligopolies.

Importantly, vote-with-our-fork solutions can also too easily reinforce the idea that the only power people have to effect change in the food system is confined to *mere* consumption. This limiting narrative is one that many corporations will happily support. It reinforces what Korten in 1995 termed the "elitist ideology of individualism." The more that people identify as mere consumers, rather than active, informed participants in society and policy, the more corporations can expand their reach. Indeed, through buyouts of organic and health food companies, corporations are already profiting from niche markets. But the collective power of people to rebel against the corporate status quo should not be reduced to buying organic arugula or cooking heirloom squash soup. Rather, balancing the scales of power between people and corporations will require a great deal more than shopping and eating differently. Achieving food justice will involve confronting powerful elite corporate actors who control our food system and demanding change through social movement organizing and political struggle.

The third prevailing narrative we interrogate with this book is the idea that the organizing and political struggle involved in attaining food justice can be confined to a "food movement." We argue that the term "food movement" is often used easily and uncritically and has been too loosely conflated with shopping and eating differently. Moreover, we submit that building a social movement to combat corporate power in the food system will involve not simply changing prevailing food systems alone. Rather, it must involve diverse, intersectional alliances and coalitions with other groups that are also experiencing injustices and threats to their livelihoods by corporate power. In much the same way that we cannot reduce the food movement to changing what is on our individual plates, we also cannot confine a movement to challenge corporate dominance and achieve more democratic decision-making to food systems alone. We suggest that in this particular political moment, people engaged in changing the injustices of the food system must also ally and organize with social movement efforts to battle corporate power *outside* the "food movement." These alliances necessarily involve centering the lived experiences of those who are most marginalized by corporate domination: Indigenous Peoples, persons of color, and people with limited financial means, to name only a few.

Many of these efforts have been successful and inspiring. From groups such as Occupy, to those engaged in Fight for $15, to coalitions fighting against the American Legislative and Exchange Council (ALEC), to critical battles for racial justice like Black Lives Matter and gender equity through #MeToo, people are standing up to corporations and the powerful elite who control them, and they are achieving victories. While not advocating the elimination of corporations, these groups have worked to reduce undue and unregulated corporate influence over our democracy and our lives in order to achieve greater collective prosperity. The successes described by the authors of this book aim to inspire advocates to work for more structural change *within* the food system, but in ways that also forge productive alliances with those outside of it.

With the examples they share in each "part," or section, of *Bite Back,* the authors propose a counternarrative to the inevitability and vote-with-your-fork narratives, and we aim to add to the many early and incisive analyses of corporate power by presenting this counternarrative in detail. The case studies demonstrate success in *biting back*—winning policy or programmatic changes that balance the outsized influence of food corporations over our democracy. They also interrogate the notion that food systems organizers can attain policy or campaign victories without alliances that intersect with other efforts to impede corporate power. The descriptive accounts of each victory provide critical organizing tools for advocates. These successes provide a persuasive argument that the struggle against corporate power is not only possible—it has been successful. The case studies provided by the authors herein demonstrate how people who organize *can, have,* and *will* reduce corporate control over our democracy and our food system to increase equity, sovereignty, and sustainability.

As we highlight these examples, we endeavor to make several contributions with this book. First, each part of the book unites scholars and activists in a format that invites productive, collaborative conversations between the two groups. We seek to highlight both the voices of those who study and analyze the food system and the voices of those directly engaged in changing it. Importantly, we also recognize that the categories of "scholar" and "activist" are not tidy, narrow identities. Instead, we see exciting potential for breaking down often-entrenched boundaries between academies and communities through new conversations in which scholars also advocate for change and advocacy groups engage in robust research and the dissemination of knowledge. In this book, we celebrate the fact that the authors do not speak with a single, uniform voice. Rather, each of the nearly two dozen contributors to this book offers a rare and irreplaceable perspective on food systems, reflecting the diverse set of skills, abilities, insights, and commitments that will be necessary to achieve food democracy.

Second, this book is structured topically to highlight particular agrofood sectors where corporate influence is evident and victories have been achieved. With the topical arrangement of the book—seeds, pesticides, extraction, labor, health, hunger, and trade—we intend to show a range of strategies for combatting corporate power throughout food systems. While this case-study approach presents an overview of several key food system sectors, the subjects highlighted herein are not intended to be comprehensive. For example, some of our topics represent timely, specific challenges to food and farming—such as the rapid trends in seed industry consolidation or the swift advance of unconventional natural gas drilling (a.k.a fracking) into rural communities in nearly half of the states in the US. Other topics represent broad, ongoing challenges to food justice—such as the corporate influence in international trade and anti-hunger efforts. We have prioritized sharing cases for which there are key successes in combatting corporate power while also recognizing there is no standardized prescription for success. Social movement organizing is not a one-size-fits-all proposition. Moreover, though we highlight some food sectors where significant gains or successes have been achieved in combatting corporate power and influence, we recognize that there are many food system sectors in which successes are forthcoming, or for which the fight against corporate domination is particularly challenging and entrenched and will involve sustained efforts or new approaches.

Finally, each part of the book is structured in a unique call-and-response style. The first chapter in each part is devoted to presenting problems and injustices linked to corporate power in a particular part of the food system: wage inequities, environmental destruction, and corporate bullying, to name a few. The authors of these chapters detail ways that corporations have influenced the very boards and bodies intended to regulate them. They describe new forms of corporate collusion and consolidation resulting from now-widespread takeovers and rebranding, as well as the consequent illusion of choice and competition perpetuated by food firms. But the story does not end there.

The second chapter in each part highlights a particular story of success—how organizers, activists, and community members have combatted injustices—and describes strategies that have been successful. Within these case studies there are also lessons that show how people can effectively oppose this corporate power, even without the financial clout and privileges enjoyed by powerful corporate elites. The authors of these chapters share successful stories of resistance and strategies that people in coalitions have employed to organize together and win.

So, for example, in the first of the two chapters focusing on seeds, Phil Howard details how agribusiness firms have increasingly and methodically consolidated the seed sector through buyouts and takeovers, resulting in the mere appearance of choice for farmers seeking diverse seed inputs. In the second chapter on seeds, Kiki Hubbard of the Organic Seed Alliance describes how alliances supporting organic seed and public plant breeding are working to combat the trend of corporate privatization of genetic resources.

In the next section of the book, on pesticide drift, Jill Harrison describes the way that corporations control the decisions about what, how, and where pesticides will be applied to our food crops, such that they frequently drift into nearby communities, sickening residents. Emily Marquez, Marcia Ishii-Eiteman, and Kristin Schafer with the Pesticide Action Network then describe the organized citizen science work of those who document pesticide drift using the Drift Catcher air-monitoring device in an effort to hold corporations accountable for the way that these chemicals pollute vulnerable communities.

Next, Kathryn De Master and Stephanie Malin tell the story of Pennsylvania dairy farmers—one echoed in many agricultural communities today—who face a "devil's bargain" between two corporate sectors, energy and agriculture, as the widespread march of unconventional natural gas extraction fuels a rapid transformation of rural landscapes and livelihoods. Wenonah Hauter and Seth Gladstone then describe their successful campaign to keep fracking companies out of New York State just across the border. They show how farmers and community organizers mobilized to effect political and regulatory change in spite of powerful opposition.

In the labor chapters, Joann Lo and Jose Oliva document worker exploitation in the food system, while Saru Jayaraman details how exploited workers are successfully pushing back against corporate domination by organizing for higher wages, benefits like paid sick days, and health and safety concessions on the job.

In the section on health, Kristine Madsen and Wendi Gosliner show how the industrial diet that corporations have created disregards the health of those who consume their products. Anna Lappé and Kelle Louaillier then show inspiring ways to combat the corporate diet, as they describe Corporate Accountability's successful campaign against McDonald's assault on America's health, and in particular the "Happy Meal," which targets children.

Next, Andy Fisher writes about the corporate production of hunger in America, showing how corporations through philanthropy have increasingly influenced anti-hunger organizations. Jim Araby then provides an inspiring example of how to bite back against corporate influence in anti-hunger work, describing the successful work of the United Food and Commercial Workers Union partnering with food advocacy and other community groups to achieve multiple statewide policy victories in California.

Finally, as Raj Patel and Maywa Montenegro de Wit detail in our concluding section, international trade agreements such as the Trans-Pacific Partnership reflect the enmeshed relationship between corporate power and global economic trade. Yet as small-scale farmer Ayumi Kinezuka and coauthor Montenegro de Wit show us, Japanese smallholder farmers—members of the increasingly powerful international food sovereignty movement—are mobilizing to resist corporate power's involvement in international trade.

It is notable that this final section is the only one describing challenges and organizing occurring outside of the United States. Of course, the growth in power and influence of multinational corporations is a global phenomenon that has resulted in the exploitation of people and the planet for corporate profit worldwide. However, this phenomenon is experienced differently around the world, and these differences are especially notable with regard to each nation's regulation of corporate activity. We focus mostly on the United States in this book not only because it is where we live and work, and where many agrofood corporations are headquartered, but also because the United States provides an extreme example of deregulation and corporate influence over democratic practice. Organizing to bite back against corporate power can be difficult everywhere, and is also growing increasingly difficult in the United States as corporations wield increasing power over electoral campaigns, the media, and public institutions. The examples provided here illustrate biting back against corporate power in the face of eroding democratic principles.

Not all of the authors in this book detail the same kinds of organizing campaigns. Some involve legislative policy advocacy. Others involve direct confrontation and focus on campaigns to change particular corporations' practices. Others show the importance of links to larger social movements, policy change, shifts in trade regimes, and efforts to transform entire agrofood sectors. But all reflect some form of social movement organizing practice as defined by a vast social movement literature: mobilizing a base of directly affected individuals with limited resources to engage in contentious direct action (protest activity) targeted at those with power over their lives (in this case, corporations and the elected officials they control) for concrete improvements in the food system and in people's lives.[20] As the case studies in this book illuminate, subsequent steps toward agrofood system transformation will involve sustained, engaged, and targeted organizing efforts.

Historically we know that people create social movements to achieve transformational change through sustained, collective actions that target those in power. Effective social movements radically disrupt the status quo in our political systems, society, and economy. They often create coalitions with unlikely partners aligned in their dedication to intersecting values and priorities. People in social movements recognize that their power is collective and collaborative, not atomized. Social movements also *demand* change—and they *achieve* it.

What would organizing an effective social movement in food systems look like? If we revisit the Goliath analogy—inspired by the diverse campaigns described in this book—we imagine it will look like felling stones from countless slingshots. These stones may entail, for example, people organizing to increase antitrust regulation and then holding policymakers accountable for that enforcement through public pressure. This organizing could look like direct actions in front of corporations seeking to consolidate, or in front of meetings of regulatory bodies tasked with enforcing antitrust regulation in the moment of a proposed merger. It might look like large numbers of affected people—small producers, community members, workers, and others—engaging in direct actions against corporations that hurt people and the environment. These direct-action protest activities could occur in corporate boardrooms, at factory farms, and in the political spaces in which these corporations attempt to change regulations in their favor.

Ultimately, an organizing vision for food democracy would include a diverse coalition of affected peoples targeting corporate power collectively, with a unified set of demands. Each chapter of this book shows ways that some of this activity is already beginning to emerge and take shape. But much more sustained action is needed to bite back and rebel against the corporate status quo and to fight for equity, sustainability, and collective prosperity. As you read the stories presented here in *Bite Back,* we hope they will inspire you to join us in this effort.

PART ONE

Seeds

CALL TO ACTION—
HOW CORPORATIONS CONTROL OUR SEEDS

Philip H. Howard

COLLECTIVE RESPONSE—
TAKING BACK OUR SEEDS

Kristina "Kiki" Hubbard

How Corporations Control Our Seeds

Philip H. Howard

IN OCTOBER 2016, Mike Wallace, an Arkansas farmer, was shot and killed by a man who worked for a neighboring farm. Just prior to this encounter, Wallace had argued with his killer over the phone, asserting that his soybean crop had been damaged by the herbicide dicamba after it had been applied to nearby fields and drifted to his farm. Wallace's neighbor had planted a new variety of soybean seed on his farm, released by the seed and chemical corporation Monsanto in 2016. Unlike Wallace's soybeans, this new soybean variety was genetically engineered to be resistant to damage from dicamba. Though a new and supposedly less drift-prone formulation of dicamba was approved for use for the 2017 growing season, for Wallace this was obviously too late. And it might not have helped in any case: even newer versions of dicamba (from Monsanto, as well as BASF and DuPont) were suspected of causing damage to millions of acres of nonresistant soybeans and other crops throughout 2017, just like the damage Wallace experienced. Some farmers and weed scientists have reported impacts from dicamba more than a mile away from its application, and they suspect that certain weather conditions allow the chemical to move long distances.

Although banned only in one state (Arkansas) during the 2018 growing season, dicamba was still being used illegally. Therefore, nearly all soybean farmers were under pressure to buy dicamba-tolerant seeds to prevent damage to their crops. This was true even for those farmers who preferred to grow non-GE (genetically engineered) crops. Farmers who plant crops other than soybeans or dicamba-tolerant cotton do not even have the option of purchasing dicamba-tolerant seeds, increasing the likelihood of conflicts between neighbors over damage from drifting dicamba. Monsanto has deflected blame for this crisis toward the farmers that buy their seeds, accusing them of not following the label instructions for applying this herbicide. Critics, however, have pointed out that the corporation took the unusual step of refusing to allow university researchers to fully test its new dicamba formulation, including testing its potential to vaporize and drift away from the application site, until after it was approved by the Environmental Protection Agency.

Why is this case important? Corporate control of the seed industry has continued to increase each year, as measured by both market share and political power, resulting in fewer and fewer people making decisions about the future of our food supply. Given that nearly all of the foods humans consume are derived directly from plants grown from seeds or indirectly via animals that consume plants, seeds arguably represent the most critical agricultural resource.

In the 1970s, the seed industry in the United States was composed of thousands of small, mostly family-owned companies in the United States.[1] At the time, Monsanto did not even sell seeds. By 2011, however, there were just a few hundred independent commodity seed companies remaining in the US, and one firm, Monsanto, was estimated to control more than one quarter of proprietary seed sales for the entire world.[2]

Here, I explore three questions related to increasing corporate involvement in the seed sector. I ask first, what changes have occurred in the industry as a result of corporate involvement? Second, what are the negative impacts of these changes? And finally, what factors are driving these trends?

WHAT CHANGES HAVE OCCURRED?

The inner workings of the seed industry are relatively hidden from public view. The majority of people in industrialized nations do not buy or plant seeds. People who do buy seeds directly typically obtain them from gardening-focused retailers, a highly competitive niche within the seed industry. As has been the case in many other sectors of the economy, however, dominant seed corporations have significantly increased their market share at both national and global levels in recent decades, and smaller firms have either been acquired or gone out of business.[3] Most corporations that make acquisitions do not disclose ownership ties on their packaging or marketing materials, making these consolidation trends difficult to notice and follow, even for those who work in the seed industry (see figure 1). Two additional trends include increasing corporate control of all types of seeds, in contrast

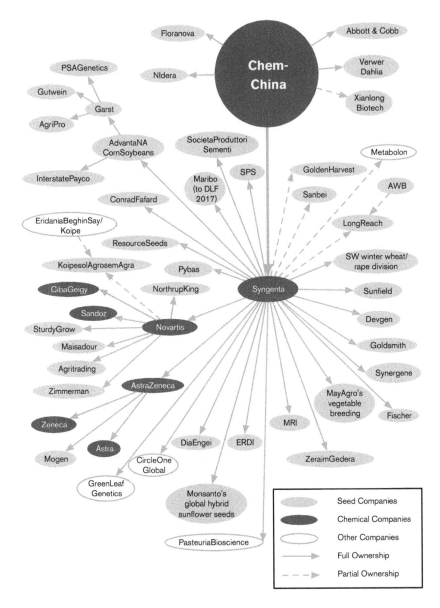

FIGURE I. Seed company ownership changes involving ChemChina and subsidiaries from 1996 to 2019. Credit: Philip H. Howard.

to an initial focus on just a few commodities, and increasingly tighter ties between the remaining, dominant firms.

Increased Market Share

Market share data from 2013 indicated that 55 percent of the global commercial seed market was controlled by Monsanto, DuPont, and Syngenta.[4] Notably, these are all agricultural chemical companies that expanded into seeds. Until 2017, these firms were part of the "Big Six" chemical companies, which together accounted for more than three-quarters of the global market for pesticides. In 2017, the Big Six was reduced to the "Big Four," when DuPont and Dow won US antitrust approval and completed a merger, renamed as Corteva. ChemChina also took ownership of the Swiss firm Syngenta in 2017, followed by the 2018 acquisition of US-headquartered Monsanto by a German firm, Bayer. The remaining firm, BASF of Germany, had previously focused on research and development of seed traits, but acquired a number of seed divisions from Bayer to enable regulatory approval of the Monsanto buyout.

This seed market concentration trend began in earnest in the 1970s, when corporations moving in from other sectors acquired scores of seed firms. Oil companies and grain traders were some of the first to expand into the seed industry, with the expectation that commodities like corn would become more profitable. By the late 1990s, these firms had largely been replaced by companies that manufactured and sold pesticides and fertilizers. The agricultural chemical industry was experiencing slowing rates of growth in industrialized countries as a result of environmental concerns that discouraged increasing rates of application.[5] Although the industry sought additional markets in developing countries, farmers in these countries lacked sufficient income to buy proprietary chemicals, and they also preferred less profitable generics. One corporate strategy in response to this dilemma was acquiring or merging with other firms in the industry. This allowed firms to essentially buy their way to increased market share.

This strategy eventually reduced the number of global agricultural chemical corporations; thirty firms in the 1970s had been combined into just six corporations by 2001.[6] However, such mergers failed to increase growth rates enough, when compared to other sectors of the economy. Corporations compete to increase their power relative to other firms, even though they may strenuously avoid competing in other arenas, such as lower retail prices.[7] In their efforts to escape the increasingly limited growth opportunities in the chemical industry and find other markets in which to expand their power, agricultural chemical corporations viewed seeds as a promising frontier. Technologies for herbicide-resistant crops were being developed, along with the possibility of tying the chemical corporations' proprietary chemicals to seeds. Oil companies and grain traders soon exited the industry because they did not have the patented technologies that would allow them to increase their market share to the same extent.[8]

These changes also triggered a number of defensive mergers and acquisitions involving remaining independent seed firms, as the rapidly growing number of farmers purchasing herbicide-tolerant corn and soybeans motivated independents to have access to these technologies. One example is the holding company American Seeds Incorporated, formed by Monsanto to buy regional corn and soybean companies. The subsidiary made more than two dozen acquisitions between 2004 and 2007, which allowed the smaller firms to incorporate Monsanto's patented traits into their seeds and also gave Monsanto control of their locally adapted germplasm.[9] Together, Monsanto and DuPont were estimated to account for 69 percent of corn seed sales and 58 percent of soybean seed sales in the US by 2010.[10] In recent years, with fewer independent firms left to acquire in the US, buyouts and joint ventures have increasingly focused on firms based overseas, particularly the rapidly growing markets of India, China, and Brazil.

Increased Control of All Seeds, Not Just a Few Types

Initial seed company acquisitions by larger corporations focused on government-subsidized commodity seeds like corn, soy, and cotton in the United States, which have very significant markets. Without subsidies, many farmers would lose money on these crops, but planting is encouraged by direct subsidies under previous farm bills, and via insurance subsidies under the current farm bill.[11] More recently, corporations have expanded their focus to acquire fruit and vegetable seed firms. A Mexican billionaire, Alfonso Romo Garza, who formed a company called Seminis to eventually subsume eight different field fruit and vegetable specialists, anticipated this trend. He then sold the firm to Monsanto for $1.4 billion in 2005. Monsanto subsequently acquired De Ruiter Seeds in the Netherlands, which also specialized in greenhouse fruit and vegetable seeds, for $863 million in 2008. Monsanto has since formed collaborations with other firms to develop new vegetable seed varieties, including the world's largest producer of fruits and vegetables, Dole Food Company Inc.

Other dominant seed firms have also increased their emphasis on acquiring more diverse seed producers. Syngenta, for example, purchased the lettuce seed companies Pybas and Synergene in 2009, followed by the cucumber-, pepper-, and tomato-breeding programs of MayAgro (Turkey) in 2013. Bayer acquired four fruit and vegetable seed specialists in 2007, as well as the US melon seed firm Abbot & Cobb in 2012. Although the sale prices for these transactions are not always disclosed, giant corporations have demonstrated a willingness to pay much higher prices for acquisitions than was typical in the seed industry just a few decades ago. For example, Syngenta paid fourteen times estimated annual sales to buy DevGen (rice seed) in late 2012, and analysts expect it to take many years for this investment to be paid back.[12] Clearly Syngenta remained confident that there would be a return on this investment, likely because of increasing retail seed prices, as will be discussed further below.

Increased Ties between Dominant Corporations

Although the top seed/chemical firms once engaged in a number of lawsuits against each other, claiming infringement on their numerous patents, they have ended most of these. Instead, leading firms have increased their collaborations. One example is the web of cross-licensing agreements they have formed to exchange genetically engineered seed traits (see figure 2). This allows them to insert multiple traits into a single plant, such as SmartStax, with eight different traits (six for insecticidal toxins and two for herbicide tolerance). Such partnerships also create a strong barrier-to-entry for seed firms that want to sell the patented traits that are desired by farmers, such as the ability to spray herbicides without killing the crop, or the production of insect-killing compounds in the plant itself. Seed firms outside of the web have less access to these technologies unless they are willing to pay the high licensing fees that are demanded by this cartel.[13] Monsanto and BASF had a particularly strong connection via a joint venture to develop stress-tolerant crops, for which the firms invested a total of more than $2 billion.

Five of the original Big Six seed/chemical corporations (excluding Syngenta) have signed an agreement called the AgAccord, which is supposed to address issues with off-patent organisms, particularly the responsibilities for regulations that apply to transgenic seeds. Although the AgAccord is

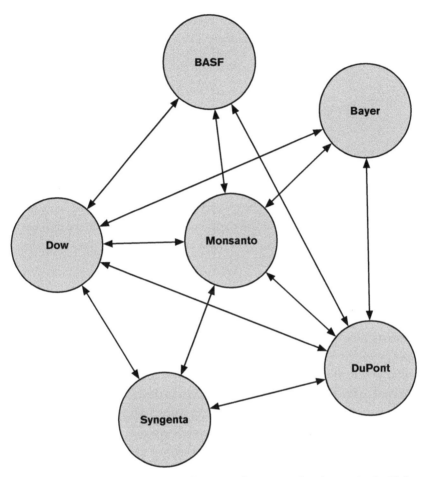

FIGURE 2. Cross-licensing agreements for genetically engineered seed traits. Credit: Philip H. Howard.

described as an effort to reduce barriers to access for farmers, the fine print may have the effect of maintaining market dominance rather than allowing smaller seed companies access to these varieties.[14] All members of the current Big Four also closely collaborate on public relations strategies to increase public acceptance of genetically engineered seeds. The Council for Biotechnology Information, an industry association funded by these corporations, distributes coloring books for children to promote these technologies, for example. Another area of collaboration is the spending of tens of millions of dollars on successful efforts to defeat initiatives to label transgenic foods. These include the states of California (2012), Washington (2013), Oregon (2014), and Colorado (2014), some of which lost by small margins.

WHAT ARE THE NEGATIVE IMPACTS?

Increasing corporate control of the seed industry has resulted in a much smaller number of people making decisions about most of the seeds that are produced. Moreover, these decisions tend to prioritize profits over other goals, such as ecological integrity, resilience, and human health. Some of the negative impacts that are already apparent include (1) a reduced number of seed varieties, (2) reduced rates of innovation, (3) higher prices for farmers, and (4) reduced rates of seed saving.

Reduced Number of Varieties

Maintaining seed diversity is important to protect crops against pests, disease, and climate change. Monocultures of genetically uniform plants are more susceptible to these issues, as demonstrated by the potato blight in Ireland in the mid-1800s and the corn blight in the US and Canada in 1970.[15] In recognition of these problems, plant breeders have made efforts to ensure that a reservoir of diversity remains available in seed banks. Because these seeds are not replanted on a frequent basis, however, they may be less viable, and less locally adapted, than seeds that continue to be selected in response to changing climates, pests, and pathogens.[16]

Corporations are reducing seed diversity by eliminating varieties from their seed catalogs as a cost-cutting measure. Seminis, for example, dropped 2,500 fruit and vegetable varieties from its offerings just before Monsanto, in order to boost profits and reduce debt incurred from financing previous acquisitions, acquired the seed company.[17] Large firms have also influenced government decisions to outlaw the sale of specific seeds, as the European Economic Community (now the European Union) did for two thousand vegetable varieties in 1980.[18]

In addition, farmer choices are reduced by local seed dealer incentives that steer farmers toward more profitable varieties. Dominant seed firms have made it difficult to acquire non-GE varieties in some parts of the Corn Belt, as well as reducing access to cheaper, single-trait GE varieties; dealers instead

22 · SEEDS: CALL TO ACTION

push stacked traits even if a farmer may not want them all. Trisler Seed Farms in Fairmount, Illinois, for example, offered thirty-three conventional corn varieties in 1994. By 2009, a few years after being acquired by Monsanto, they were offering just three.[19] In this same year, 42 percent of farmers surveyed in Illinois reported they could not access high-yield, nontransgenic corn.[20] Even the number of corn and soybean brands available has dwindled, with more than fifty-seven regional and local seed brands (including Trisler) eliminated as a result of consolidation since the late 1990s.[21]

Reduced Rates of Innovation

Large corporations tend to have complex bureaucracies that stifle the rate of innovation.[22] In addition, innovations that are selected for commercialization are typically limited to those with the potential for blockbuster profits. Scholars Rachel Schurman and Bill Munro, for example, found that Monsanto carefully calculated the potential profitability of products in their research and development efforts, frequently to the exclusion of goals touted in their advertising and public relations efforts.[23] A trait that would only be useful in countries where farmers were poor and could not pay higher prices for seeds, for example, would not receive the same investment as a trait favored by wealthy farmers.[24] Food scientist Paul Stitt reported similar consequences in efforts to reduce hunger when working for food corporations.[25]

One result of this narrow focus is that new seed varieties are less likely to be adapted to low-input forms of agriculture (such as organic) or to local regions (especially those with lower average incomes). After Dow Chemical acquired the North American seed division of Cargill, for example, the firm discontinued research efforts in southern states to focus on the more profitable Corn Belt region.[26] There is also decreasing emphasis on "orphan crops" that can make important contributions to diets in the Global South but are not viewed as being as profitable as heavily subsidized commodities.[27]

Public-sector innovation has also been affected by increasing restrictions on research, as well as shifting funding sources. In 2009, for instance, a group of scientists complained anonymously to the EPA that they could not legally carry out independent research on the impacts of genetically engineered seeds due to the intellectual property protections those seeds were granted by the government. An attempt to address this problem lifted some restrictions on commercialized seeds, but not for those that were still in development. Public funding for seed research has declined in recent decades, and many scientists

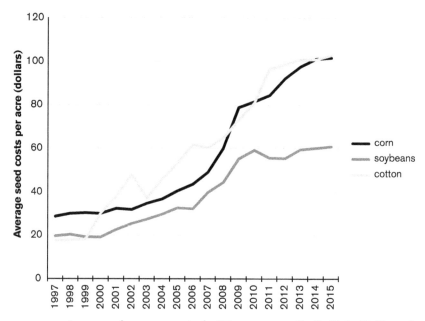

FIGURE 3. Average seed costs per acre in the US, 1997 to 2015. Credit: Philip H. Howard. Source: USDA, "USDA Economic Research Service—Commodity Costs and Returns," May 2, 2016, www.ers.usda.gov/data-products/commodity-costs-and-returns.aspx.

have sought to make up these shortfalls with corporate funding. Such a trend may result in significant restrictions, as well as conflicts of interest.[28]

Higher Prices for Farmers

In the last twenty years the prices of commodity seeds have increased dramatically, and at rates much faster than other agricultural inputs, such as fertilizers and machinery. Between 1997 and 2015, the average cost per acre of corn and soybean seeds increased more than 300 percent; for cotton seeds, more than 500 percent (see figure 3). Price increases are perhaps the least surprising of negative impacts, as the firms that increasingly control the industry are under pressure to continually increase their profit margins.

Farmers pay not only the direct costs of seeds themselves, but also indirect costs when they purchase proprietary chemicals that are "bundled" with seeds for crop application. When Roundup Ready seeds were introduced, farmers who purchased these seeds entered into an agreement with Monsanto whereby they were required to use Monsanto's Roundup herbicide, which was more expensive than equally effective generic versions. Six years after the patent on this herbicide expired, Monsanto still maintained an 80 percent market share, despite prices that were three to four times higher than generic glyphosate.[29] In 2016, Monsanto agreed to pay an $80 million penalty to the US Securities and Exchange Commission for improper accounting on farmer rebates that had incentivized dealers to increase their sales of more expensive Roundup in 2009 and 2010.

Another example of bundling involves selling seeds that are already coated with pesticides and fungicides. The most controversial of such treatments are neonicotinoid; companies claim neonicotinoids reduce crop losses from insect pests, but they are also likely contributors to the decline of numerous bee species.[30] More than 90 percent of corn seed in the US and Canada is pretreated with these pesticides, and farmers have few options to buy untreated seed. This tactic has effectively increased chemical sales, even though most studies suggest pretreated seeds do not actually improve yields.[31]

Reduced Rates of Seed Saving

Since the 1930s, seed companies have used the technical or biological means of hybridization to discourage seed saving.[32] Since hybrids do not uniformly express the characteristics of the parent seed when replanted, farmers who plant hybrids are effectively encouraged to purchase new seeds each year. Corn was one of the first crops for which breeders were able to increase yields for hybrids, and sorghum followed in the 1960s. Rates of seed saving for these crops quickly fell. Other important commodity seeds, such as soybeans, have been more biologically resistant to hybridization efforts, but changing intellectual property protections, discussed further below, have provided a legal-political means of discouraging saving.[33]

Corporations have been increasingly aggressive in the enforcement of restrictions on seed saving and replanting in recent years. Monsanto has hired Pinkerton detectives and advertised anonymous tip lines to identify farmers suspected of infringement. This tactic resulted in more than 142 lawsuits and $23.7 million in recorded judgments paid to Monsanto by 2012.[34] Because thousands of additional farmers threatened with litigation quietly settled out of court, however, total payments are likely to have been more than $100 million. At least one farmer in Tennessee, Kem Ralph, was sentenced to eight months in prison, as well as more than $1 million in fines, despite claiming he had never signed a technology agreement, and that his signature had been forged.[35] Technology agreements, even for conventional hybrid seeds, now increasingly prohibit seed saving or on-farm breeding efforts.[36]

Even the infrastructure for seed saving is being dismantled, reducing the potential to save seeds in the future. Most counties previously employed a seed cleaner to help them save their own seeds and prepare them for replanting. One of the last remaining soybean cleaners in the US was a man named Moe Parr in Lafayette, Indiana. As described in the 2008 documentary *Food Inc.*, Parr was sued by Monsanto and then ordered by a judge to disclose his customer list and send samples from every load to be tested for the presence of Monsanto's patented traits. This drove Moe out of the soybean-cleaning business.[37] The rate of soybean seed saving declined from well over 50 percent in the mid-1990s to less than 10 percent by 2001.[38] These trends are likely to affect an increasing number of crops.

WHAT IS DRIVING THESE TRENDS?

Increasing corporate control of the seed industry is driven by a number of factors, but some of the most important include government actions in the form of reduced antitrust enforcement, as well as increased intellectual property protections. Although these policy changes have been, unsurprisingly, influenced by corporate demands, governments have been exceedingly willing to favor corporate interests over those of the public.[39] In a vicious cycle, this government influence leads to greater corporate power, followed by even more government influence; one indicator is that the number of industry lobbyists relative to public interest organizations has increased dramatically in recent years.[40]

Reduced Antitrust Enforcement

A number of antitrust laws were passed in the United States in the late 1880s and early 1900s. This rule-making was a result of public concern about the negative consequences of a few corporations dominating key industries, such as railroads, meatpacking, and supermarkets. While these laws were selectively enforced, proposed mergers and acquisitions of large firms were frequently blocked by federal agencies and court decisions through the 1970s.[41] Since the 1980s, however, the interpretation and enforcement of these laws by heads of agencies and federal judges has changed dramatically, and the scale of consolidations continues to increase as a result. A series of workshops, held jointly by the Department of Justice and the Department of Agriculture in 2010, reported that changes in food and agriculture industries, including consolidation of the seed industry, have led to numerous concerns (such as reduced diversity and higher prices for farmers, as noted above). Their report concluded, however, that federal agencies have little power to stop proposed mergers and acquisitions in the future.[42]

Concurrently, the Department of Justice was conducting an antitrust investigation involving Monsanto, after receiving reports that the firm requested that its competitors charge higher seed prices. The investigation quietly ended, however, even though Monsanto's competitor DuPont supported this investigation in its early stages.[43] DuPont even funded activist groups calling for more regulation of Monsanto, such as the Organization for Competitive Markets and the American Antitrust Institute.[44] Some analysts suspect that greater cooperation in off-patent agreements and the recent resolution of the two firms' legal disputes may have reduced DuPont's interest in drawing attention to higher seed prices.[45]

Antitrust enforcement efforts have also become more difficult due to the increasingly transnational scope of markets, and the more limited jurisdictions of nations. In addition, other countries have also relaxed their antitrust laws in the face of corporate pressure. For example, although the South African government initially opposed DuPont's purchase of a majority stake in Pannar Seeds because it would result in DuPont and Monsanto controlling most of the country's seed market, DuPont's efforts to overcome this opposition were eventually successful.[46]

Increased Intellectual Property Protections

Stronger intellectual property protections for seeds have in most cases originated in the United States via changes in legislation or judicial decisions, and then been extended to other countries. Some key legislative changes that increased the power of seed companies are the Plant Patent Act of 1930, the Plant Variety Protection Act (PVPA) of 1970, and the Amended PVPA in 1994.[47] One of the most important judicial changes was the narrow decision in *Diamond v. Chakrabarty,* in which the US Supreme Court ruled that living organisms could be patented. More recent decisions have extended this precedent to non-GE seeds, and restricted how seeds are used after purchase.[48] The European Union (EU) has similarly strengthened intellectual property protections over time; the EU is beginning to follow the US in granting patents on seeds produced by conventional breeding.

Activities once protected through exemptions that the US Congress deliberately placed in the PVPA are now routinely prohibited under utility patents and strictly enforced, such as seed saving, the very practice that helped establish much of the tremendous diversity of domesticated crops and varieties we rely on today. To illustrate, farmers immediately enter into a contract with the patent holder when they open a bag of patented seeds. These fine print licenses are printed on the bags—think of a shrink-wrap license on software—and are known in the industry as "bag tags." Utility patents are expensive, too. Only companies of a certain size find them economically feasible. Not surprisingly, the top two industry leaders that have profited tremendously from intellectual property rights on seeds are also the top two owners of utility patents on plant varieties. Between 2004 and 2008, Monsanto and DuPont accounted for 60 percent of utility patent applications.[49]

Trade agreements have also been an important tool for strong-arming other countries into increasing their intellectual property protections and reducing the rights of farmers to save and exchange seeds. Monsanto and DuPont were part of the Intellectual Property Committee, an "ad hoc" coalition of thirteen corporations working to increase restrictions on buyers of their products via multilateral trade negotiations.[50] Some countries have resisted and remain subject to the 1978 UPOV (International Union for the Protection of New Varieties of Plants), which allows farmers to save and exchange seeds. The texts of a number of recent trade agreements, including the Trans-Pacific Partnership, require member countries to adopt the more restrictive 1991 version of UPOV or enact similar patent regimes.[51] These trade agreements are negotiated with a high degree of secrecy: although hundreds of corporate executives have access to trade agreement details, affected citizens (and even members of Congress) only learn the details when drafts are leaked or the deals are presented as a fait accompli.

．　．　．

The market share of seed/chemical corporations and the ties between them have accelerated in recent decades. Their focus was once limited to commodity crops, but this focus has since expanded to all seeds, including those of fruits and vegetables. The negative impacts of this increased corporate control of the seed sector include a reduction in the number of seed varieties, reduced rates of innovation, higher prices for farmers, and reduced rates of seed saving. Seed industry changes have been aided by the government actions of increasing intellectual property protections and reducing antitrust enforcement. These changes have been continually resisted, with varying degrees of success. In the next chapter, Kiki Hubbard describes this resistance and how we can achieve more democratic control of our seed supply.

Taking Back Our Seeds

Kristina "Kiki" Hubbard

IN 2005, WHEN MONSANTO PURCHASED SEMINIS, the largest vegetable seed company, organic farmers found themselves facing an ethical quandary. Should they continue purchasing seed varieties they had relied on for years from what was now a multinational biotechnology giant, or should they scramble to find alternatives?

Count Judy Owsowitz of Whitefish, Montana, among those farmers who chose to abandon Seminis. It took years for Owsowitz to replace an estimated 20 percent of varieties that she dropped following the acquisition. But the gap, it turned out, provided fertile ground for new opportunities.

"The biggest losses," she says, "were varieties that have a short growing season and traits for cold tolerance and cold soil emergence. Alternative varieties I came across did nothing for Montana's organic farmers."

Owsowitz saw herself as part of the solution to the worsening trend of consolidation in the seed industry, having seen competition and variety options dwindle even before Monsanto entered the vegetable scene.

"That's why I took seed into my own hands," Owsowitz says.

Owsowitz began saving and reproducing seeds for dozens of vegetable crops on her farm, varieties that fit northwestern Montana's short growing season and cool temperatures. In this way she maintains control over her seed supply while actively contributing to the conservation and improvement of crop genetic diversity. Each year she selects seeds that demonstrate desirable traits on her farm. Each year she sees more advantages.

"Learning to grow seed has been one of the most gratifying aspects of farming, and having Organic Seed Alliance as a resource has been an integral part of gaining that knowledge," Owsowitz says.

Organic Seed Alliance is helping farmers like Owsowitz build their skills in growing and adapting seeds to their changing environments and to the needs of society. We are also facilitating the distribution and exchange of seeds through regional grower networks and enterprises. For example, in 2014, we supported Owsowitz and seven other Montana growers in launching the state's first organic seed cooperative, a mission-driven enterprise that now sells hundreds of vegetable varieties. The cooperative is committed to improving and selling seeds adapted to Montana and other northern latitudes, and all of their seeds are grown using organic practices. The founders believe that to build a secure regional food system, we need to return control of our seeds back to the growers.

We at Organic Seed Alliance have joined a variety of partners in building an alternative to the dominant system by fostering decentralized models of breeding, growing, and sharing seeds, while pushing back against corporate control of our seeds. We are a small but mighty organization made up of scientists, educators, and policy advocates. Our work is collaborative, closely engaging farmers and university breeders, seed and food companies, chefs and consumers, and other policy advocacy groups. We envision seed systems that are democratic and just, support human and environmental health, and deliver genetically diverse and regionally adapted seeds to farmers everywhere. We take pride in helping farmers like Judy Owsowitz grow seeds for the common good.

Our research program involves plant-breeding projects conducted in collaboration with farmers and university breeders. We teach organic plant-breeding principles and techniques to further this scientific field, and work to put new varieties into the hands of farmers. We also teach farmers how to grow seed as a crop and how to breed their own varieties, providing them more independence from the consolidated market, and more seeds that are better adapted to their specific climate and farm conditions. Our advocacy promotes the benefits of organic seeds, public research, and farmers' rights as seed stewards, while challenging policies and practices that threaten to further privatize our seed supply. Though our work primarily focuses on the needs of organic farmers, the seeds we develop, policies we promote, and the education we provide have far-reaching benefits for all of agriculture.

As director of advocacy for Organic Seed Alliance, I present direct-action strategies for addressing unjust practices and policies, as well as proactive solutions that allow us to collectively resist corporate control through the development of democratic seed systems. The issues and policies surrounding seeds are decidedly complex—and our strategies honor and reflect that complexity. We do not do this work alone. That is why you will find a diversity of stories and stakeholders within each strategy described below, told through the lens of Organic Seed Alliance. Collaboration with these stakeholders is a bedrock principle of our advocacy, and is essential to resisting corporate control of our seeds.

Owsowitz's story demonstrates that seeds are the embodiment of potential, of hope. It is not too late to take back control of our seeds. Indeed, in important ways, we already are doing just that.

CHALLENGING THE BIGGEST SEED MERGER OF OUR TIME

Combatting corporate power involves a diversity of strategies, and political organizing around mergers is one strategy in this fight. When the chemical and pharmaceutical giant Bayer announced its intent to purchase Monsanto (as Phil Howard describes in the preceding chapter), advocacy groups of all kinds mobilized to challenge this merger. Because these industry consolidations involved the biggest manufacturers of agricultural pesticides and seeds, they were met with resistance from environmental groups concerned about the ecological and human health impacts of pesticides. Groups that took action included conventional agriculture groups representing farmers who were already suffering high seed and pesticide costs, as well as fewer seed options in the market. They also included organic farming organizations like ours that feared the further proliferation of chemical agriculture, more genetically engineered (GE) crops, and higher hurdles to achieving policies and investments that support sustainable agriculture.

Over the course of two years, Organic Seed Alliance joined these groups in coordinating strategies and resources to form a unified front against the mergers. When the Dow-DuPont and ChemChina-Syngenta deals were finalized quickly in 2017, organizing efforts zeroed in on challenging Bayer's purchase of Monsanto. Friends of the Earth, a well-established international environmental advocacy group, took the lead on much of the organizing. They engaged groups that represented farmers most affected by the mergers, including some unusual partners, such as the National Farmers Union and the Organization for Competitive Markets. These groups represent conventional farmers who sometimes disagree with other positions the environmental group takes. Yet convening these organizations with environmental, consumer, and organic farming groups made for a potent alliance.

This ad hoc coalition's activities were forceful and frequent, and included coordinating meetings with congressional members, state attorneys general, and the US Department of Justice (DOJ); collaborating on messaging, petitions, organizing tools, public comments, and press releases; conducting opinion polls of farmers and consumers on the pending merger; and hosting informational hearings on Capitol Hill. In all, these organizing efforts resulted in the delivery of more than a million signatures to the DOJ in opposition to the merger—not a small feat—and much needed pressure on Congress and state attorneys general to act. Twenty-seven members of Congress called on the DOJ to oppose the merger, as did five state attorneys general.

Although the DOJ eventually green-lighted the Bayer-Monsanto merger, the organized public resistance was successful in two ways. First, the DOJ gave a conditional approval, requiring Bayer to divest its vegetable seed business, Nunhems, in addition to its wheat research platform and some of its herbicide products. Would these divestitures have been required without public pressure? Not likely. Second, resistance efforts were successful in bringing national attention to antitrust issues in the seed industry through traditional and social media, so much so that policymakers were compelled to act. Shortly after Bayer and Monsanto announced that DOJ would allow their merger to proceed, Senator Cory Booker of New Jersey introduced a bill that would put a moratorium on major mergers in the food and agricultural sectors. The bill would also establish a commission to study ways to strengthen antitrust oversight of the food and farming sectors and recommend improvements to merger enforcement. This legislative action was a direct result of the extensive organizing and public awareness generated in previous months, and the eighty-four organizations endorsing the bill further underscore the impact of alliances representing a wide diversity of interests and stakeholders.

LAYING THE GROUNDWORK
FOR ANTITRUST ACTION

In important ways, the groundwork for the collaborative efforts described above began eight years earlier, when the US Department of Agriculture

(USDA) and DOJ jointly hosted five workshops across the country to explore competition concerns in agriculture. The historic listening sessions resulted in written comments from more than eighteen thousand food and farming stakeholders representing a diversity of interests. Hundreds of farmers showed up at each event to share compelling stories of how they were being impacted by unchecked market power.

On March 11, 2010, a day ahead of the first workshop, which was held in Ankeny, Iowa, a group of national and local organizations—National Family Farm Coalition, Food and Water Watch, and Iowa Citizens for Community Improvement—hosted an antitrust rally. The sense of urgency in the room was palpable as Organic Seed Alliance joined other advocacy groups, farmers, environmentalists, independent businesses, and social justice activists to collectively call on the DOJ to take swift action to restore competition to US agriculture.

A declaration from Missouri farmer Wes Shoemyer, who took to the podium that evening, is still with me: "We've waited a long time for justice in the heartland." This particular workshop included a focus on the seed industry. Shoemyer, a rancher and grain grower who had seen his crop variety choice go down as his seed prices skyrocketed, was hopeful that these historic listening sessions signaled a new era of antitrust enforcement in agriculture. He was not alone—eight hundred people, many of them farmers, attended the workshop the next day.

An ongoing challenge to addressing corporate power in the seed sector is the limited public opportunities to resist anticompetitive mergers and other decisions that lead to industry consolidation. But, if the USDA and DOJ workshops demonstrated anything, it is that the food and agriculture community is eager to speak up about the impacts of concentrated power when given the opportunity. Since that time, resistance has only grown louder and more diverse, as evidenced by the resistance to the Bayer-Monsanto merger.

Advocating for the enforcement of antitrust law is just one strategy for pushing back on corporate power. Driving the Bayer-Monsanto and other seed mergers is the profit potential that acquiring more intellectual property through these deals can deliver. In this way, consolidation and intellectual property rights are two sides of the same coin. Therefore, the second piece of our strategy is to push back on the intellectual property regime that facilitates the concentrated ownership of our seed supply.

In the words of Dr. Bill Tracy, a public plant breeder at the University of Wisconsin, Madison: "Placing the responsibility for the world's crop germplasm and plant improvement in the hands of a few companies is bad public policy."[1] Just as seeds adapt to changing environments, so must policies evolve to fit modern circumstances. In the context of seeds, intellectual property (IP) rights are one area in dire need of reform.

A tension exists between IP and antitrust policy, as both legal frameworks are presumed to support innovation. IP that provides exclusive ownership over seeds—without any exceptions for research, seed saving, and further plant breeding—brings this tension into sharp relief. At the time of the 2010 antitrust workshops, fourteen state attorneys general agreed that there should be resolution between IP and antitrust policy in the seed sector.[2] Even the assistant attorney general for the DOJ's antitrust division spoke to this tension in her remarks in Ankeny: "Patents have been used in the past to create or extend monopolies," Christine Varney said. "We will be looking closely at any attempts to do so via abuse of the patent laws." This statement drew loud applause. This tension demands further academic and legal inquiry, and emphasizes the need to challenge restrictive IP rights on seeds.

As Phil Howard described in the preceding chapter, seeds were once managed primarily as a public resource, but are now one of the most privatized agricultural inputs. A number of IP mechanisms used by the seed industry facilitate privatization. One of the most restrictive forms of IP available, utility patents awarded under the US Patent Act, are especially problematic in the seed sector, as they are broad in scope and provide extraordinary control over protected products. Utility patents on GE traits in major crops quickly led to increased concentration of financial and genetic resources. Resistance to increased corporate control of our seed supply via the patents associated with GE seeds continues to grow.

There have been several victories on this front. Earlier in my career I worked for the Center for Food Safety (CFS) in Washington, DC, which employs a number of attorneys who regularly challenge the USDA on the introduction of new GE organisms. I recall how, between 2002 and 2004, these attorneys worked closely with farmer-led organizations in the Northern Plains to successfully resist the introduction of GE wheat, citing the economic ramifications for farmers who export to countries that adamantly reject GE wheat. To this day, GE wheat is not sold commercially thanks to the organizing of regional organizations like the Western Organization of Resource Councils and their state chapters. Together, the groups commissioned economic studies on the market impacts of introducing GE wheat, data that showed grim consequences for US wheat growers if GE wheat were to be introduced. CFS brought legal expertise to the strategy and fight. Armed with this data, farmers took to the front line of the resistance. Under this grassroots pressure, Monsanto announced in 2004 that it was pulling its petition to USDA for regulatory approval of GE wheat.

CFS has enjoyed other successes, too, including stopping GE crop plantings on wildlife refuges in the US; supporting county-level bans on GE crop plantings; and halting the approval of GE alfalfa between 2007 and 2011, which forced the USDA to conduct a full Environmental Impact Statement (EIS) on a new GE organism for the first time. In 2008, Organic Seed Alliance joined a CFS-led lawsuit as a plaintiff in challenging the introduction of GE sugar beets. Most sugar beet seed is grown in the Willamette Valley of Oregon and Washington, a region known for commercial seed production. We joined the case on behalf of organic seed growers who produce seed for table beets and chard, relatives that easily cross with GE sugar beets. These growers were rightfully worried about the genetic integrity of their seed given this new threat.

In September 2009, the federal district court in San Francisco agreed with us and other plaintiffs—which included High Mowing Organic Seeds and the Sierra Club—and ordered the USDA to prepare an EIS as required by the National Environmental Policy Act (NEPA). In the end this court battle delayed the introduction of GE sugar beets, allowing time for seed growers in the region to prepare for their introduction, and forced the USDA to publish another assessment of the potential environmental, economic, and social impacts of GE crops.

Two court cases have sought to overturn the validity of patents themselves. The first case, *Bowman v. Monsanto*, went all the way to the Supreme Court. In this case, Vernon Hugh Bowman claimed that utility patents associated with GE soybeans he purchased should no longer apply after the first planting under the doctrine of patent exhaustion. The court unanimously disagreed, concluding that "patent exhaustion does not permit a farmer to reproduce patented seed through planting and harvesting without the patent holder's permission."[3]

In another case, the Organic Seed Growers and Trade Association sued Monsanto in a challenge to some of its patents on GE seed. The plaintiffs sought to leverage patent law through this legal challenge to address Monsanto's products trespassing into their organic and other non-GE crops. The issue of whether two very different production systems can coexist is increasingly contentious. Ultimately it is up to farmers who do not grow GE crops to protect their seeds and crops from contamination. In the end, the court sided with Monsanto by dismissing the case; however, a decision at the court of appeals in September 2013 legally bound Monsanto to a courtroom assurance that the company would not "take legal action against growers whose crops might inadvertently contain traces of Monsanto biotech genes (because, for example, some transgenic seed or pollen blew onto the grower's land)."

While these two patent cases involve GE seeds, even more egregious examples of utility patents on plant genetics are arguably not "novel," as required under the US Patent Act. Increasingly, utility patents are awarded for general traits also found in nature and selected for in crops through traditional breeding methods. A few examples include "red lettuce," "brilliant white cauliflower," and "heat-tolerant broccoli."

Plant breeders are rightly concerned about the growing list of utility patents on plant varieties and genetic traits. Dr. Jim Myers, a vegetable breeder at Oregon State University, had been working to select for heat tolerance (among other useful traits) in his publicly bred broccoli varieties years before he heard about the heat-tolerant broccoli patent. "If my broccoli meets the claims in the patent for heat tolerance," Myers shares, "then I probably can't go forward with those varieties."[4]

The heat-tolerant broccoli patent broadly covers broccoli plants that produce a "commercially acceptable broccoli head under heat stress growth conditions."[5] The patent potentially covers any broccoli plant that produces a head size similar to that described in the patent and that grows well under the stated temperature range. The progeny of the protected broccoli plants is also claimed, and the patent explicitly denies other breeders the right to develop new varieties from this protected material.

Myers works on crops for both the processing industry and the fresh market, including tomatoes, broccoli, snap peas, peppers, and winter and summer squash. His main interest is to improve vegetable varieties for disease resistance and human nutrition while maintaining quality and productivity. In recent years he has focused some of his breeding on the needs of organic farmers and regularly collaborates with these growers as well as chefs to improve culinary quality and flavor. Myers has identified a number of other patents that potentially impact his breeding work. He is not alone.[6]

These and other examples of patent abuse could potentially be challenged. A successful utility patent challenge in 2008 is instructive. In 1999, the US Patent and Trademark Office (USPTO) issued a utility patent claim for a common yellow bean (the Enola bean) that was genetically identical to a preexisting Mexican variety. The immediate effect was a plummet in production and US-Mexican trade of this bean. The Rural Advancement Foundation International (RAFI), a nonprofit based in North Carolina, launched a campaign in 2000, through sustained organizing and media engagement, to bring the Enola bean to the public's attention as an example of "biopiracy." A nonprofit advocacy group based in Canada, the ETC Group, joined these efforts the following year, as did the Consultative Group on International Agricultural Research (CGIAR). CGIAR filed a legal challenge in 2001 that eventually led to the USPTO reversing the patent—an important victory.

This example highlights the importance of pushing back on the misuse of IP on seeds in the private sector. Importantly, Supreme Court decisions that allowed for the practice of patenting seeds—including *Diamond v. Chakrabarty*, described in the preceding chapter—also left the door open for Congress to change patent law (or create new legislation) to address conflicts involving living organisms. But what about plant varieties coming out of the public sector, from universities charged with serving the public good? How do they handle IP on seeds? Next, we explore a third strategy that brings together academics and advocacy groups to effect change in this area from the inside out—from within our public institutions.

PUBLIC PLANT BREEDERS GET ORGANIZED

When I attended my first Seeds & Breeds for 21st Century Agriculture meeting in 2014, I was struck by the diversity of stakeholders in the room: public plant breeders, seed companies, policy advocates, and farmers representing multiple regions, crops, and scales. RAFI, the group mentioned above, convened the event to discuss the state of our seed supply and develop recommendations for strengthening our public breeding infrastructure.[7] It was August, and what had brought everyone to Washington, DC, during the busy growing season was a powerful truth: the public research sector is critical to the future of food and farming.

RAFI launched the Seeds & Breeds initiative in 2001 with the support of other organizations and plant breeders to build support, awareness, and a national road map for reinvigorating our public seed systems. A primary goal of the initiative, and key to fostering agricultural resilience, is ensuring that farmers have more choice in plant varieties adapted to their regional climates, environmental conditions, and market needs. The meetings that followed in 2003, 2007, and 2014 helped monitor the adequacy of funds available to the public plant-breeding community to meet these seed needs and train the next generation of plant breeders.

Casting a shadow over the 2014 summit was an alarming statistic. The US had lost more than 30 percent of its public plant-breeding programs over the last twenty years.[8] This meant that our national capacity to respond to the needs of US growers, develop new crop varieties, and train the next generation of seed experts was deteriorating even as consolidation continued in the private sector. In other words, public plant-breeding programs were disappearing at a time when we needed them most. Dwindling public funding was identified as a key driver of this trend.

As public support of university programs steadily decreased over the years, industry-funded research at universities increased. For example, the contributions of just three corporations—Monsanto, Cotton Inc., and Pioneer Hi-Bred—to the Texas A&M Department of Soil and Crop Sciences made up 56 percent of the department's research grants between 2006 and 2010.[9] Private donations now provide nearly a quarter of the funding for agricultural research at land grant universities.[10]

Public researchers often welcome private investment, especially in an era of diminished public funding. But private investment often comes with strings attached that dictate the terms and direction of research, ultimately compromising the independence of public research.[11] As several scholars have shown, university research has become increasingly privatized.[12] The shift in US policy toward stronger rights for IP owners fostered the privatization of public research, as did the 1980 Bayh-Dole Act, which encourages universities to patent and license public research as opposed to placing that research in the public domain.[13]

The 2014 Seeds & Breeds participants were united in staying true to the mission of public universities by resisting the privatization of public research and keeping seeds in the public domain, meaning without restrictions on research or seed saving. They also see their role as filling gaps that the private sector is not filling: underserved markets, like organic and other low-input production systems, and "orphan" crops and regions (those no longer receiving adequate attention and investments). Examples include cover crops or field corn for regions outside the Corn Belt, such as the Southeast.

Coming out of the 2014 summit was a road map for reinvigorating our public breeding infrastructure. These pathways included policy needs for the next Farm Bill, recommendations for keeping public seed collections robust and useful, and next steps for addressing hurdles created by inconsistent IP policies across institutions. In fact, IP concerns came up so frequently that there was unanimous support for a separate meeting to unpack challenges and identify solutions.

Subsequently, in August 2016, in conjunction with the National Association of Plant Breeders annual conference, the University of Wisconsin, Madison hosted a meeting in Raleigh, North Carolina, titled "Intellectual Property Rights and Public Breeding." Outcomes from the meeting included a statement of best practices for the use of IP tools in the public seed sector and effective strategies for using royalties or other funding sources to support public plant breeding.[14] These best practices serve as a code of ethics that should underpin publicly funded breeding: encouraging the free exchange of seed between researchers, eliminating any restrictions on a farmer's right to save seed, and directing financial returns back to plant-breeding programs. Plant breeders now have these best practices and funding strategies—and a cohort of colleagues—to help them educate their respective institutions so there's more consistency in policies and efficiency in sharing seeds across breeding programs.

At Organic Seed Alliance, we believe that increasing public funding for plant-breeding programs is essential. Corporations profiting most from utility patents and other forms of IP rights say that innovation and shared access to protected seeds are in conflict. But innovation and open access are mutually *inclusive,* and IP rights can be designed and used in a manner that incentivizes both. Therefore, promoting appropriate uses of IP tools is a strategy for protecting open access to seeds and furthering innovation in plant breeding.

For example, at this IP meeting in Raleigh, Organic Seed Alliance's Micaela Colley described the commercial release of organically bred varieties in a presentation to participants. A sweet corn variety was released to a seed company through a license that returns a royalty that is shared between the breeding partners (including the farmer partner) to help fill important funding gaps in their programs. The license does not restrict seed saving or research, and in this way, serves as an example of furthering the principle of open access to seeds through a traditional IP tool.

We see that advocates are using approaches that repurpose existing IP tools within their institutions to keep seeds as freely available as possible. Other models have emerged that bypass IP law altogether. The Open Source Seed Initiative (OSSI) takes a different approach to keeping seeds in the public domain, and their tireless efforts have provided lessons for fostering open-access models.

Inspired by the open-source software movement, Jack Kloppenburg, a sociologist at the University of Wisconsin, Madison who has long been an authority on the politics of seed, organized a group of plant breeders, seed companies, and nonprofits to try to create a "protected commons" for seeds. Out of these efforts grew OSSI, a nonprofit organization that promotes shared access to plant germplasm, recognizes and supports the work of plant breeders of all kinds, and supports a diversified and decentralized seed industry.

Early on, OSSI attempted to develop a license that could provide a contractual framework for viral sharing. Due to various legal, pragmatic, and cultural challenges, the group abandoned the license, and with it, an approach focused on repurposing existing IP tools. Instead, OSSI developed a pledge based on a social contract, one that could be affixed to seed packets to encourage four essential freedoms:

1. Freedom to save or grow seed for replanting or for any other purpose.
2. Freedom to share, trade, or sell seed to others.
3. Freedom to trial and study seed and to share or publish information about it.
4. Freedom to select or adapt the seed, make crosses with it, or use it to breed new lines and varieties.

Today, OSSI includes thirty-eight plant breeders who have released 415 varieties of more than fifty different crops under the pledge. Sixty-two seed companies sell OSSI-pledged varieties in seven countries, and the diversity listed in the OSSI database grows each year. OSSI provides a platform for protest and serves as a powerful rallying cry that seeds belong in the hands of the people, not the patent holder.

Utility patents and other anticompetitive restrictions on seeds must continue to be directly challenged. It is as important to continue fostering democratic models for developing—and protecting—new crop varieties that involve a diversity of decision makers, ensure shared benefit, promote ethical practices, and support sustainable agriculture. These models return growers to their rightful role as stewards of our seeds. Decentralizing our seed system in this way is our fourth strategy to resisting corporate control of our seeds.

TAKING BACK OUR SEEDS

Marko Colby and Hanako Myers of the Midori Farm in Port Townsend, Washington, shared a strong interest in seeds when they started farming. They integrated seed production into their business plan from the start, in part to be less dependent on a consolidated seed market. They knew that ongoing consolidation in the seed industry could leave farmers in the lurch when varieties unexpectedly disappeared from catalogues. They saw the effects on farmers when Seminis cut 2,500 of its nearly six thousand varieties in one year.[15]

"The seed industry is centralizing on a macro scale, and at the same time, and perhaps in reaction to this trend, is now sprouting more small farm-based, regional seed companies," Colby explains. "There is more interest in organic seed and more farmers growing seed."

Colby and Myers are evidence that seed industry trends are not all doom and gloom. Increased demand for organic seed, and new regional seed companies, are providing farmers both an alternative to the seed oligopoly and a chance to take seed into their own hands. This includes new economic opportunities to grow seed commercially. They are also "farmer breeders," and, helped my research team at Organic Seed Alliance, developed and commercially released a new organic spinach variety called "Abundant Bloomsdale." Midori Farm conducts breeding projects each year and grows organic seed under commercial contracts as well.

There is a growing movement of farmers who are empowered to save, improve, and produce seed at a larger scale—and these growers are getting organized. For example, in California, Montana, North Carolina, and Washington, organic seed growers developed their own formal networks to offset the costs and risks associated with seed production. Organic Seed Alliance has helped some of these networks purchase shared equipment for harvesting and cleaning seed. We also helped create email lists and website forums to allow these seed growers to more easily troubleshoot production challenges and share seeds with one another. Most of these networks coordinate annual variety trials to identify which crop varieties perform well in their region and which need improvement through plant breeding.

The resurgence of farmer breeders, seed growers, and seed savers is supported by other seed conservation, education, and research organizations across the country. These groups include the Farm Breeding Club (a project of the Northern Plains Sustainable Agriculture Society), Seed Savers Exchange, Native Seeds/SEARCH, Indigenous SeedKeepers Network (a project of the Native American Food Sovereignty Alliance), Seedshed, Rocky Mountain Seed Alliance, and others.

A national survey confirms that organic farmers are growing more seed each year.[16] This interest in seed has spawned a number of new regional seed companies across the US, most of which were started by organic farmers.[17] For this reason, many of these new regional companies primarily sell organic seed. There is a lot of room for growth, since the supply of organic seed is still catching up to demand.

CREATING DECENTRALIZED SEED SYSTEMS

Among the new companies emerging in response to seed industry consolidation is Adaptive Seeds, based in Sweet Home, Oregon. Farm operators Andrew Still and Sarah Kleeger saw how a variety of factors, including corporate control of seeds, contributed to the erosion of agricultural biodiversity and the decline in quality seeds. "And we realized that this was a problem that we could do something about," Still says.

Still and Kleeger decided to grow seeds exclusively on their organic farm. They sell more than five hundred varieties of seed for vegetables, flowers, herbs, grain, and cover crops online and through a print catalog. They say their business is growing at a rate that is hard to keep up with, even as other regional seed companies emerge.

Adaptive Seeds and their newer competitors operate on a relatively small scale, yet these companies—including farmer-led seed cooperatives—are expanding choice in the market. More importantly, these companies are committed to conserving crop genetic diversity, protecting open access to seeds, and supporting organic agriculture.

The rapid increase in seed libraries is part of this positive trend, inspiring a revived movement in backyard seed saving. Though these community seed exchanges operate outside the commercial trade, they demonstrate a growing awareness among the public that seeds are a vital resource that should be collectively managed. There are at least three hundred seed libraries operating in the US.

Still says the ongoing concentration of market power in the private seed industry also underscores the need for more public plant breeding. He says land grant universities should conduct more plant breeding that engages regional growers, emphasizes underserved markets and crops, and releases new varieties into the public domain. In his backyard, plant breeders at Oregon State University (OSU) provide inspiring examples.

Dr. Myers, the OSU broccoli breeder mentioned earlier, is the project director for the Northern Organic Vegetable Improvement Collaborative (NOVIC). NOVIC is a USDA grant-funded project through the Organic Research and Extension Initiative (OREI) with the goal of breeding new vegetable varieties adapted to organic agriculture across the Northern Tier of the US. The collaboration involves three land grant universities (OSU, University of Wisconsin, Madison, and Cornell), the USDA, my team at Organic Seed Alliance, and more than twenty organic farms. These researchers adhere to participatory plant-breeding methods, where farmers and formal breeders collaborate on farm-based breeding projects to identify varieties that do well for organic production through variety trials and to breed new varieties. Farmers are equal partners, from setting breeding goals to evaluating results.

One of the most important contributions of any public plant-breeding program is to get useful varieties into the hands of farmers. In 2014, NOVIC partners released "Who Gets Kissed?" sweet corn. It was one of the first organically bred, open-pollinated varieties developed using participatory plant-breeding methods. Because it is open pollinated, farmers can save seeds from their harvest to replant (which is not as easy with hybrids). In fact, the breeding team encourages farmers to save seeds so they can adapt the variety to their local conditions and market needs. NOVIC partners have hosted eighty events in twenty-one states to teach farmers these skills. NOVIC has also supported the release of ten additional varieties of four crops, and an additional twelve varieties of seven crops are in the pipeline. Notably, the project has trained thirteen graduate students in plant breeding and organic production. Several of these students have already gone on to work in the field of organic seed.

Another example of collaborative public plant breeding is the Eastern Sustainable Organic Cucurbit Project (ESOcuc). Like NOVIC, ESOcuc is funded by a USDA-OREI grant. Partners include Auburn University, North Carolina State University, and Organic Seed Alliance. Farmers, extension agents, and seed companies along the East Coast play an important role. Though focused on different crops and regions, the objectives and approach of ESOcuc are similar to those of NOVIC—evaluating and breeding new varieties for organic systems (with an emphasis on disease resistance), training the next generation of plant breeders, and hosting educational events for farmers.

Organic farmers who grow cucurbit crops—such as cucumbers, zucchini, and winter squash—are extremely challenged by diseases that emerge and evolve quickly, especially in warm and humid climates. One of these diseases, downy mildew, can obliterate a farmer's entire crop. While conventional growers rely on pesticides (including neonicotinoids, now understood to cause persistent harm to pollinators, birds, and other organisms), organic growers instead rely on protecting crops from the inside out: through plant genetics resistant to diseases.

As part of ESOcuc, Cornell University breeder Michael Mazourek released new downy mildew resistant cucumber varieties developed in close partnership with organic farmer Edmund Frost in Louisa, Virginia. Frost helps operate a regional cooperative called Common Wealth Seed Growers. In recent variety trials up and down the East Coast, one particular slicing cucumber variety, DMR401, stood out as the best. It even outperformed varieties from the biggest vegetable seed company in the world: Monsanto's Seminis. Because Monsanto and other dominant players prioritize chemical pesticide sales that aim to combat diseases, they do not prioritize disease-resistant varieties for the marketplace. Mazourek says pesticide costs are going up as their effectiveness, in the case of downy mildew, is going down.

"The beauty of our success is that these high-yielding, disease-resistant varieties are as beneficial to conventional growers as they are to organic," Mazourek says. "The great arc of continued public plant-breeding funding is crucial so that we can keep developing new varieties like DMR401 that have characteristics farmers urgently need."

Still and Kleeger of Adaptive Seeds say projects like ESOcuc and NOVIC are essential to supporting decentralized seed systems and training farmers in breeding and seed growing: "We haven't yet reached a critical mass of farmers engaging in seed work," Kleeger says, adding that seed is the most important thing she could be doing with her time. Still agrees: "I would characterize our work with seed as the most powerful way to create the world we want, from the bottom up."

As the number of seed stewards like Still and Kleeger increases, so does the security of our seed and food supplies. By supporting more democratic seed systems, farmers take back control over their seed while actively conserving and improving global crop diversity. Many of these farmers are also helping to fill gaps in the organic seed supply at a time when demand outpaces what the market offers.

Seeds are powerful; they represent profound potential for improving our food and agricultural systems. Organic Seed Alliance is working to embrace this potential—from farm to fork—through collaborative research, education, and advocacy. To support organic farming, plants can be bred to thrive without the help of pesticides. We can adapt seeds to naturally resist disease. Plants can also be bred to make our food supply more secure in the face of climate change. We can adapt our seeds to warmer and drier conditions. Plants can be bred to improve the quality of our food, too. We can breed for improved nutritional content. But to realize all of this potential, we must create structural changes to how seed is managed and shared.

Creating structural change in the seed sector will require ongoing resistance to deep-seated trends, including anticompetitive mergers, to preserve competition in the market. Regulators must enforce antitrust laws as they were originally intended: to fight the concentration of economic and political power. Therefore, restructuring our seed systems to be more democratic and just requires advocating for antitrust law enforcement and changes to patent law, while simultaneously challenging the increased privatization of seed. But, as explained in this chapter, we do not have to wait for all of this change to come from Washington, DC.

Consider Marko Colby and Hanako Myers of the Midori Farm and Edmund Frost of Common Wealth Seed Growers—and all the farmer breeders, seed savers, Indigenous SeedKeepers, and public plant breeders in between their coasts who are fostering decentralized seed systems. These dedicated individuals are keeping the diversity of our seeds alive, available, and adaptable so that future generations will have the plant genetics they need to respond to their changing climates and the needs of society. Underpinning this work is the conviction that seeds are a living, natural resource that requires careful stewardship.

At a June 2016 event in Washington, DC, titled "America's Monopoly Problem," Senator Elizabeth Warren of Massachusetts provided a compelling case for restoring antitrust enforcement. Her recommendations were many, among them to "[revive] the movement that created antitrust laws in the first place."[18] I agree, and believe that tending to these seeds of resistance is not only possible—it is necessary.

In my nearly twenty years working in seed policy, no single issue has brought together a stronger and more diverse group of affected and concerned stakeholders than that of corporate control of our seed supply. Back in Ankeny, Iowa, at that first 2010 USDA and DOJ workshop, I saw firsthand how the dichotomies we create—Republican and Democrat, organic and chemical, grower and consumer—quickly vanish when we are confronted with shared challenges. Those of us in attendance who came to resist business-as-usual practices and policies spoke with one voice. We asked our regulators and policymakers for justice in the Heartland and beyond. We indicated that we were not going away. We demonstrated that we had the ability to concentrate our own power.

PART TWO

————

Pesticides

CALL TO ACTION—
PESTICIDE PURVEYORS AND CORPORATE POWER

Jill Lindsey Harrison

COLLECTIVE RESPONSE—
DRIFT CATCHERS COMBATTING PESTICIDE POWER

*Emily Marquez, Marcia Ishii-Eiteman,
and Kristin Schafer*

Pesticide Purveyors and Corporate Power

Jill Lindsey Harrison

TOXIC ENCOUNTERS

ONE NOVEMBER EVENING IN 1999, over 170 residents of the small agricultural community of Earlimart in California's Central Valley experienced a frightening and inexplicable set of symptoms: vomiting, impaired breathing, dizziness, and burning eyes and lungs. Emergency crews responding to the multiple calls for help did not speak Spanish and thus could not effectively communicate with the residents. Moreover, they could not identify the source of the illness and were unsure of how to advise the victims, telling some to stay indoors while directing others to leave the vicinity. Eventually, later that night, emergency crews evacuated some of the most sickened residents to a nearby middle school, and instructed them to strip. They then proceeded to spray them down with fire hoses, all in view of their neighbors and television crews. A subsequent investigation revealed that a poisonous cloud of a soil fumigant called metam sodium, a known carcinogen as well as reproductive and developmental toxicant, had volatilized more quickly than anticipated from an agricultural field one-quarter of a mile away, drifted into the town, and poisoned the residents. Victims were left fearful, with lingering illnesses, and medical bills they could not afford to pay. What happened that night is called *pesticide drift*—the off-site movement of pesticides away from sites where they are applied and into other spaces, where they harm people and other creatures.

Unfortunately, emergency response to pesticide drift incidents did not improve quickly. In 2000, after the highly toxic soil fumigant chloropicrin drifted from a field into the California town of Lamont, at least twenty-four residents suffered a range of acute toxicity symptoms, including nausea, vomiting, and blurred vision, as well as impaired, painful breathing. Emergency crews responding to the scene decided that the symptoms were not severe or persistent enough to warrant further investigation, and they instructed residents to return home and air out their houses. Consequently, the second half of the pesticide application proceeded the following day, again drifting into the same residential area. This time the drift sickened over two hundred additional residents. On this second day, some victims were evacuated to a nearby parking lot. There they waited for several hours without food, water, medical treatment, or access to bathrooms. Barricades were set up on the edge of town, and emergency response crews prevented residents from leaving the area. One woman told me about her friend's harrowing experience that day: "Emergency crews came into their house, where my friend and her husband were having difficulty breathing, where the children were on the floor throwing up. And the crew said, 'Nothing's wrong here, we don't smell anything.' The ambulance was across the street, and she said she didn't know if she was going to live or die. No one helped them. She said that their neighbor chased the ambulance, but they laughed at him and drove away."

The issue of pesticide drift has garnered considerable attention since that time, and emergency response procedures have arguably improved. Yet pesticide drift incidents continue to occur regularly throughout the world. Indeed, in May 2017, over fifty farmworkers were exposed to the highly toxic insecticide chlorpyrifos, which had drifted from a neighboring orchard. Moreover, people working on and living near farms report that pesticide drift and exposure are a part of everyday life.[1]

In this chapter, I address the ways chemical pesticides harm human health and the reasons US agriculture uses extraordinary quantities of dangerous chemicals. I focus in particular on the agrichemical industry, which is dominated by a handful of large corporations who use their massive financial resources and their limited competition to cover up the harms their products cause, keep them on the market, compel farmers to use high amounts of them, and hide their own nefarious business practices.

PESTICIDE USE, ILLNESS, AND DRIFT

While large-scale pesticide drift events like the ones described above make the news, agricultural pesticides are apt to drift any time they are applied. In

California alone, there are over one million agricultural pesticide applications every year. Chemical pesticides come in various formats: liquid sprays, powders, and fumigants that quickly turn into gasses. Farmers use them to control insects, weeds, plant diseases, and other things that harm crops and livestock health. They are applied by helicopter, airplane, and tractor, through irrigation lines, and manually with backpack sprayers.

Exposure to pesticides can produce serious acute illness at the time of exposure, leading to nausea, vomiting, eye and skin irritation, and difficulty breathing. Pesticide exposure also contributes causally to many chronic diseases, including asthma and other lung diseases, cancer, birth defects, immune system suppression, behavioral and learning disorders, and neurological disorders.[2] Research has demonstrated that official statistics greatly underestimate the full scope of pesticide exposures.[3] Complicating these statistics is the fact that the acute symptoms of pesticide exposure mimic common ailments, so diagnoses can be challenging. Nevertheless, toxic pesticides poison workers who are applying them, as well as children and others who encounter and handle pesticide equipment on farms. They affect they health of consumers who eat food containing pesticide residues; they contaminate ground and surface water; and they kill bees, birds, fish, amphibians, and other wildlife.

Studies show that pesticide concentrations at the edge of farm fields during and shortly after pesticides are applied regularly exceed levels of health concern.[4] Pesticides travel many miles from where they are used. For example, environmentally persistent chemicals have been shown to travel through atmospheric air currents and be deposited in the colder regions of the globe thousands of miles from where they are applied.[5] US government test results show that 85 percent of food is contaminated with pesticide residues.[6] Although most of these studies detect pesticides at levels that some government agencies claim are safe, those "safe" levels are hotly contested by scientists in academia, the government, and the private sector.[7] Additionally, studies show that the US government does not always test produce for the pesticides actually used by farmers growing those crops, in turn misrepresenting the actual extent of pesticide residues on food.[8] With over six billion pounds of agricultural pesticide active ingredients used worldwide and as little as 0.1 percent of all pesticides applied effectively reaching their target pest, the risks and frequency of pesticide exposure and illness are extraordinarily high.[9]

How did this pervasive use of toxic agricultural chemicals come to be? Scholars have shown that there are many answers to this question. For example, historians have shown that public university agricultural research has long devoted the majority of its agricultural research and extension resources to developing pesticide-intensive production designed to maximize yields rather than protect human health and the environment.[10] Chemical pesticides are now such a central component of mainstream approaches to researching and managing weeds, insects, and diseases that pesticide-intensive agriculture is widely characterized as "conventional." Following historian Christopher Bosso, I use the term "pesticide paradigm" to characterize the central role of chemical pesticides in agricultural pest management and the "unspoken and almost unconscious assumption" by researchers, farmers, and others that chemical pesticides are absolutely necessary, safe, and effective.[11]

Another reason toxic pesticides are so widely used is that many factors limit scientists' abilities to document the full scope of risks pesticides pose to human health. Risk assessments of pesticides rely on toxicological studies of the effects of chemical exposure on animals and then must estimate how those results translate to humans, who have much longer life spans, have different physiologies, and can be exposed to a chemical in many different ways, in varying quantities, and for different lengths of time. Moreover, risk assessments do not account for the health effects of chemical mixtures, the wide range of human bodies and susceptibilities to harm from chemical exposure, the health effects of so-called inert ingredients in pesticide formulations (i.e., those not designed to kill the target pest), or the health effects of a given pesticide's breakdown ingredients.

The extensive use of toxic pesticides also stems from the ways that agencies regulate these chemicals. First, as with many other areas of US environmental law, the Federal Insecticide, Fungicide, and Rodenticide Act that serves as the basis for federal pesticide regulation requires that all pesticide regulatory decisions be based on a cost-benefit analysis. That is, regulatory restrictions on a chemical must outweigh the costs associated with the regulation. However, the benefits of restrictive regulations are typically conceived of very narrowly because most impacts of pesticide use are uncertain, long-term, diffuse, and thus nearly impossible to quantify. Second, the burden of proof for challenging a registered pesticide rests with the public—pesticides are presumed innocent, and widely used, until proven guilty. In contrast, public health and environmental advocates argue that pesticides should be regulated according to the "precautionary principle"—the notion that when current data and analytical techniques indicate that hazards likely pose serious risks to human health or the environment, agencies must take action to reduce those risks, even without full scientific certainty.[12] Third, because their own research funding is severely limited, government agencies conduct very little monitoring of air and water for evidence of pesticide drift. They also rely on pesticide manufacturers' own data about the safety of their products. Yet, as I discuss further below, these corporations hide evidence that their products cause harm.

The widespread use of toxic pesticides is also rooted in the fact that those most frequently and seriously exposed to pesticides—farmworkers and their families—are vulnerable in ways that limit their ability to report pesticide exposures. This diminishes how seriously officials take their pesticide exposures and concerns. Most farmworkers are immigrants from Mexico and Central America; their average income falls well below the poverty level, they experience job insecurity because of the seasonal nature of agricultural work and competition for jobs, few are covered by union contracts, and at least half are unauthorized and subject to the racialized surveillance, risks of arrest, and other consequences of heightened immigration enforcement.[13] Farmworkers, their kin, and their peers are often reluctant to report pesticide exposures. They fear employer retaliation, losing their jobs, and interacting with law enforcement. Most cannot afford to take time off work or to pay for medical care and the legal assistance required to report and document their exposure.

In the following, I focus my attention on one of the foundational pillars of the pesticide paradigm: corporate concentration in the agrichemical industry, the companies that manufacture and sell agricultural pesticides. I first describe this concentration, and then I identify how it enables corporate actors to engage in practices that weaken pesticide regulations, construct pesticides as normal and respectable among farmers, and otherwise entrench the harmful hegemony of pesticide-intensive agriculture. I end by introducing a group of pesticide activists who fight these corporate actors and their practices that damage human and environmental health.

DEGREES OF CORPORATE CONCENTRATION IN THE PESTICIDE INDUSTRY

As historian Edmund Russell has detailed, the US chemical industry flourished during World War I and World War II, largely through the development of chemical technologies for warfare that were later adapted to other purposes.[14] During those wars, the US chemical industry produced explosives, poison gases, dyes, and pesticides on government military contracts. After the war effort, chemical companies successfully adapted many pesticides to agricultural uses.[15] The US government fostered this process through various means, including directing and funding the development of aerial pesticide application technologies, along with conducting large-scale campaigns to eradicate public health pests such as mosquitoes and lice with chemical controls. Government contracts for chemical industry products during wartime thus facilitated the development of the US chemical industry, which then used its accumulated capital, skills, and continued government contracts to expand into new markets—notably, home and agricultural pest control.

The agrichemical manufacturing industry has continued to grow in size over time, with annual sales of $54 billion in 2013.[16] Importantly, pesticide manufacturing has become an extremely concentrated sector, in which only the most highly capitalized firms can compete. In recent years, three-quarters of all pesticides sold globally have come from just six multinational corporations—Bayer, Syngenta, BASF, Dow, Monsanto, and DuPont— the same six companies that dominate the seed sector and that are also major players in pharmaceutical and other manufacturing sectors.[17] As Phil Howard notes in the first chapter of this volume, this concentration is becoming even more acute. DuPont and Dow merged in September 2017, Bayer is attempting to acquire Monsanto, and ChemChina (which was seventh in size among agrichemical companies) has acquired Syngenta. Following these mergers, the new top four corporations—Bayer CropScience-Monsanto, Syngenta-ChemChina, DuPont-Dow AgroSciences, and BASF—will control an unprecedented 84 percent of the agrichemical market.[18]

HOW PESTICIDE MANUFACTURERS USE THEIR POWER

With their massive and concentrated financial power, pesticide manufacturers use various techniques to help secure the pesticide paradigm of agricultural pest management, despite its toxic legacy.

Advertising

Pesticide manufacturers use their immense resources to advertise their products in ways that promote pesticide-intensive agriculture among farmers and other pesticide users in the US and abroad. These corporations spend tens of millions of dollars per year promoting routine ("preemptive") pesticide applications, which violates the sustainable farming approach of carefully monitoring pest populations and using pesticides only when and where needed.[19] In their advertisements, corporations also frame "healthy" farms as free of weeds and insects, rather than as free of toxic chemicals. Additionally, they extol the productive virtues of herbicide-resistant genetically modified seeds and other new products that usher greater use of highly toxic herbicides. Such advertising effectively naturalizes the pesticide paradigm among farmers, who have been shown to widely view chemical pesticides as essential for not only farm productivity but also their own status as modern and respected members of their communities.[20]

The pesticide industry also legitimizes pesticides by framing them as environmentally beneficial.[21] Even as public concern about the environmental impacts of pesticides has increased, so too have industry actors' claims proliferated about the environmental sustainability benefits of pesticides in their advertisements, annual reports, and websites.[22] The promotional materials of CropLife America are particularly revealing. Billing itself as the "national trade association that represents the manufacturers, formulators and distributors of pesticides," the organization claims on its website that pesticides "contribute to stronger environmental and human health, sustainable growing practices and ecological diversity."[23] The same website posts and answers the following powerful question to frame pesticides—and pesticide corporations—as beneficial: "Would the world be a better place without pesticides? We believe that without them, our overall quality of life would diminish . . . Today's agricultural tools, including pesticides, enable growers to conserve and protect our water, air and soil."[24]

These claims by pesticide corporations are misleading. For example, they obscure ways that farmers are encouraged to adopt unsustainable practices such as routine applications of highly toxic pesticides, despite the availability of less toxic alternatives. This messaging also neglects to mention industry organizations' vehement rejection of nearly all environmental regulations. Additionally, researchers have found that pest control corporations widely use false and misleading statements in their advertisement to portray pesticides as "safe."[25]

Corporate industry advertisements and other promotional materials also make sweeping humanitarian claims, presenting current pesticide products and the rates at which they are used as essential to the production of food.[26] For example, Bayer CropScience's website showcases employees on a page titled "Careers That Help Feed Our Growing Population" and explains that "without crop protection, nearly half of the world's harvest would be lost to pests and diseases. To play our part so we are able to feed not only today's population but [also] the estimated 9 billion people in 2050, Bayer CropScience continues to develop innovative crop protection solutions to help safeguard harvests and increase productivity from existing arable land."[27] Such arguments are deceptive, however, since they frame hunger as a function of absolute quantities of food produced in the world rather than a function of poverty. In fact, millions of people suffer from chronic hunger in the United States, the land of agricultural plenty.[28] Such claims also ignore the evidence that organic agriculture and other less-toxic forms of farming are nearly as productive as pesticide-intensive agriculture, are more environmentally sustainable, are more profitable, and generate safer food and other social benefits.[29] Industry leaders obscure or even belittle such evidence, instead tapping into contemporary fears as the basis for making misleading connections between current pesticide use patterns, food security, and food safety.

Research

Corporate pesticide manufacturers, like other major industry groups, devote considerable resources to producing scientific knowledge that serves their own interests. Indeed, private-sector research and development budgets for agrichemicals and seeds far outweigh those of major public-sector institutions' budgets for such work.[30] These corporations fund trade organizations, think tanks, and "independent" experts to conduct research. The corporate funders then disseminate the particular results that represent pesticides as benign or beneficial, obscure manufacturers' role in funding such studies, and refrain from disseminating studies that show their products to be unsafe. Critical observers have shown that industry-funded studies often contain egregious and deliberate design errors that cause the results to show that industry products are safe despite other evidence to the contrary.[31] Industry-funded experts also defend company interests in chemical liability lawsuits and regulatory proceedings, and write letters to the editor of newspapers in defense of the industry. Such work contains the illusion of impartiality despite being paid directly to serve chemical industry interests. In one current example of such practices, investigative journalists have shown that Monsanto wrote research papers that discredit health concerns about its herbicide glyphosate, presented them as independent studies, issued public statements that ignore the overwhelming majority of studies that find glyphosate to cause cancer, and cast as "independent" the Monsanto-funded scientists who vouch for the safety of glyphosate.[32]

Agrichemical corporations also fund think tanks to disparage organic and other forms of less-toxic pest management as unproductive and harmful. Dennis Avery's research from his Hudson Institute, funded by major pesticide manufacturers (including Monsanto, DuPont, and Dow), is notorious for such practices.[33] In his self-published book, *Saving the Planet with Pesticides and Plastic,* as well as in other publications, presentations, and interviews, Avery disingenuously argues that organic agriculture is contaminated with dangerous levels of bacteria and threatens wildlife, concluding that conventional agriculture is better for the planet.[34]

Agrichemical firms also directly fund and control research conducted at public universities, selectively disseminating those results that legitimize industry investments and expand market opportunities while suppressing findings that indicate their products are harmful.[35] In a particularly notorious case, Syngenta conspired to discredit biology professor Tyrone Hayes of the University of California, Berkeley when Hayes's Syngenta-funded research showed that the company's widely used herbicide, atrazine, pervasively contaminates groundwater at dangerous levels and disrupts proper functioning of the human endocrine system.[36] Syngenta disputed and misrepresented Hayes's findings, emphasized other research (all Syngenta-funded) that found no relationship between atrazine and endocrine disruption, and obscured glaring methodological problems with those other studies. Public-private research relationships are increasingly common in an era of declining funds for public education, with private companies funding 25 percent of research conducted in some public university departments.[37] Although the actual terms of any given contract determine to a large extent how much control the donor firm has over the research process and results, researchers have shown that scientists receiving industry funding tend to be biased toward industry interests even in cases where the industry sponsor does not actively pressure the researcher. For example, Als-Nielsen et al.

found that pharmaceutical researchers were more likely to conclude that the drug they were testing was effective when for-profit corporations, as opposed to nonprofits, funded them.[38]

Regulatory Capture

Agrichemical corporations are also able to use their financial power to "capture" the agencies that are supposed to regulate them—that is, to control regulatory and legislative decisions about pesticides so that government agencies protect industry investments rather than act in the public interest.[39] Agrichemical corporations make campaign contributions to political candidates who have experience as industry leaders or support industry interests from the public sector. In a context in which candidates cannot win without significant financial resources, such contributions play a key role in getting industry actors into office. Observers often critically characterize these types of relationships between industry and government as a revolving door through which individuals in leadership positions rotate between industry and the public agencies that regulate them, providing "insider know-how and friendly connections through which rules can be bent and loopholes exploited."[40] One of the most recent examples was President Donald Trump's appointment of Scott Pruitt, a former Oklahoma attorney general known for his legal challenges to the US Environmental Protection Agency (EPA) and other federal agencies, to lead the EPA.[41] In his first few months in office, Pruitt, who proudly stated that he strove to "combat unwarranted regulation and overreach by the federal government," reversed the EPA's decision to ban the neurotoxic pesticide chlorpyrifos (which was introduced by Dow Chemical, still its primary manufacturer) and rolled back many other environmental protections.[42]

Pesticide manufacturers also hire professional lobbying firms to pressure decision makers at the local, state, federal, and international levels. In recent years, agricultural input firms spent between $20 and $37 million per year on lobbying.[43] Such firms provide special access to policymakers and regulatory officials in part because of lobbyists' past work experiences within the policy and regulatory arenas.[44] Pesticide manufacturers also pressure agencies to craft scientific advisory boards that protect the industry's interests. In addition to insisting that such boards include industry representatives, they also pressure agencies to remove scientists who have raised concerns about the health effects of certain pesticides.[45]

Industry actors come together in corporate-funded think tanks and policy institutes to identify their shared interests and strategies for capturing regulatory agencies. Such strategies include funding ballot initiatives that support their own interests and defeating ballot measures and proposed regulations that would increase restrictions on pesticides. Pesticide corporations and other agribusinesses develop reports, opinion pieces to newspapers, and public hearing testimony that frame pesticides as beneficial and regulations as dangerous.[46]

Specifically, they often frame regulatory restrictions on agricultural pesticides as pushing family farmers out of business. As the vice president of the Western Growers Association stated at a legislative hearing in 2009 on proposed soil fumigant regulations, "The many regulatory mandates and costs associated uniquely with California—and our separate and lengthy process for crop protection registration is one of them—are combining to force small farmers into consolidation with large farms and increasingly motivating farmers to look elsewhere for future operations." There is certainly some truth to this statement. In particular, many environmental regulations pose financial burdens on growers, and these burdens are often felt most acutely by small farmers who are already disadvantaged in the marketplace and operate on lower profit margins. That said, such framings obscure a few important facts: many other factors further marginalize small-scale farmers (including corporate consolidation among input manufacturers, processors, and retailers that enables them to charge high prices for farm inputs products and pay low prices for farm products), and chemical manufacturers and distributors stand to lose little by farm structural change. These corporations invoke the idealized notion in the United States of the family farmer largely to protect their own investments in agricultural chemicals.

Violating Laws

Chemical manufacturers also protect and bolster their profits by violating labor and environmental laws, which enables these corporations to reduce their costs. Environmental damage and social exploitation are thus a hallmark of pesticide corporations' business practice, even while their advertisements make claims about environmental sustainability and human welfare. Companies are particularly apt to violate labor and environmental regulations when the benefits of doing so are greater than the associated fines or other sanctions, as is true throughout much of the world and which is an easy option for mega-corporations. It is for these reasons that chemical manufacturers are responsible for committing innumerable egregious acts. For example, Dow Chemical has failed to assist the tens of thousands of victims of the chemical disaster at a factory of its subsidiary (Union Carbide) in Bhopal, India, and sued victims who peacefully protested outside its corporate headquarters.[47] As another example, community activists are suing Dow for contaminating the water around its corporate manufacturing plant in Michigan, where the EPA found the highest levels of the carcinogenic chemical dioxin recorded in US history, and where women have disproportionately high rates of breast cancer.[48] Additionally, all pesticide corporations globally distribute and promote products that have been banned in the United States.

·   ·   ·

The agrichemical industry is dominated by a rapidly shrinking handful of large corporations. Their power stems both from their massive financial resources and their limited competition. Through advertising, research, regulatory capture, and violating laws, they wield this power to define pesticides as essential and beneficial. They fight regulatory and research efforts that would facilitate sustainable agriculture, while protecting their existing and toxic pesticide investments. While they reap the financial rewards of this system, the public loses. Toxic pesticides in food, water, and air regularly poison farmworkers, farmers, residents of agricultural communities, and wildlife. Yet farmers feel unprepared to transition to alternative forms of pest management, as pesticide corporations actively normalize the pesticide paradigm.

A group of pesticide activists is working to bring this corporate concentration to light and combat these corporate actors' undemocratic and toxic practices. They direct their critiques at the regulatory arena, pursuing state-, federal-, and international-level regulatory restrictions on pesticide use as rights-based protections from pesticide exposure for all people. These pesticide activists allege that officials drastically underestimate the scope of pesticide pollution and illness, do not adequately regulate pesticides, and must confront the dangerous and undemocratic practices agrichemical industry actors use to shore up their profits. Pesticide Action Network (PAN) is one of the organizations leading this work. In the next chapter, staff members of PAN describe some of the work they do to combat corporate concentration in the pesticide industry and help foster a more sustainable and just food system.

Drift Catchers Combatting Pesticide Power

Emily Marquez, Marcia Ishii-Eiteman, and Kristin Schafer

ON A COOL SUMMER MORNING IN 2018, Iowa farmer Rob Faux stepped off the front porch and set out to check on his Drift Catcher device. Part way through the twelve-hour monitoring period, he checked that the air tubes attached to the simple air-monitoring tool were still firmly connected and in place. When it was time to change the air tubes, Rob carefully logged the wind speed and air temperature, then moved on to his usual morning chores.

Rob had attended a training a few months before, so he knew exactly how to set up and operate his Drift Catcher. He signed up to be trained after he and his wife lost their organic certification the season before, when pesticide drift from a neighboring farm contaminated their crops and exposed Rob to a mixture of pesticides. This year, he wanted to document the drift himself, so that if problems occurred again he would have direct evidence. Rob's sampling detected the insecticide chlorpyrifos, one of the pesticides that had drifted onto him and his farm the year before.

For more than a decade, Pesticide Action Network (PAN) has worked with farmers like Rob and their rural communities to document pesticide drift with this passive air-monitoring device. The Drift Catcher, developed by former PAN scientist Dr. Susan Kegley, is a community-based monitoring tool modeled after air-monitoring equipment used by the California Air Resources Board. Dr. Kegley developed the Drift Catcher to put air-monitoring equipment in the hands of community members interested in documenting otherwise invisible exposures to pesticide drift.

The Drift Catcher has been deployed in thirteen states to date, and has captured fumigants, fungicides, and insecticides drifting onto farms and into homes, playgrounds, and schools—in many cases at levels well above what is considered safe by the Environmental Protection Agency (EPA). This direct evidence of exposure can be an effective counterweight to combat the pesticide industry's assertions that bystander pesticide exposures will not happen if the chemicals are correctly applied.

The organophosphate insecticide chlorpyrifos is a widely used, drift-prone chemical that has been measured by Drift Catchers across the country. This pesticide is of particular concern, as a strong body of scientific evidence has linked prenatal and early childhood exposures to impaired brain development and function, including lower IQ, reduced motor skills, and increased risk of attention-deficit/hyperactivity disorder and autism. Use of the Drift Catcher through organized, community-based documentation of chlorpyrifos exposures has been a powerful tool for change in combatting corporate pesticide power.

At the national level, evidence of drift submitted by PAN scientists helped set in motion new EPA rules about bystander exposures. This strengthened the legal petition—filed in 2007 by PAN and its partners at the Natural Resources Defense Council and Earthjustice—calling for removal of the dangerous insecticide from the market. As a result of this petition, EPA's scientists reviewed the health impacts of chlorpyrifos, finding that it could not be used safely and should be withdrawn. After years of delay, the court recently ordered the agency to act on these findings.[1]

At the state level, community-generated evidence of drift from agricultural applications of chlorpyrifos and other pesticides was key to winning protective buffer zones around rural schools and day-care centers in California and Hawaii, as well as cancellation of chlorpyrifos use in both states.[2] Concerned community members were able to bring on-the-ground evidence of drift exposures to policymakers and the media, highlighting the urgency of the problem. In Iowa, community monitoring has contributed to a new public conversation about pesticides and children's health, including farmer engagement in press events, learning circles, and social media campaigns.

For more than a decade, PAN has been using the term "grassroots science" to describe our work challenging corporate ownership of science. The grassroots science hub focuses on enhancing public engagement in science and science-related public discourse, including community monitoring as well as "translation" of scientific research and findings from public institutions. In the case of chlorpyrifos, data generated through PAN's grassroots science program directly challenged the assertions by the pesticide's maker, Dow, that when "applied as directed" exposures would not occur—and if they did, they would certainly not be at levels of concern. PAN's experience with the

Drift Catcher clearly illustrates that data in the hands of informed, concerned members of frontline communities is a powerful, effective tool for challenging corporate control.

COMMUNITY MONITORING, COMMUNITY DATA

There is no single approach to community-based participatory action research (CBPAR), as the practice itself involves researchers determining how to proceed in a cooperative process with community partners. However, CBPAR does include some common key characteristics. One central theme of CBPAR is consciously "blurring the lines between the researcher and the researched," leveraging knowledge and experience that community members bring, and acting on the new knowledge co-created by research partners to bring about social change.[3]

PAN's Drift Catcher work differs from typical CBPAR approaches in that the community partners already have the "why" of the project defined. Community groups already know they want to tackle the health risks they face from ongoing pesticide exposure, and have contacted PAN requesting support. The details of the main research activity (the "how" of the project) is defined together with the community members—though some parameters are defined from the outset, because PAN uses the Drift Catcher exclusively for air-monitoring work. In some cases, air monitoring may not be the most appropriate approach, and PAN will work with community members to identify alternative methods (e.g., water monitoring, health surveys, etc.).

PAN's approach to CBPAR includes assessing the project's viability according to certain criteria that help PAN staff determine whether the conditions for a successful project are met, based on previous experiences as well as on current PAN campaigns. A core criterion, for example, is that community members are interested in using Drift Catcher data to press for locally defined solutions, such as a health-protective policy outcome.

Other basic criteria developed by PAN for CBPAR projects involving PAN's Drift Catcher include the following:

- Community members should be affiliated with a local group or other organization.
- Community members want to know whether pesticides are drifting in the air at the chosen monitoring site.

- Community members are willing to be trained to do air monitoring.
- One or more community members are willing to be a spokesperson.
- Community members want to work toward a policy change locally, or on a state or national basis.
- A monitoring site is available near where people live or frequent.
- Air monitoring projects are aligned with an ongoing PAN campaign, either state based or national.

DRIFT CATCHER DATA ARE UNIQUE

To understand why community-generated Drift Catcher data are significant in the policy process, it must be understood that most of the data used by EPA are from studies commissioned or conducted by pesticide registrants; for example, the pesticide manufacturer provides data that are used in assessing the risk of their own products. EPA's risk assessment framework has specific requirements that favor industry studies, as the pesticide registrant will conduct the study according to EPA's requests and specifications. It has become a commonplace tactic of industry to challenge the science behind a public health or environmental regulation proposed in the US, because the "manufacturing [of] uncertainty," as studies have shown, influences public opinion.[4] Journals and other publications can use additional improvements in guidance to authors regarding disclosure of conflicts of interest, as some authors fail to properly disclose funding conflicts.[5] However, the burden should not fall to journals alone to ensure the integrity of research, as public health agencies also have an interest.[6]

Pesticide registrants do not document pesticide drift into people's homes for pragmatic reasons; it is not required by the EPA, and such studies would not serve their interests. Air monitoring by pesticide registrants generally consists of air monitoring at a field edge or close by within mandated (if any) buffer zones, and typically lacks adequate analysis of potential implications for human health.

The only other air-monitoring studies on pesticide drift of which PAN is aware (other than a few conducted by independent research scientists) are conducted by the state of California, through the Department of Pesticide Regulation and the Air Resources Board. While this work does include community sites, the state conducts ambient air monitoring rather than targeting the air-monitoring work to specific times coinciding with known application of drift-prone pesticides.

In contrast, PAN targets air-monitoring projects to coincide with known applications, which, when pesticides are detected, give data on when and what the highest bystander exposures to a nearby pesticide application might be. The data provide a snapshot of what exposures are occurring, but only during the time of monitoring. Pesticide applications are variable in terms of type of pesticide applied, the time of day, the weather and the time of year—all of which can vary from year to year based on a farmer's needs. Because the air-monitoring work is targeted, PAN partners are vital to the Drift Catcher work. PAN would not be able to conduct air monitoring without partners who live near (or at) monitoring sites, for the simple reason that PAN partners decide when to begin monitoring based on their observation of pesticide application activities.

Partners do not play a role in laboratory or data analysis, but they do share in campaign work afterward. PAN and community partners share ownership of the data. Once laboratory results are obtained, the partners are updated via phone, and sent a packet that includes copies of the raw data, the partner's data log sheets, and a written explanation of the final results, including context in terms of agency levels of concern and context from PAN that may include critiques of agency levels of concern.

As part of the follow-up in policy work, PAN might provide data summaries or information sheets in the form of "issue briefs" that a community member might use for campaign work, either locally or to meet with a policymaker (e.g., agency officials or local, state, or national representatives).

Though PAN is not able to monitor every day at a given location throughout the year, the data are sufficient to address a community member's initial questions about exposure. The main question Drift Catcher data have addressed for most of PAN's community partners is "Am I, or is my family, exposed to pesticide drift while at home?" The limitations of monitoring are explained to partners, such as the possibility of "nondetects" when pesticide drift may have occurred, but not at a level detectable by the Drift Catcher. PAN and partners have also conducted a limited number of monitoring projects at sites other than residences, such as playgrounds and schools.

PAN's rationale for targeting Drift Catcher air monitoring at the time of pesticide applications is that the aim of the projects should be to document higher exposures, based on the logic that if regulations were to protect against the worst exposures for vulnerable populations (such as fence-line communities, children, and farmworkers), most individuals would be protected by that rule. A secondary consideration is that air monitoring is expensive, both in terms of community participant time and monetary expense. Partners sometimes go through the training and certification process only to find that they do not have enough time to do air monitoring.

FROM RESEARCH TO ACTION

Once data is collected and analyzed, PAN supports the community partner and the group they are affiliated with in advocacy work. The PAN organizer, partner organization, and community partners discuss next steps, including determining strategies for campaign work. This includes identifying an achievable goal, policy processes that could be initiated or are in motion, potential allies and opposition, and key targets to be influenced. Social and traditional media tactics are also important components of campaign planning.

One key decision is whether or not a technical report and/or an issue brief for policymakers would be strategic. Technical reports are often used as a way to draw greater attention to the results—and the broader problem they represent—through a press release and event, often timed to influence a specific policy process, such as regulatory review of or comment period on a particular pesticide. The technical report is meant to stand apart from the advocacy pieces (e.g., press release and issue brief), because the report summarizes the data without advocating for a policy recommendation, and may be broadly useful to agencies that are interested in air-monitoring data.

Connections with other groups in the state or locally may be made through the PAN organizer or other groups PAN networks with. Support can include communications materials or other communications work, including media and spokesperson training, travel support, joint participation in press events, and answering any questions they may have when they speak about their data publicly.

CASE STUDY: THE DRIFT CATCHER IN IOWA

"What does it take to recruit a group of Iowa farmers and rural residents to an all-day, indoor training on one of the first beautiful days of spring? An issue as serious as pesticide drift," writes Lex Horan, PAN organizer.[7]

After assessing the landscape of state-based organizations when we opened our Minneapolis office in 2012, PAN's Midwest organizing director, Linda Wells, reached out to groups in Iowa that focus on food and farming to explore their interest in working with us around pesticide drift.

Practical Farmers of Iowa (PFI) is a well-established group that provides information and technical assistance to farmers across the state. Many PFI members are small farmers, and the group is composed of many growers who farm without pesticides, are organic certified, or are using pesticides as a last resort in an integrated pest management approach. PFI's interest in pesticide drift was due to concerns over the financial impacts of drift on specialty crop and organic growers in Iowa, most of whom farm in a landscape surrounded by commodity crops that are heavily reliant on pesticides.

PFI's horticultural farmers, some of whom are organic certified, identified two major concerns. If a farmer is organic certified, pesticide drift from neighboring fields threatens their organic certification, a costly process that allows farmers to get a premium market price for the labor and time they invest in farming organically. In addition, when herbicides applied to herbicide-resistant GE crops drift onto non-herbicide-resistant crops (not necessarily organic), the drift can result in a damaged product that can't be sold at market.

After working with PFI to identify member farmers who might be interested in drift catching, PAN organizers set in motion a simple application process, and screened applicants over the phone. Criteria for screening included having an adequate location on their property to site the Drift Catcher (within 350 yards of the neighboring field's edge); being able to do monitoring at a site that is somehow significant to people, such as at a residence; and being able to attend a one-day Drift Catcher training, followed up by testing and certification of their ability to operate a Drift Catcher. Five participants were selected for our first year of drift catching in the state.

Partners then attended a group training in the winter months, when farmers are less busy and before spray season began. Some participants drove for up to four hours to attend the session, gathering in a room reserved at a local college. The training began with a discussion about individuals' experiences and concerns about pesticide drift, followed by a hands-on training where partners would learn how to attach the air tubes to the Drift Catcher, log in the air flow through the air tubes, fill out the data log sheet, and discuss siting considerations.

In the group discussion, several drift-catching partners shared that their concerns about drift were often dismissed by other community members.

Therefore, the training itself provided an important space for drift-catching partners to be heard and to network, creating a cohort of Iowa farmers and other community members taking action to document pesticide drift. Following the training, a PAN organizer and/or scientist visited partners at their farm or monitoring site to check the Drift Catcher siting and certify the participant's ability to appropriately operate the tool.

Drift-catching partners determined exactly when to monitor based on their observations of pesticide application activity in the area. After samples were collected, they were shipped to the PAN office, where a few initial samples were selected by a PAN scientist and sent to a certified analytical laboratory. If the initial samples came back positive for pesticide residues, then the rest of the samples were sent in for analysis.

Once all the data were collected, data analysis and reporting back to partners were done via phone, followed by a letter and copies of the data. Though the herbicides of concern have proven difficult to monitor, partners in Iowa have detected chlorpyrifos drift over the past few years of drift catching at five sites, including one that has had detections every year for the three years that monitoring has been done.

In the early days of PAN's work in Iowa, drift catching allowed PAN to connect with partners and gain public recognition as a resource on pesticide issues in the state, building vital relationships for ongoing organizing. Though collecting evidence of herbicide drift using the Drift Catcher proved difficult, the fact that chlorpyrifos—a neurodevelopmental toxicant that is especially harmful to children—was so widely found opened the door to conversations about the impact of pesticides on children's health. This early community monitoring thus laid the groundwork for PAN's continued campaign work on drift with Iowa partners, highlighting the concerns about the impacts of pesticide drift on health and livelihood across the state.

CHALLENGING CORPORATIONS
WITH GRASSROOTS SCIENCE

In one of PAN's *GroundTruth* blogs, Midwest organizer Lex Horan speaks to the value of the Drift Catcher to Iowa farmers: "Why does Drift Catching matter? Drift happens, and Midwest farmers and rural residents know it. They smell pesticides in their air, notice withered crops and damaged treelines. But drift is hard to prove. There are no public agencies monitoring the air for pesticides in the Midwest, and when people speak up about the problem, they're often dismissed by decision makers and pesticide applicators."[8]

Collecting air-monitoring data at targeted sites counters the story told in the research results industry submits to EPA and other agencies; specifically, the assumption that significant amounts of pesticides are not drifting into places where people live or where children attend school. Although there is no legally enforceable standard for pesticides drifting in the air, pesticide drift is supposed to be illegal, so direct evidence of drift is a powerful tool for change. This is why Drift Catcher data spurred new national rules protecting bystanders from drift-prone pesticides and has been key to winning first county-level and recently statewide buffer zone policies in California.

Drift Catcher work challenges corporations' monopoly over science when community members participate in collection of scientific data. Participation in Drift Catcher projects grants ownership of scientific data to community members, who gain expertise in a scientific protocol and are thus empowered by that knowledge. Further, collecting data confirming that drift happens is empowering, as participants finally have some of their questions about drift answered by doing the scientific work themselves.

Drift catching can be deeply personal, as partners often monitor at their homes or at a site that has some personal significance to them in terms of their family and community. The insecticide chlorpyrifos is a powerful case in point. This widely used neurotoxicant—which science clearly shows can undermine brain development—has been detected at drift-catching monitoring sites from Iowa to Washington State, from California and Florida to Minnesota. Community-generated data was critical in supporting the legal action described above, which led to recommendations from EPA scientists to pull the pesticide from the market. In the spring of 2017, the new EPA leadership ignored those recommendations after a meeting with Dow Chemical executives, deciding to postpone the planned ban indefinitely. Follow-up legal action from PAN and several partners led the court to order EPA to take action on its own scientific analysis, a ruling the judges reaffirmed after the agency appealed.[9]

With the current focus at the federal level on rolling back the most basic health and environmental safeguards, grassroots science can serve not only to continue to document exposures, but also to energize and empower communities with on-the-ground evidence that challenges corporate influence on policymaking. Again, chlorpyrifos provides a case in point.

The removal of this pesticide in California and Hawaii was driven in large part by science-based pressure from affected communities, and—in turn—built momentum for health-protective action in other states. New York voted to ban chlorpyrifos in spring 2019, and similar policies are in motion in Oregon, Connecticut, and Maryland.

It takes on-the-ground evidence like that from Rob Faux's farm. Rob and his wife Tammy had to wait three years for Genuine Faux Farm to be recertified organic after the initial drift incident that brought them to PAN. Organizer Lex Horan reflects on the Drift Catcher certification visit with Rob Faux: "After we watched Rob set up his Drift Catcher in the garage, we initialed his paperwork and handed over his certificate. He was officially ready to join the cohort of concerned Iowa residents who monitor their air for pesticide drift. We hope there are no more issues with drift on his organic farm. But if drift happens, we all agree: let's document the problem."[10]

Devil's Bargain

FRACTURED FARMS OR FREEDOM?

Kathryn De Master and Stephanie A. Malin

AS WE SAT AT HIS KITCHEN TABLE, an exasperated Pennsylvania dairy farmer described the painful decision he faced: should he sign a lease giving a petroleum corporation unfettered access to his land, to tap the natural gas reserves there, and thereby receive a royalty check that might save his farm? Or, should he continue to endure ongoing financial strain and face losing his livelihood? He explained his predicament: "Farmers now, especially dairy farmers, we are really, really hurting. So a lot of us are looking for any way out. We're doing what we love, and it costs us money to farm. So we finally break down and say 'I'll sign the damn lease. It's a way to save my cows.' And that's been happening more and more."

This dairy farmer is not alone. Many other farmers today face this devil's bargain: sign leases with energy corporations that might lead to windfall profits, but in so doing, risk lasting environmental damage to their farms and communities if they allow drilling to proceed unabated. But if they refuse to sign, many farmers risk losing their livelihoods within increasingly economically vulnerable agricultural sectors, marked by corporate consolidation and intense competition.

These impossible choices are being fueled by corporate power through an unprecedented transformation occurring on many working landscapes in the rural United States. From Pennsylvania dairy farmers to West Virginia organic vegetable growers, from Ohio soybean farmers to Colorado cattle ranchers, farmers and rural producers throughout the US are finding their landscapes and livelihoods radically disrupted through the swift advance of unconventional natural gas drilling, or "hydraulic fracturing." As drilling expands rapidly, many rural producers—especially farmers and ranchers in Western states—have not even been given the difficult choice of signing a lease or receiving a royalty check. Through "split estate" laws that give the federal government or energy companies access to subsurface mineral rights, or through "compulsory pooling" regulations, even farmers and ranchers who might otherwise refuse to sign leases with natural gas corporations may find themselves without the freedom to make that choice. As a result of this large-scale national corporate energy transition, they face enormously difficult choices about their land, farming and ranching operations, and the future of their families.

The rapid expansion of unconventional natural gas drilling is being driven in part by a revolution in new drilling and natural gas extraction technologies, including refinements to directional drilling and hydraulic fracturing techniques. Though these technologies have been in practice on a smaller scale since the 1960s, they were previously cost-prohibitive. Technological developments that began in the 1990s have catalyzed the swift utilization of hydraulic fracturing by energy corporations in and around hundreds of US rural communities in over twenty states.[1] These novel drilling technologies extract previously inaccessible deposits of petroleum and natural gas in shale formations at a scale unmatched in the modern era.[2]

As a result of this unparalleled drilling expansion, the US is now the largest producer of natural gas in the world.[3] Some of the major oil and natural gas "plays," or fields, where that natural gas is produced include the Marcellus Shale (Pennsylvania, Ohio, New York, and West Virginia); the Niobrara Shale (Colorado, Wyoming, Kansas, and Nebraska); the Eagle Ford and Barnett Shales (Texas); and the Bakken (North Dakota), though many other substantial plays are in production or preproduction by oil and gas companies.[4] Natural gas can be accessed after oil wells have been played out, so many petroleum companies are reaping the benefits from wells—and rural communities—they had previously abandoned.

In the last decade, many believed that accessing untapped natural gas reserves would offer economically marginalized US rural agricultural communities a way out of their enormous financial troubles. American rural communities today endure widespread unemployment and underemployment; rates of poverty (15.8 percent) that outpace those of many metropolitan areas; and food insecurity that affects approximately 15 percent of rural households, underscoring the stark irony that many of the nation's food producers face hunger themselves.[5] In the early days of the natural gas boom, national politicians, economists, and even some prominent national environmental organizations spoke of natural gas as the "clean" or "bridge" fuel of the future that would assure US economic development and energy independence. And as the Pennsylvania dairy farmer above explained to us, many rural American producers have signed leases in the hopes of finding "*any* way out."

FRACTURED FARMS

The story we share here is drawn from a study we conducted in the early years of the natural gas boom in 2012. We explored the impacts of unconventional natural gas production on farmers in three rural US counties in Pennsylvania—Bradford, Susquehanna, and Washington—where agriculture and drilling activity overlap intensively. In Pennsylvania's Marcellus Shale region, at the start of the natural gas boom, over half of Pennsylvania well pads were situated on agricultural land.[6] Though the experience of the farmers we interviewed is particular to Pennsylvania, it is one that resonates in many US communities today, where many rural producers face similar choices and challenges. In fact, nearly three-quarters of American farms are geographically situated in shale basins, active shale plays, or regions where sand is mined for hydraulic fracturing.[7] As oil and natural gas corporations eye many of these basins for hydraulic fracturing development, farmers and ranchers in these communities grapple over questions that carry with them the weight of generations before them, of children and grandchildren after them, whose lives and livelihoods center on their land. To learn more about the experiences of farmers in the midst of the roaring growth of hydraulic fracturing, we visited the farms and kitchen tables of forty-one primarily small and mid-sized Pennsylvania farms. We asked farmers about their operations and their positive and negative experiences with the leasing process and natural gas production on their land.

Nearly everyone we interviewed experienced natural gas activity directly on their farms, and around 75 percent of the farmers we interviewed owned their mineral rights. Theoretically, farmers who own their mineral rights have more decision-making power over what happens on their farms than those who do not.

However, as we spoke extensively with these rural producers, we realized that the choice about what to allow on their land was far more complicated than it appeared at face value. Farmers toiled over how to respond to pressure to lease their land and minerals to natural gas corporations; they vacillated about how to best assure that they honored their family's legacy while preserving the chance to hand something of value and meaning down to future generations. There were no clear or easy paths toward a secure future. In interview after interview, we spoke to farmers struggling to balance their commitments to sustainable farming practices with tenuous livelihoods, pressing debts, and the risk of foreclosure or loss of their farms. In this context, opening their land to unconventional natural gas development presented farmers with some economic security, albeit temporarily, where few other opportunities existed. As one Susquehanna County farmer described it, "Oh geez, I can [only] make $200 per acre on a corn crop, and in all likelihood, you're going to make a hell of a lot more on a well pad."

Profits received from energy leases have allowed some of these farmers to expand their operations, pay off farm debts, or transition out of farming altogether. A handful—typically those with larger, more capital-intensive operations—may have even received big payouts in the form of royalties and large signing bonuses. The stories of these farmers, dubbed "shaleionaires" by the popular press, have fueled an "energy lottery" narrative.[8] And it is clear that in the aggregate, payments by energy companies to farmers have been substantial in many cases. For example, some studies indicate average payouts of $104,000 to recipient farms.[9] But most farmers we interviewed were not "shaleionaires."

In Pennsylvania—as is the case in many US rural communities—many small and mid-sized farmers already contend with persistent poverty and economic marginalization, unstable agricultural markets, and increasing costs for farmland and other inputs.[10] Some own farms tethered to antiquated petroleum lease arrangements that give natural gas corporations unfettered access to their land, even if they technically own their mineral rights. Others signed leases reluctantly, agreeing only under intense community pressure or corporate bullying, perhaps convinced by false assurances of minimal disruption to their farms. And while farmers with larger, more capital-intensive operations may have a range of choices available to them, most small and mid-sized farmers were particularly vulnerable to misleading corporate promises.

Farmers struggle with decisions about signing leases because they could threaten the very integrity of their operations. The risks they were taking by signing a lease rarely left their minds. Farmers we spoke with shared stories of neighbors' spills that made livestock sick, or tales of polluted water from drilling operations that had leaked onto rural county roadways and into nearby streams, and they described permanent changes to once-valuable pastureland. Organic and sustainable farmers we interviewed expressed anxiety over how to balance their environmentally responsible approaches to farming with the environmental risks that can accompany unconventional natural gas production. They also lamented their perceived vulnerability to losing certification. These descriptions of risks and impacts all became a sort of folklore that we heard over and over again from farmers. We wondered: why would farmers invite these risks?

We learned that the answer to this question is complex and multifaceted and goes far beyond the simple rationale of the "energy lottery" narrative. It is embedded, in part, in the structural conditions created by both the corporatized agriculture and energy sectors. These structural conditions have paved the way for energy corporations to flourish in Pennsylvania's rural agricultural communities with few obstacles, while farmers find their freedoms diminished. We also learned of ways that natural gas corporations and their contractors exercised power not only structurally but also through strategic direct actions: obfuscation and lack of transparency, delay tactics and broken promises, and direct bullying of farmers.

STRUCTURAL FACTORS FACILITATING CORPORATE POWER: BOOM AND BUST AND DAIRY CONSOLIDATION

Structurally, unconventional natural gas corporations in Pennsylvania have benefited from the fact that many rural agricultural counties in the state have already been weakened economically by a legacy of boom-and-bust cycles associated with the petroleum sector, combined with consolidating agricultural sectors (particularly dairy).

The farmers in our study hailed from Pennsylvania's Marcellus Shale region, host to some of the most prolific natural gas extraction activity in the nation. This 104,000-square-mile formation also extends into New York, Ohio, and West Virginia, and produces over 16,000 cubic feet of natural gas per day.[11] Many Marcellus communities historically built their economies on forestry, agriculture, tourism, coal, and oil. In fact, during the early Pennsylvania oil boom in the nineteenth century, Bradford County had the "first billion-dollar [oil] field."[12] Ongoing dependence on the natural-resource sectors in Bradford and Susquehanna Counties has fostered repeated boom-and-bust cycles. Scholars have widely documented that these cycles occur predictably as resources are depleted, supply outpaces demand, or as once-burgeoning markets falter or shift to new frontiers. This can precipitate the reorganizing of rural economies.[13] Some scholars have identified the extra-local power of extraction industries over communities as a key mechanism in rural impoverishment.[14] Indeed, boom-and-bust cycles have helped structure the persistent poverty of Bradford and Susquehanna Counties, making the region one of the most chronically poor pockets of Pennsylvania.[15] Though Washington County has a more diversified economy today, it still relies on coal extraction and agriculture, and is increasingly reliant on wet natural gas production.[16]

Situated at the epicenter of the natural gas production boom, these counties have experienced uneven environmental and economic impacts from hydraulic fracturing and its associated industrial development. Drilling operations are often situated near homes, hospitals, and schools, complicating the financial benefits of the boom with environmental and health risks.[17] As the economy of these three counties has shifted toward unconventional natural gas extraction, it became clear that the recent natural gas boom is not simply another iteration of a long line of petroleum leases on or near farmers' land.

In addition to the predictable boom-and-bust cycles that the Marcellus region has faced historically, within these rural communities small and mid-sized farmers especially find it challenging to remain viable. The corporate control of supply chains and increased concentration in agricultural input and processing sectors, as well as competition from global commodity markets, make it increasingly difficult to compete. Nationwide, this constellation of factors has precipitated a seemingly relentless decline in commercially viable small and mid-sized farms.[18]

US dairy farmers—including many small and mid-sized operations in Pennsylvania—find it especially difficult to remain afloat. Most US dairy producers today face a narrowing set of options to market their milk, since nationally the dairy sector ranks as one of the more volatile and concentrated agricultural sectors. Between 1997 and 2007, for example, the US lost around five thousand dairy farms, as the average herd size grew rapidly. According to *Hoard's Dairyman,* a mere ten thousand US dairy farms (around 20 percent of total dairy farms) now produce 80 percent of US milk. Twenty-five hundred of the largest dairies dominate, producing close to 50 percent of total milk. Between 2000 and 2006, farms with over two thousand cows more than doubled, with more than 25 percent of the nation's milk coming from industrial "mega-dairies."[19] This process depresses wages for farmers and workers, rendering the surrounding communities vulnerable to economic development that might otherwise be unwelcome: private prisons, polluting industries, and—in the case of rural Pennsylvania—unconventional natural gas extraction.

Most of the farmers in our study had small or mid-sized operations, and over half were dairy farmers; many others had some direct economic connection to dairy, through raising feed crops or participating in small value-added enterprises. Though Pennsylvania's dairy farms rank fifth nationally in milk commodity sales and fourth in overall production, the state's dairy farmers face competition from larger and more capital-intensive national operations in states such as California, Arizona, New Mexico, and Wisconsin.[20] They endure fluctuating and fickle hundredweight prices for fluid milk, with prices set by antiquated government formulas and controlled by a small cadre of commodities traders.[21] Concomitant with the surge in hydraulic fracturing, Pennsylvania dairy farmers also experienced falling milk prices, with feed and fuel costs rising precipitously.[22]

The result of these inherent structural barriers found in natural resource dependent communities (NRDCs) and in the dairy sector mean that many small and mid-sized dairy farmers in rural Pennsylvania find themselves caught in a double bind between two increasingly corporatized sectors— energy and agriculture—that vie for the same geographic spaces for radically different land uses. For corporations to succeed in this instance, they need not pursue overt collusion or backroom brokering to reduce competition. Yet the effect of corporate power is the same: small and mid-sized Pennsylvania farm enterprises are rendered susceptible to the business interests of energy corporations due to their preexisting economic vulnerability. Farmers embedded in these geographic spaces now act as ambivalent gatekeepers to the land and minerals natural gas companies need to survive, all while corporate power advances in a familiar, predictable cycle of boom and bust.

CORPORATE POWER IN ACTION: OBFUSCATION, BROKEN PROMISES, AND BULLYING

While structural conditions in the dairy sector in rural Pennsylvania help explain how natural gas corporations eliminate impediments to expanding hydraulic fracturing operations on private farmland, we also found that these companies exercised corporate power through several specific strategies in farming communities: (1) obfuscation and an overall lack of transparency, (2) delay tactics and broken promises, and (3) direct bullying.

First, lack of transparency and obfuscation was a consistent theme in our interviews with farmers. This finding is not surprising, given the fact that the oil and gas industry notoriously lacks transparency. We know very little, for example, about precisely how many new wells in these regions use unconventional technologies such as directional drilling and hydraulic fracturing.[23] Neither states nor industry operators are required to report uniform data about their operations or the extent of them, so hydraulic fracturing has spread widely, speeding ahead with little uniform oversight.[24]

In our conversations with farmers, we found that energy corporations had showered many of them with lavish promises regarding lease benefits. However, most farmers had difficulty obtaining transparent and precise information about how drilling operations would impact their farming enterprises. While most farmers with whom we spoke knew that signing leases with energy corporations would entail some environmental risk, few had a sense of the scale and scope of the complex web of industrial infrastructure required for operations to proceed, including drilling apparatus, well pads, natural gas storage facilities, and pipelines that transport natural gas to processing and trade hubs. Farmers we interviewed often felt that natural gas companies took advantage of their lack of understanding. As one small-scale dairy farmer described for us, in typical fashion, "As for the companies themselves, I think the bigger frustration is, they don't tell you what's going on . . . Yes, we signed the lease, we signed the agreement, but you're [natural gas company] not going to trash my farm." As another farmer explained, "Well, we believed what they [their lease holding company] said. We believed they would do what they said, and honor the agreements [leases]. And it's just through time and experience and talking to neighbors, that we see that they don't mean a thing that they say."

Second, in addition to obfuscation and lack of transparency, many farmers faced delay tactics in which corporations failed to deliver on initial promises. Often these farmers were given seemingly ironclad assurances regarding disruption to their farm operations, damages to their land prior to signing leases, and timing and amount of lease and royalty payments. Later, however, after drilling had begun, they found natural gas companies less forthcoming. As one farmer explained:

We have friends that . . . haven't gotten paid yet . . . and their unit has been in production for almost a year. . . . Every time we have a question, it's like, "Oh you didn't send in this form," or "We haven't received this or that." . . . It's big money, big corporations. These people have a whole room full of lawyers sitting around with nothing else to do but think of ways to get one over on somebody.

Such descriptions were typical of the experience of many farmers in our study. While initial leases were negotiated with one company representative, such as a "land man" contracted by the company pursuing a lease, subsequent interactions with natural gas companies involved farmers dealing with layers of corporate bureaucracy and subcontractors to simply receive payment or lodge complaints about operations on their land. Additionally, in spite of assurances before they signed leases that they would face minimal environmental risks, we heard numerous stories about how energy companies failed to deliver on those promises. Nearly 85 percent of the farmers with whom we spoke experienced damage to their farmland, in many cases far beyond what they anticipated. As one farmer explained:

We understood that when you go in an area and you're extracting natural resources, that there is destruction, there's an inconvenience, and, yes, there are going to be accidents. Things will happen . . . We knew some water was going to be contaminated, that's the nature of the business . . . And we were assured and saw the land man's charts, the graphs, the literature and everything else. But it's been completely, completely opposite [of what we were told].

Describing the extent of damage to his land, another farmer offered,

I'll take you up and show you where they put in the pipeline . . . it's our hay-field. You should see the disgrace. They put in a temporary waterline down here one year. And it broke. We had frack water all over the friggin' place. They completely destroyed our land.

The land damage this farmer described, as well as the failure to deliver on promises, is consistent with what many researchers are now learning about hydraulic fracturing impacts in many US rural communities. For example, air pollution researchers are increasingly concerned about natural gas leaks throughout the drilling and piping infrastructure, as well as the resulting methane releases that have occurred across the US.[25] Recent United States Geologic Survey studies have shown that new processes such as reinjecting the water produced from hydraulic fracturing have increased the likelihood of earthquakes and other impacts to seismicity, especially in states such as Oklahoma.[26] Public health researchers have observed worrisome outcomes across multiple categories of human health, including increased rates of birth defects among babies who live in close proximity to natural gas wells utilizing hydraulic fracturing technology.[27] Social scientists have shown that living in close proximity to hydraulically fractured wells can lead to experiences of collective trauma and disempowerment.[28]

Finally, in addition to a lack of transparency, delay tactics, and broken promises, many farmers reported being pressured or bullied by corporate representatives. One farmer described the bullying this way:

> They're just trying to bulldoze right over us. It was all permission before, and now it's just, "We're going to buy it from Talisman"—our lease—"and then do whatever we want." That's what they said . . . basically Chief [the natural gas company] is bulldozing right over top of us, and going to do whatever they want no matter what we say.

Farmers also described how this bullying extended to public meetings that were intended to address conflicts related to leases and land impacts, associated with the industry's rapid growth in Pennsylvania. One small-scale dairy farmer described the scene at a meeting at a local church:

> The meeting, it was filled to capacity. And Chesapeake was supposed to give a presentation and answer people's questions. Instead they were a little less polite about it. Basically they were giving veiled threats, their security guards were there—armed . . . The meeting was a dismal failure.

Such veiled threats made it clear to some farmers that they had been clearly misled—a fact some described bitterly. As one farmer put it, "It's the principle of it. It's the deception, the principle and the bullying . . . by corporations, corporate bullying."

FUTURE REPAIR AND RESISTANCE

Until recently, the "shaleionares" energy lottery narrative, replete with stories that highlight Pennsylvania's economic boom, has emphasized ways that farmers have benefited from the Marcellus Shale boom.[29] Such a narrative resonates in economically vulnerable rural communities across the nation.

And some farmers do benefit financially, at least initially. Natural gas lease monies and royalty payments helped some of the Pennsylvania farmers in our study supplement modest incomes or pay off debts—a welcome financial relief for financially strapped farmers. Yet most farmers we met also spoke about ways that energy corporations failed to be transparent, broke promises or engaged in delay tactics, or even bullied them directly.

And as often as farmers we spoke with described the welcome relief that lease monies may have delivered, they also described feeling that they felt forced to make a "deal with the devil." As they experienced ongoing inequities and corporate threats, or wrangled with company representatives to receive royalty payments, or faced new environmental impacts and risks, some regretted their decision to sign leases—even if they saw no other way out.

Today some farmers are beginning to recognize ways that they are now locked into a long-term commitment with a new and very volatile commodity: natural gas. Energy corporations attain access to land, mineral, and gas reserves, and farmers can be paid to "put up and shut up" for a relatively small price. Much like the new strains of Green Revolution rice, planted by economically vulnerable farmers of the Global South, natural gas represents a new kind of "crop" that generates apparent benefits at the same time that it fosters structural dependencies. Those dependencies then foreclose other potentially less risky or destructive rural development options.

Given the disproportionate harms and unevenly distributed benefits farmers experience when they sign a lease to allow hydraulic fracturing on their land, we suggest that Pennsylvania rural farmers experience rural environmental injustice, fostered by procedural inequities. Gerald Leventhal described procedural equity as a process that is characterized by "consistency, accuracy, ethicality, and lack of bias," in which people feel they "have a voice."[30] Farmers in Pennsylvania who experience delay tactics, a lack of transparency, and corporate bullying are recognizing that after leases are signed, they no longer have a meaningful seat at the negotiating table with energy corporations. They may have been lured to that table with appealing promises designed to garner their support, only to be ignored or betrayed later.

Moving forward, demanding a seat at that negotiating table will be challenging for Pennsylvania farmers, as it will be for farmers and ranchers throughout the US. Indeed, in other regions, particularly Western states in which farmers and ranchers may own their land but typically not their mineral rights, some obstacles may appear insurmountable. Nevertheless, even more problematic than the energy lottery narrative is the "inevitability narrative"—in which corporate power is presumed inexorable. As Wenonah Hauter and Seth Gladstone detail in the story that follows, a New York coalition demonstrated specific ways that the corporate power of the oil and gas industry can be successfully challenged.

In spite of the New York victory, however, much more work is necessary. Addressing entrenched corporate power, including the structural interdependencies between the corporate agriculture and energy sectors, will involve organizing and mobilizing broad coalitions that not only address unconventional natural gas production but also attend to the profound needs of rural agricultural communities. Coalitions must therefore act with sensitivity, attentiveness, and responsiveness to the needs of farmers, ranchers, and rural people in NRDCs throughout the US who contend daily with various devil's bargains.

Food and Water over Fracking

Wenonah Hauter and Seth A. Gladstone

MAKING RURAL AMERICA A PLACE where farmers and farmworkers can earn a fair living will require many changes in our politics and economy. Bringing people together to prevent rural areas from simply becoming sacrifice zones for corporate resource extraction or other destructive activities is critical for building a truly sustainable future.

The battle over "fracking" in New York State offers many of the lessons for how a large and politically powerful movement can be built to include farmers and food professionals among broad constituencies mobilized for action. Rather than the usual weak demands for regulation, our campaign had a strong and visionary goal: to ban fracking across New York State. We believe the strategies used in New York can be duplicated in other areas and as applied to other organizing efforts to address corporate power in the food system. The New York case provides important lessons about how people can come together, work incredibly hard, and achieve success, particularly when they are inspired by a vision of a healthy future for their communities.

BANDING TOGETHER FOR THE BAN

One of the most important steps in the movement to ban fracking in New York State was the 2012 creation of a broad-based coalition, New Yorkers Against Fracking (NYAF), which was comprised of more than 225 groups. Coordinated by a steering committee of its founding members—Food and Water Watch, Frack Action, Water Defense, Catskill Mountainkeeper, New York Citizen Action, and others—the coalition developed a detailed, statewide, goal-oriented tactical campaign to hold Governor Andrew Cuomo accountable to the people of New York State. NYAF was cofounded by noted author and biologist Sandra Steingraber, who donated a significant portion of her 2011 Heinz Foundation Award for environmental work to underwrite the formation of the coalition.

In addition to NYAF, many nonprofit organizations, scientific experts, businesses, elected officials, political parties, labor unions, thought leaders, faith groups, celebrities, artists, and entertainers came together collaboratively to build the political power needed to make the governor ban fracking. Most importantly, this campaign was driven by the many thousands of volunteers, most of them New Yorkers, who gave of their time and energy to resist the controversial fossil fuel drilling and extraction method being considered for implementation in New York.

Importantly, NYAF explicitly demanded a *ban* on fracking at a time when many statewide environmental groups preferred a regulatory approach. Having a broad, statewide coalition calling for a ban gave this demand— which grassroots groups had been making at the local level for years—new credibility and opened up new political space in the state. Where the political debate had often focused on how to regulate fracking, this new coalition called into question whether the practice should be allowed at all. Because grassroots energy was already behind the ban position, groups across the state quickly came together under the NYAF umbrella. This focused the pressure around fracking toward the governor as the key decision maker.

In the years leading up to the formation of NYAF and afterward, concerned individuals from across New York State attended community meetings, forums, public hearings, film screenings, rallies, and protest marches. They educated their neighbors, organized their communities, joined with statewide and national groups, formed coalitions, yelled, screamed, chanted, and sang. They submitted more than two hundred thousand public comments opposing fracking. They wrote letters to editors, called the governor's office, signed petitions, and voted for anti-fracking candidates. Perhaps most importantly, they came out at every possible opportunity to Governor Cuomo's public and private events in an attempt to engage directly with him and make their opposition to fracking known. He simply could not appear in public without encountering dozens, hundreds, or even thousands of loud, animated "fractivists" holding ban-fracking signs and shouting ban-fracking chants.

Once the coalition mobilized a large movement to ban fracking, many mainstream environmental groups made notable contributions to the effort, despite the fact that they do not work to ban fracking in other states. National organizations like Credo Action, 350.org, and others joined the coalition, strongly advocating for a ban.

The movement to ban fracking in New York was ultimately an unequivocal success. Governor Cuomo announced at a public cabinet meeting on December 17, 2014, that his administration would act to prohibit fracking statewide, out of concern for suspected human health risks. For anti-fracking activists worldwide, this was a watershed moment in what is generally considered to be a defining environmental issue of this decade.

The success was not simply an environmental one, either. A broad coalition of constituencies and causes that actively engaged on the issue was critical to winning the ban. Good-government groups, faith-based groups and statewide religious councils, small business owners, hunting and fishing groups, and many other organized interests all contributed significantly to the movement. The public health aspects of the campaign, particularly, and the active involvement of numerous medical doctors, biologists, researchers, health professionals, and their associated academic institutions and professional associations, cannot be understated. In its explanation of the decision to ban fracking, the Cuomo administration focused primarily on volumes of data pointing to fracking's negative human health effects. In fact, at a key point in the campaign, the movement in New York pivoted its framing of fracking from primarily an environmental issue to primarily a public health issue. This was ultimately decisive. In addition to the public health community, however, one constituency in particular stood out as indispensable to the anti-fracking movement in New York: food, beverage, and agriculture interests.

FOOD OVER FRACKING

The New York farmers, farmworkers, suppliers, food workers, restaurateurs, and chefs whose livelihoods depend on the health and safety of the food supply understood they had much at stake in the movement to ban fracking. From organic dairy farmers to celebrity Manhattan chefs, from food co-ops to craft beer brewers, from name-brand yogurt producers to small-town market proprietors, food producers and preparers played an integral part in achieving New York's fracking ban. Given the nature of fracking, it is no surprise that those closely associated with food and agriculture would find the process so alarming.

New York's growing wine and beer industry played a particularly critical role in the campaign to ban fracking. New York's vintners and brewers immediately understood the dire threats that fracking posed to New York's clean water, one of their essential resources, and were early and persistent in their clear demand for a ban on fracking. This was crucial to the success of the campaign, as Cuomo saw the local beverage industry as a key economic asset to the state. Both wine and beer production have greatly expanded during the governor's tenure, and he often touts this success as evidence that his upstate job creation program is working. New York's wine and beer industry worked with NYAF to turn these summits into key moments to highlight the industry's widespread opposition to fracking, as this process directly threatens the water cycle so critical for agriculture.

Due to the strong agricultural presence in New York's Southern Tier, the threat of fracking in the region was felt acutely by food and farming interests throughout the state, and by organizations such as Food and Water Watch that are heavily engaged in both the anti-fracking and food safety movements. Food and Water Watch first became involved in the fight against fracking in 2009, when evidence of fracking's threat to water resources began to emerge. Local activists and concerned residents in affected communities around the country were already raising the alarm about fracking's impacts, from chemical spills to truck traffic accidents, even lighting tap water on fire to demonstrate gas leakages into water sources.

Meanwhile, many prominent national environmental organizations were celebrating natural gas as a "bridge fuel"—an energy source improvement from coal, which is widely known to be a dangerous and unsustainable driver of fossil fuel emissions and climate change. Communities already suffering from fracking, or those like New York's Southern Tier, were about to face a growing onslaught from fracking companies, felt betrayed and abandoned by the mainstream environmental movement.

Coming to those communities' defense, Food and Water Watch produced a report in 2010 titled "Not So Fast, Natural Gas" that raised serious initial questions about the safety of fracking. Evidence of harm continued to mount, and in 2011 Food and Water Watch became the first national organization in America to call for a complete ban on fracking.

Since our ban demand in 2011, more than 150 additional studies have been conducted on a range of issues—from water pollution to climate change, air pollution to earthquakes—reinforcing the case that fracking is simply too unsafe to utilize. Finally, in the face of continuously emerging science, a consensus is emerging among many local, state, and national groups working against fracking that complete bans on fracking are the only reasonable solution.

This is the conclusion that many New York food and agriculture interests came to years ago.

One of the first food institutions to speak out against the threat of fracking in New York was the Park Slope Food Coop in Brooklyn. Formed in 1973, it is one of the oldest and largest food cooperatives in the United States, boasting over sixteen thousand active members who spend almost $50 million at the store annually. The co-op spends more than $3 million each year on food products grown and produced in New York State.

More than its buying power, though, the Park Slope Food Coop is known for its social activism and ability to generate attention and collective action within the highly engaged, politically influential, and wealthy community of "brownstone Brooklyn," where it is based. During the apartheid era, for example, goods from South Africa were banned from the store, as were goods from Chile during the Pinochet regime. More recently the co-op has organized boycotts of Coca-Cola products and stopped selling bottled water.

In 2010 the Park Slope Food Coop officially endorsed a ban on fracking in New York after a certifying vote from its membership. Publicity of the vote brought the issue of fracking into focus for many in New York City for the first time. In December of that year, the co-op followed up with a letter from its general manager, Joe Holtz, to then governor-elect Cuomo:

> We are very responsive to the needs of our shoppers. If hydrofracking is allowed to go forward, our shoppers are certain to be asking us if the fruits, vegetables, dairy products, eggs and meats from New York State are produced in areas where hydrofracking is taking place . . . Please insure that we are not wondering about whether the grass-fed cows we buy were drinking contaminated water and breathing the air fouled by numerous enormous trucks that will support the hydrofracking process . . . I guarantee that our members will not want the fruits and veggies that come from farms in an industrial area. They will ask their employees to look elsewhere and we will.

In subsequent interviews, Holtz made it clear that the co-op would stop carrying any items sourced in New York towns where fracking was instituted. "We would have stopped buying from them. There is no doubt in my mind," he said, after the ban was finally enacted. Holtz then went on to highlight the role the Park Slope Food Coop could likely have played in a large-scale boycott of food produced in a New York fracking zone, an action he threatened repeatedly in letters to public officials and in remarks to reporters. "Just a few years ago, we were the first store to remove products from our shelves produced by a company that was ignoring a ruling by the National Labor Relations Board. Over a hundred other stores followed us. The same would have happened with fracking in New York, only much bigger."

FARMERS' RESISTANCE

To resist fracking hundreds of miles away from where it would actually occur is important, of course. To resist it from the midst of a potentially affected community, one dominated by a rural, agricultural landscape most easily exploited by the fracking industry, with known, plentiful deposits of shale gas directly below one's feet, is another matter entirely.

Farmers, whose livelihoods depend on the health of their land, face especially stark choices. As discussed by Kathryn De Master and Stephanie Malin in the preceding chapter, many farmers throughout the Marcellus Shale region leased their land to natural gas corporations with the promise of huge gas royalty payments and nominal ecological impact. The promises they were given were made by "land men"—agents who typically seek out landowners willing to sign fracking leases, often sharing with them exaggerated estimates of recoverable gas and royalty rates, as well as grossly minimizing fracking's impacts.

Kathie Arnold, a third-generation dairy farmer running the 140-cow Twin Oaks Dairy Farm in Truxton, New York (an area well within Marcellus Shale coverage in the Southern Tier), experienced this firsthand. She was approached by a "land man" about leasing her land to gas drilling in 2006. The employee of Fortuna Energy (later Talisman Energy) made no mention of fracking. "We just assumed their interest was in traditional vertical drilling, which had been happening throughout the region for a long time," Arnold explained recently. She signed a five-year lease.

In the months and years that followed, Arnold learned a lot more about fracking. Reports of serious agricultural and environmental degradation began migrating north from Pennsylvania and elsewhere. She learned how cows exposed to fracking fluids have experienced higher rates of stillborn and deformed calves. In Louisiana, for example, sixteen cows died after drinking water tainted with fracking fluid,[1] and in Pennsylvania, only three of eleven calves born from a group of cows exposed to fracking fluid survived—an alarmingly low survival rate.[2]

The more Arnold heard about fracking, the more she became motivated to act. She attended community meetings and spoke at public hearings. But that was not enough. In 2008 she ran for a seat on the Cortland County legislature and was elected. This gave her the platform she sought to educate, empower, and organize her community against fracking.

While in the county legislature, Arnold was introduced to a burgeoning organization called Elected Officials to Protect New York (EOPNY), a sign-on group of mostly rural New York State elected officials opposed to fracking. Working with EOPNY, Arnold was uniquely poised to advocate both on behalf of her constituency and on behalf of her cows. She participated in local press conferences, published opinion pieces in New York's capital city newspaper, and organized workshops for community members looking to ensure termination of expired gas leases.

In a letter to Governor Cuomo in April of 2012, shortly before closing out her second and final term in the county legislature, Arnold wrote:

> As a landowner of many acres of farm and forest land, [fracking] in Cortland County could bring many riches to my family and me. However, no amount of money can fully compensate for contamination of our groundwater, that of our neighbors, or that of our community . . . No amount of money can compensate for ill health effects. As my husband, who has Parkinson's, answers in a heartbeat, the choice is health, not money . . . I would rather work for my living, work in a beautiful, unspoiled green region that is noted for its pristine, abundant water . . . Given today's drilling techniques, the risks are too great that profiting from that gas will jeopardize the health and wellbeing of my family, my neighbors and the greater community.

Years later, and after the ban on fracking in New York was finally achieved, Kathie Arnold still has disdain for the deceitful land men that preyed upon unsuspecting residents of her community. "When our lease was finally up, I went about confirming the actual termination. I received a letter back from Talisman that they were fine with the termination, but Chesapeake [another oil and gas company with leases in the area] now owned a piece and they wouldn't let us out. But the county clerk's office had no record of Chesapeake owning any of my lease," she said. "Also, my sister and brother-in-law had a land man simply forge their signatures on a lease document."

Overall, dairy farming played a key role in resisting fracking in New York State, due in no small part to the simultaneous emergence of the state's yogurt industry. From 2000 to 2012 the number of yogurt-processing plants in New York grew from fourteen to twenty-nine, and the amount of milk used in those plants grew from 158 million pounds to about 1.2 billion pounds. While the fracking question simmered and steamed, New York's daily business progressed into a real economic and political force.

In August of 2012, Governor Cuomo convened in Albany his first annual "yogurt summit," an economic development event to promote and further enable the industry. The summit was a golden organizing opportunity for Food and Water Watch and New Yorkers Against Fracking, the statewide coalition of hundreds of anti-fracking groups that Food and Water Watch helped create. Outside the summit, NYAF held a press conference featuring dozens of dairy farmers and dairy product producers from throughout the region, all highlighting fracking's threat to the industry Cuomo was seeking to elevate.

"I'm excited about what the growth of New York's yogurt industry could mean for agribusiness and farms like mine," Kathie Arnold, who was present, stated. "But Governor Cuomo needs to realize that fracking would be a detriment to the very industry he's trying to promote. Fracking would act as a hand brake on the milk production just as we have this new opportunity to rev up our businesses to meet the burgeoning demand for yogurt."

"Dairy cows require thirty to forty gallons of water a day to stay healthy and produce good quality milk," added Tim Stoltman, a third-generation dairy farmer from Conesus, New York. "Imagine if all that water was tainted with toxic fracking chemicals. Yogurt makers utilize great amounts of milk from farmers like me, and I require clean groundwater for my cows. Fracking would jeopardize all of this."

THE BAN PREVAILS, WITH MORE WORK TO BE DONE

The irony of Governor Cuomo's simultaneous courting of both the dairy and fracking industries in New York was not lost on activists in the movement or among the media covering state news. This was just one of many unexpected developments amidst years of determined organizing by anti-fracking activists and concerned constituencies that ultimately led to Cuomo's ban decision.

Over the years, the education and advocacy efforts of the entire anti-fracking movement, particularly those of NYAF and its food and dairy allies, succeeded in shaping and shifting popular opinion in New York State. From 2012 to 2014, polling on the fracking issue gradually but consistently moved from an almost even split on the issue to consistent pluralities of polled voters voicing opposition to fracking throughout the state. After the ban was announced, a Sienna College poll found that 57 percent of New Yorkers approved of Cuomo's decision, compared to 23 percent that opposed it. In the end, the movement's laser-like focus on Cuomo as the sole political target was critical to his decision to ban fracking. The framing of fracking by the movement as first and foremost a human health threat was also critical. The education, activism, and organizing among New York State's food and dairy interests remained a third key element of the eventual successful ban on fracking statewide.

Today the fight to resist continued fracked gas importation and infrastructure development in the state is still very much alive. In the years since the 2014 ban was achieved, environmental activists throughout the state have largely turned their attention to resisting a plethora of fracking-related projects—including new gas-fired power stations and the complex pipeline networks needed to supply them—that exist or may soon exist due to the prevalence of imported fracked gas from just across the border in Pennsylvania. The continued and even expanding utilization of fracked gas in New York in recent years has directly contributed to the ongoing fracking boom—and all its accompanying hazards—elsewhere in the region. However, the initial success of our coalition has helped to build a movement of ongoing activism. With more work to be done in many regions, we hope our story of success will inspire others to meet the ongoing challenge of combatting corporate fracking.

Food Workers versus Food Giants

Joann Lo and Jose Oliva

MARIA GONZALEZ WORKS at Tyson Foods Inc. in northwest Arkansas.

Maria, whose real name is being withheld, explained in an interview that she is from Guerrero, a state in southern Mexico.[1] She came to the United States when she was twenty, searching for work to help her impoverished family. As the eldest of nine, Maria felt obligated to help support the family. At first, she worked in Mexico with her mother selling refreshments and drinks at a small shop in the town marketplace. But when her father became ill and needed help, Maria left for the United States to earn more income for the family.

Maria reported that she came to the United States with nothing but the clothes she wore. Soon after she left Mexico, her father died, and like so many immigrants, Maria was unable to return to attend the funeral. Her sister was working in northwest Arkansas; Maria's first job upon arrival was to take care of her sister's children. After some time, Maria obtained documents to work legally through her husband, and she began working at a metal works factory. In 2008, Maria was laid off from the factory and began working at a restaurant across the street from Tyson Foods. Tyson Foods Inc. is the world's second largest processor of meat and poultry and was the world's sixth largest food producer in 2017.[2] Established in 1935, Tyson employs 122,000 people at more than three hundred facilities worldwide.[3] In addition, the company contracts with eleven thousand farms.[4] The majority of Tyson's processing plants are located in the southern and midwestern regions of the United States, and the company's headquarters are located in northwest Arkansas, where Maria lives.[5] A couple of years after she began working at the restaurant across from the Tyson factory, a friend who worked at Tyson told Maria that the company was hiring for full-time work. She applied and said that within a week she was working at Tyson.

Maria described starting at $7.25 per hour, working forty hours per week as a de-boner. She cut chicken wings all day, about one hundred wings every minute, nonstop, for more than three years. It was a tiring job, Maria said, and the day-long repetitive motion was hard on her body. The company kept the processing plant refrigerated at all times, so Maria's fingers would get very cold as she cut the meat off the bone. She was eventually transferred to the gutting department, where she cut chickens open so that a machine could then remove the chicken guts. During the 2017 interview, Maria insisted she was still working in the gutting department.

On June 27, 2011, Maria was present during a chemical spill at the Tyson processing plant in which she worked.[6] She said it was a bad spill, and many people were impacted. When the spill occurred, no one—no supervisor, no manager—told Maria or any of her coworkers what was happening. Another worker informed Maria and her peers that the spill had occurred; Maria recalled that at that point, the entire department's workforce panicked, each person aware they would all have to flee through a single, narrow door. Maria and her coworkers were stuck behind others as each worker filed out the narrow exit. Lacking warning or information, Maria explained, the entire group fled toward the chemical spill rather than away from it.

The experience was harrowing for Maria. Above all else, she said, it affected her health. Tyson's managers took the workers to health clinics, Maria conceded, but Tyson management would not allow her to consult any doctors except for the company doctor. Each worker, according to Maria's account, received a limited amount of time with a company doctor. Over six years later, Maria said in the 2017 interview that she was still struggling with her health as a result, she believes, of the spill. Maria's respiratory system has been the most affected, including her lungs and her throat, although her entire body, she insists, has been compromised. Tyson did not cover any additional doctor visits, treatments, or medicines for ailments potentially caused by the chemical spill, said Maria. She receives no company assistance in paying for these treatments and visits. She continues going to work, even now, while sick. If Maria feels too ill and calls in sick, the company gives her "points," or a negative marking on her employment record, and she does not receive pay for days she misses.[7] According to Maria, the only way she can take time off and not accumulate points is if she claims her FMLA (Family Medical Leave Act) right to leave. To claim this right, she reported, Tyson requires Maria to show proof of a doctor's appointment in order to not accumulate points and to forfeit pay for the time missed.

At the time of our interview, Maria said she had two children, both born in the United States—one was already in college and another would soon graduate from high school. When asked what she would want Tyson to understand, Maria replied,

> I would want [them] to understand that we are not machines. We are human beings with hearts, and we want to live, we want to see our kids grow up. I would want them to take the same interest in the well-being of their workers as they currently have on their machines. If a machine breaks down, they quickly get someone to fix it. Just like that, they should make sure their workers are whole. After all, we are human beings, just like them. My goal used to be to work and save up to go to school, but now because of the accident and the debt I am in, my dream is on hold.

CORPORATE INFLUENCE IN THE LABOR SECTOR

Maria Gonzalez is one of twenty million workers in the United States who not only process our chicken but also plant and harvest our food, breed livestock, process food and meat, transport food, cook it, sell it, and serve it.[8] In fact, the food system is the largest source of jobs in the US. Food system workers constitute one in five private-sector workers and one-sixth of the nation's entire workforce.[9] Internationally, millions more are employed in food system work.[10] These workers labor in five major sectors of the food chain: production (farms and fisheries), processing (slaughterhouses and food factories), distribution (warehouses), retail (grocery), and service (restaurants and cafeterias).

The food system's workforce is a significant driver of the US economy. The food production, processing, distribution, retail, and service industries collectively produce over $2.2 trillion in goods and services annually, accounting for over 14 percent of the US gross domestic product (GDP).[11] The wages and work conditions of food workers, therefore, affect not only the workers and their families, but also their communities and the economy as a whole. Unfortunately, more than 86 percent of workers in the food system earn low- to poverty-level wages.[12] Ironically, food workers face higher rates of food insecurity, or limited or uncertain access to adequate food, than any other workers in the United States. In fact, food system workers use food stamps at more than one-and-a-half times the rate of the rest of the US workforce.[13] They also report working in environments with severe health and safety violations, long work hours with few breaks, and lack of access to health benefits.

Today it is almost impossible for the typical US resident to procure a meal that does not involve some form of labor exploitation. A recent example of this exploitation was unearthed in a December 2015 investigative report by the Associated Press revealing that enslaved workers were forced to peel shrimp in Thailand for up to sixteen hours a day for little or no pay, and were locked in production facilities for months and even years on end. The shrimp then made its way to US retailers and restaurants, including Walmart and Olive Garden.[14]

Corporate consolidation exacerbates food worker exploitation. Large-scale corporate farms now control approximately 75 percent of agricultural production.[15] Four corporations now control over 80 percent of the beef industry, and five corporations control 50 percent of grocery retail.[16] Tyson alone has been a party in several cases of horizontal integration, including mergers with brand-name companies such as Jimmy Dean and Sara Lee (the frozen pastry division), in addition to chicken-producing companies such as Holly Farms, Weaver Chicken, and Tasty Chicken. In the summer of 2014, Tyson won a bid to take over Hillshire Farm against Pilgrim's Pride's bid for over $8 billion.[17] This merger resulted in revenue growth in Tyson's stock and overall sales. As of 2014, Tyson owned a total of twenty-six brands. The company reports that its stake in overall production of chicken in the US market is 20 percent, followed by Pilgrim's at 17 percent and Perdue at 7 percent.[18]

The rapid consolidation of food companies such as Tyson has meant that many frontline workers like Maria in these companies are being pushed further into poverty. And as mergers and acquisitions amplify the market power of food corporations, those corporations also increase their political clout, even as they expand their business reach. Tyson, for example, is a major supplier to the federal government, receiving $4.2 billion in federal contracts from 2000 through 2012. Food corporations benefit from such government contracts while exerting their influence over policies and laws impacting workers, including wages, health and safety regulations, and discrimination laws in the legislative process. They also lobby to limit enforcement of labor and employment codes. If we are to move toward a healthy, affordable, fair, and sustainable food system, we need to directly challenge these corporations' power over our democracy.

Directly challenging corporate power involves addressing wage inequities first. Frontline workers in nonmanagerial food system positions make up the core of the food industries—86 percent of all food system jobs—yet they earn the lowest wages of all positions: a median salary of $18,889 a year. The median annual salary for US CEOs in the food system, on the other hand, is $151,833.[19] Overall, wages of US food system workers are lower than the wages of workers in other industries. In fact, when compared to statistics of all workers in the US, the median hourly wage of food system frontline workers is just 27.5 percent that of all other frontline workers. More than ten million of these frontline food system workers earn less than $28,635 per year, only slightly above the federal poverty level for a family of three.[20] According to the Food Chain Workers Alliance's (FCWA) 2011 national survey of 630 food workers, the median hourly food system wage was $9.65 per hour, and almost one in four—23 percent—of respondents claimed they were paid less than the minimum wage.[21] (Unless otherwise noted, the following statistics are drawn from these 2011 findings.)

In addition to wage inequities, food system workers lack access to benefits that would allow them to care for themselves and their families when sick or injured. Three-fifths (60 percent) of food system workers reported not having a single paid sick day, and an additional 19 percent reported not knowing whether they had paid sick days. Only 21 percent of respondents could confirm that they had paid sick days. In addition, 58 percent of respondents reported having no health care coverage; more than one-third reported using the emergency room for primary care. Given their lack of health benefits, more than half of respondent workers (53 percent) reported having worked while sick for a median of three days each year. Among workers who worked while sick, almost two-thirds reported having done so due to a lack of paid sick days. Given their direct contact with the nation's food supply, food system workers' health and safety should be of concern to consumers.

Food system workers also reported working in high-risk environments, where accidents and injuries were frequent. More than half of all workers surveyed (57.2 percent) reported that they had suffered an injury or health problem on the job. Of the workers who reported such an injury or illness to their employers, only 28.8 percent stated that they received free medical care from their employer. Almost one-third of all food system workers (32.7 percent) reported that their employers did not always provide necessary equipment to do their jobs, and more than one in nine workers (11.7 percent) reported being required to do something that put their own safety at risk. If we return to the case of Tyson, we find that the Occupational Safety and Health Administration (OSHA) and the Environmental Protection Agency (EPA) have investigated and cited the company for labor rights violations and inadequate safety measures at multiple facilities. Some of Tyson's employees are represented by a union, and their working conditions are better than those of non-union Tyson workers. Nevertheless, from 2007 to 2012 alone, Tyson was cited for 161 OSHA violations for a total of almost $7.2 million in penalties, and was also responsible for the deaths of eleven workers. One example was a fatal incident at Tyson's Nebraska processing site in 2012; following this horrible incident, OSHA charged Tyson a fine of $121,720 for repeated safety violations at the company's New York plant in 2013. On more than one occasion, Tyson has been charged with, and agreed to pay for, depriving workers of compensation for time spent putting on and taking off personal protective equipment as required by law. And yet the company continues to violate employment laws across the country, as it did with Maria. Tyson's tremendous market share and influence over lawmakers has allowed it to continue to grow even in the face of these outrageous violations of the law and inhumanely low employment standards.

Racial and gender disparities also add to the inequities faced by food workers. For example, food service workers of color are concentrated in the lowest-paying jobs in the food system. In its 2011 report, *The Color of Food,* the Applied Research Center reported that, on average, people of color earn less than whites working in the food chain. Half of white food workers earn $25,024 a year, while workers of color make $5,675 less than that.[22] FCWA survey data confirms this finding. The percentage of workers who earned a living wage did not significantly vary by race, but the percentage of workers concentrated in subminimum wage jobs was strikingly different. About one-quarter of Black and Latino workers and almost 40 percent of Asian workers reported earning less than the minimum wage, whereas 13.5 percent of white workers surveyed reported earning less than the minimum wage. However, the low number of white, Asian, and indigenous workers who participated in the survey makes the survey data for those particular groups somewhat unreliable. More study is needed on differential experiences between white workers and workers of color in the food system.

Workers of color also reported that they suffered from wage theft—employers not paying workers their full wages or overtime wages, directly stealing wages or tips, and not paying workers for all the hours they worked—at higher rates than white workers (see table 1).

There were also gender disparities in wages and reported treatment of food system workers. Women earn slightly less than men; they reported median weekly wages of $400, while men reported $421 per week. Women also reported suffering greater discrimination and harassment than men. Women

TABLE 1 Percent of Industry Cases of Wage Theft by Race

Worker group	Farm/agricultural & nurseries	Meatpacking & poultry processing	Food processing, distribution, & packing-houses	Restaurant & food services	Grocery	Warehouse	Total wage theft
Latino	92.9%	25%	68.2%	36.4%	78.6%	10.3%	57.9%
Black	0%	0%	18.2%	40.9%	14.3%	75.9%	27.8%
White	0%	0%	4.5%	4.5%	7.1%	6.9%	3.8%
Asian	0%	75%	9.1%	4.5%	0%	0%	4.5%
Indigenous	7.1%	0%	0%	4.5%	0%	0%	3%
Other	0%	0%	0%	9.1%	0%	6.9%	3%
Total	100%	100%	100%	100%	100%	100%	100%

SOURCE: Food Chain Workers Alliance survey data.

reported experiences of discrimination, such as being fired, not getting a promotion, or being scheduled for fewer hours of work at much higher rates than men (44 percent versus 32 percent). Women also reported suffering verbal abuse from employers at a higher rate than the men surveyed (16.9 percent versus 11.1 percent).

Undocumented immigrant workers are also more vulnerable to exploitation in the food system. Less than 1 percent of undocumented workers reported earning more than 150 percent of the poverty line, compared to 20 percent of documented workers. The median wage reported by undocumented workers—$7.60 per hour—was significantly lower than the median wage reported by all other workers ($10 per hour). Undocumented workers also suffered from greater wage theft. They reported losing forty-three cents per hour, on average, to lack of overtime, shaving off hours, nonpayment of wages and tips, and other forms of wage theft.

With low wages and a lack of benefits, US food workers suffer higher rates of food insecurity compared to the general workforce. These workers use public assistance programs at a higher rate than the general workforce. Public assistance programs for fast-food workers alone costs taxpayers (not the corporations) nearly $7 billion per year.[23]

The conditions faced by workers we have described can be traced to corporate control of our food system. Taken together, the low wages, lack of benefits, and race and gender inequity that workers face in the food sector result in a significant pull downward on wages and conditions for all workers. Historically, when workers have faced such injustices, they have found ways to organize and to create market-intervention tools to improve their conditions. Food workers are no exception, and have in several cases taken on corporations and won. In the next chapter, Saru Jayaraman highlights some examples.

Food Workers Taking On Goliath

Saru Jayaraman

UNTIL RECENTLY, FOOD SYSTEM WORKERS were overlooked and neglected among institutions and individuals concerned with food systems reform. A new public focus on food labor presents tremendous opportunities for a broader spectrum of food systems reform advocacy. Organizers and advocates who work on food labor issues have long argued that the food system cannot be truly sustainable without addressing the fact that it is the nation's largest and lowest-paying employer—the worst employer in the United States.[1] Among all those involved in the struggles for food system reform in the United States, food workers have been the most successful in pushing back against corporate power. Over the last ten years in the United States, in particular, food workers have won a minimum wage of $15 an hour and legislated earned sick leave in multiple cities and states;[2] they have forced major food corporations to sign codes of conduct, improving wages and conditions for farmworkers;[3] they have secured union contracts with food corporations, codifying wage and benefit standards;[4] they have secured bipartisan legislation in Congress protecting tips as the property of workers;[5] and much more. Other food system advocates who are concerned with the negative environmental and health effects of industrial agriculture can learn much from food workers' track record of taking on corporate power and winning.

The struggle between food system workers and food corporations dates back to this nation's early history, when enslaved peoples revolted on American sugar plantations. In 1811, Charles Deslondes, an enslaved person, led the "largest and most sophisticated" slave revolt in US history against the Andry sugar plantation in Louisiana.[6] Like most such uprisings, the Andry revolt was quashed, and two hundred insurgents were killed.[7] Nevertheless, such revolts paved the way to the abolition of the slave trade and initiated a long tradition of food system workers in the US standing up to abusive employers.

Over the next two hundred years, agricultural workers would repeatedly resist large food and wine corporations. In one of the most famous examples, Cesar Chavez led an iconic farmworker movement, based out of the United Farm Workers union, and succeeded in obtaining wage and working condition improvements for tens of thousands of farmworkers in California.[8] And meanwhile, tens of thousands of nearby California cannery workers stood up against powerful cannery corporations and won the right to unionize.[9] These workers turned the poverty-wage jobs of John Steinbeck's *Cannery Row* into livable-wage middle-class jobs that sustained several generations of California coast families.

Today, workers in every segment of the food chain are organizing against large food corporations. The Coalition of Immokalee Workers has won large and notable victories against major fast-food restaurant and grocery corporations, pushing these companies to sign the Fair Food Agreement, which guarantees tomato farmworkers the right to decent wages and working conditions in the fields.[10] The United Food and Commercial Workers International Union (UFCW) has led bloody battles against meat- and poultry-processing corporations, such as those featured in the book *Fast Food Nation*, in which African Americans, African immigrants, Latino immigrants, and Native Americans work in segregated plants killing, butchering, and processing most of our nation's beef, pork, and poultry. These battles have resulted in the unionization of thousands of meat- and poultry-processing workers in the South, guaranteeing them the right to a decent wage and representation on the shop floor.[11]

At the consumer end of the food chain, food workers are engaged in a massive social upheaval. UNITE HERE, a union that represents institutional food service workers (i.e., cafeteria workers in office buildings, hospitals, and universities), has won union contracts requiring livable wages and benefits for thousands of workers of the largest cafeteria corporations in the United States.[12]

OUR Walmart (Organization United for Respect at Walmart) has organized tens of thousands of employees of the single largest grocery company—and the single largest employer—in the United States. Although the fight against Walmart continues, the company has made tremendous changes as a result of these workers' persistence, including its recent announcement that it would begin paying workers more than the minimum wage.

With support from the Service Employees International Union (SEIU), since 2012 fast-food workers have been striking all over the world, demanding $15 an hour and the right to unionize. In the US, the SEIU mass protest resulted in the National Labor Relations Board ruling that major corporations no longer have the right to hide behind their franchisees in accepting liability for the rights of their employees.[13] Through these confrontations, workers have won direct changes in corporate behavior, such as raising wages, allowing for workplace democracy, and improving health and safety standards, as well as indirect improvements, such as greater government regulation of corporations and legislated minimum wage increases. Given that food corporations have spent millions of dollars lobbying to keep wages and worker benefits as low as possible, workers successfully forcing corporations—via the legislators who regulate them—to pay and provide a livable standard to their employees has been a tremendous feat. In both cases, workers and worker organizations have increased pressure and regulation on corporations to balance the undue influence that corporations have had over US democracy and residents' lives.

The following examples from Restaurant Opportunities Centers United (ROC United) illustrate precisely how such campaign victories happen, what was sacrificed to win them, and how they might occur again. These success stories are inspiring not only for workers, but also for anyone seeking to balance the power of corporations vis-à-vis the government and the general public.

ROC'ING THE RESTAURANT INDUSTRY

I cofounded ROC United after September 11th, 2001, together with restaurant workers displaced from the World Trade Center. Over the intervening years, we have grown into a national organization of 130,000 workers, restaurant owners, and consumers nationwide. Our growth also mirrors the growth of the US restaurant industry. The restaurant industry is both the largest employer within the food system and the second largest private-sector employer in the United States as a whole.[14] The restaurant industry also remains one of the nation's lowest-paying employers; every year the US Department of Labor publishes a list of the ten lowest-paying jobs in the US, and every year at least half of the ten lowest-paying jobs, including one of the two lowest-paying jobs in the country, are within the restaurant industry.[15]

What enables one of the largest, fastest-growing, and most profitable industries in the US to have the lowest-paying jobs in the country? This phenomenon is the result of the power and influence of the National Restaurant Association (NRA), which has been named the tenth most powerful congressional lobbying group, and is the most powerful employer lobby in almost every state legislature. The "other NRA" has paid millions in lobbying dollars to keep the federal minimum wage for most workers at $7.25 an hour, and at $2.13 an hour for tip-earning workers. NRA has also fought against paid sick days, health care reform, unionization rights, protection against pregnancy discrimination, and a wide swath of other legislation on employment conditions. Additionally, the group has lobbied against organic and sustainable food sourcing standards, ethical animal treatment, environmental regulations, equal pay legislation, and other issues affecting women.[16] The NRA is led by the nation's Fortune 500 restaurant corporations, from Darden, the parent company of Olive Garden, Capital Grille, and LongHorn Steakhouse, to McDonald's and Subway. Collectively these corporations set abysmally low standards for the whole industry—and the whole economy—through the lobbying efforts of the NRA.

MOVING CORPORATE POLICY

Before ROC United became a national organization, our efforts to change industry standards had a local focus. We focused our efforts on setting standards for restaurant behavior in particular localities. In New York City, the highest-profile restaurants were fine dining restaurant companies, some owned by celebrity chefs. Encouraging these corporations to change their wages and working conditions resulted in many other New York restaurants changing their behavior as well.

For example, from 2005 until 2007 we waged a campaign against exploitation in the Fireman Hospitality Group, a restaurant corporation that owned many of the restaurants surrounding Carnegie Hall and Lincoln Center in midtown Manhattan. The owner was a man named Shelly Fireman, called the "Mayor of Fifty-Seventh Street" by some and reviled by many of his employees, and even his peers, for terrible treatment of his workers.[17]

A small group of workers first approached ROC United from the Redeye Grill, an upscale restaurant across the street from Carnegie Hall. These workers reported that their tips were being stolen by management, and sought restitution from the company. Notably, these workers were mostly white; their racial privilege contributed to their confidence in speaking out against their employer.

As an organization representing workers of all different races and positions in the restaurant, we knew that tip stealing was not the only issue at the Redeye Grill, nor were these the only workers whose rights were being violated. We also knew from experience that simply suing the restaurant would not entirely solve the problem. The Fireman Hospitality Group, like many restaurant companies in the US, had been sued fairly regularly for a wide variety of issues.[18] In the case of workers' wages, cases typically take between four to six years and often result in an employer paying only a small fraction of what workers are actually owed. They almost never result in systemic corporate behavior change or industry change.

We knew the top priority was not simply litigation, but collective action that would involve a much wider group of workers and that would escalate the issue to gain widespread public interest. This broader scope would facilitate institutional change locally as well as nationally. Lawsuits had limited consequences, whereas the risk of widespread reputation damage would prove much more powerful.

Thus, we worked with the initial group of servers to increase the number of workers willing to stand up for their rights. At first, the servers were skeptical; they were sure that none of the other kitchen workers or bussers were experiencing any violations of their rights. However, as they started referring other workers to us, they learned the truth: other workers' rights were being violated even more than their rights were. Kitchen workers and bussers were not being paid for all hours worked, and were not receiving sick pay. And the company was falsifying payroll records.[19]

Almost every single worker who joined the campaign started out with similar fears: fear of losing their jobs, fear of being deported, fear of being "blacklisted" in the industry, and fear of speaking up to authority. Almost every single worker was initially skeptical that we could win against Shelly Fireman, who had a reputation for quashing all attempts for change. The workers were also skeptical that more workers would join the cause. Through increasingly numerous meetings, we talked people through their fear and into a place of courage, helping them understand that nothing would ever change if they did not take a stand. We organized 250 workers from all positions and racial groups in the seven Fireman midtown Manhattan restaurants. Among other actions, these workers engaged in protests in front of the restaurants, marches, public theater and musical performances, and much more. At one point, in solidarity with the restaurant workers, truck drivers refused to deliver goods to the restaurants.

The company feared protests in front of their restaurants far more than lawsuits; they said the protests detracted from their diners' experience and embarrassed the management. If we had kept the fight in the legal arena, the company could have quietly delayed the process indefinitely, as they had done for decades. Instead, they ended up paying their workers $4 million in stolen tips and wages, instituted a new human resources department, created a new anti–sexual harassment and anti-discrimination policy (including greater transparency in hiring and promotion), instituted a grievance procedure, and much more. Arguably they instituted these changes not for moral reasons but primarily to make ROC United stop the humiliating actions outside their restaurants. These changes affected all two thousand workers in the company, as well as the entire New York City restaurant industry. For years afterward, workers came to ROC United saying that their employer had stopped stealing their tips as a result of seeing what was going on in front of Fireman's restaurants.

Forcing this company to not only comply with the law but to also agree to many of its workers' additional demands regarding workplace respect and dignity demonstrated a balancing of power between the workers and the restaurant owners. This balancing of power is productive for all parties, not only the workers. In fact, many of our current employer partners started a practice called "Open Book Management," in which workers are involved with, and invested in, the company's success. As a result of workers' involvement and investment in the company's long-term sustainability, these companies have found that creating a healthier balance of power between workers and employers can result in greater productivity and profitability.

The Fireman campaign is an inspiring example of workers standing up against a corporation and demanding change in corporate behavior. However, to truly change the industry, we at ROC United know we need to change not only individual corporations' behavior, but also their influence over policies that set standards for the whole industry. Realizing that the source of this power was not based in New York, but in a national entity—the NRA—we grew into a national organization, with the intent to counterbalance the power and influence of that incredible trade lobby.

As a national organization, ROC United has continued to conduct campaigns—using many of the same tactics we used in the Fireman campaign—against national restaurant corporations. We have also won victories against the NRA in the public sphere. In earlier years, we helped pass legislation to make it illegal for restaurateurs to deduct credit card processing fees from workers' tips in Philadelphia, won paid sick days for restaurant workers in Pittsburgh and Washington, DC, and helped win minimum wage increases in multiple states. In 2018, we had some of our greatest victories— we worked with dozens of organizations nationally to win a bipartisan bill in Congress protecting tips as the property of workers, and won a wage increase for tipped workers in Washington, DC, New York, and Michigan.[20] We have won these fights by organizing workers, responsible restaurant employers, and supportive consumers who agree with our cause to collectively speak up at legislative hearings and town halls. Collectively we have educated policymakers, the press, and the public on the importance of these issues, presenting evidence to counteract the myths perpetuated by the NRA.

In July 2019, as a result of our organizing efforts around the country, the US House of Representatives passed the Raise the Wage Act, which calls for a $15 minimum wage and a complete wage with tips on top for all workers, including tipped workers—despite serious lobbying against the bill by the National Restaurant Association. The vote represented the first time since Emancipation that either house of Congress moved to eliminate the legacy of slavery that is the subminimum wage for tipped workers. Although the Senate will not pass it immediately, the House vote has created tremendous momentum for the issue to move in multiple states, and then ultimately to pass in the Senate, and is a great example of what can be achieved when workers organize against even the most powerful opponents. As this book goes to press, we continue to fight to eliminate the subminimum wage for tipped workers.

As mentioned earlier, the restaurant industry is one of the largest yet lowest-paying employers in the United States. Even accounting for tips, four of the seven lowest-paying jobs in the US are tipped restaurant workers.[21] Tipping as a practice originated in feudal Europe. European aristocrats gave tips to domestic and field workers as a gratuity, always on top of an existing wage. Rich Americans traveling to Europe in the 1850s and 1860s brought the practice home with them, performing a sort of cultural superiority demonstrating that they knew the rules of Europe.[22] Many Americans widely rejected the practice, supporting a populist anti-tipping movement in the late 1800s and early 1900s that claimed tipping was un-American and undemocratic.[23] This populist movement caught fire in Europe, where the labor movement fought against tipping as a vestige of the feudal system.[24]

In the United States, however, both the restaurant industry and the Pullman train company hired formerly enslaved people and managed not to pay them anything at all, forcing them to live off customer tips.[25] This idea was codified into law: the first minimum wage law, passed in 1938, required that employers provide a minimum wage that could be earned directly from the employer *or* be obtained as tips from customers.[26] Thus, the first minimum wage law passed in the United States required that employers pay no wages to their employees if those employees received tips equivalent to the minimum wage. This concept—that an employer did not have to pay workers—was a manipulation of the tipping practices of feudal Europe and a reflection of America's uniquely ugly racialized caste system, codified through slavery.

From 1938 until now, the federal minimum wage for tipped workers has risen to a paltry $2.13 an hour as a result of successful lobbying efforts by the NRA.[27] Over the last eighty years, each time the minimum wage has risen for all other workers, the other NRA has successfully lobbied at the federal level and in forty-three states to exclude tipped workers from the increase. The other NRA has argued that these workers do not need a minimum wage increase, and has painted a false picture that the typical tipped worker is a high-earning white man working in a fine dining restaurant. In fact, 70 percent of tipped workers in the US are women, the majority of whom work at casual restaurants like Applebee's and IHOP. These women experience three times the poverty rate of the rest of the US workforce and use food stamps at double the rate (see the preceding chapter). Worst of all, our research has shown that as a result of having to live off tips as the majority of their income, this largely female workforce has had to tolerate the worst sexual harassment of any industry. They are often encouraged by management to wear revealing clothing in order to increase tips, which can leave them more vulnerable to coworker and management harassment. Ninety percent of workers in this industry report experiencing sexual behavior in the restaurant that is frightening and/or unwanted.[28] Even worse, since one in two American adults has worked in this industry at some point in their lifetime, millions of young women start their work lives being encouraged by restaurant management to subject themselves to objectification in order to earn more money in tips.

Thus, this industry sets the standard for what is acceptable and tolerable for women in the workplace.

Seven states have rejected this system. California, Oregon, Washington, Nevada, Minnesota, Montana, and Alaska all require that restaurant employers pay the full minimum wage to all workers, regardless of tips. In these seven states, workers have higher incomes, restaurants have higher sales per capita, job growth is strong, even for tipped workers, and tipping rates are the same or higher than in the forty-three states with a subminimum wage for tipped workers. Best of all, these seven states have half the rate of sexual harassment of the states with a $2.13 subminimum wage for tipped workers. California, in fact, has the largest and one of the fastest-growing restaurant industries in the country.[29] In 2013, ROC United launched the One Fair Wage campaign, calling for all states and the federal government to follow the example set by these seven states and eliminate the lower wage for tipped workers.

Perhaps the greatest power corporations have over our democracy is the influence they have had on public understanding of an issue, even on advocates' understanding of an issue. It took us several years to convince even some of our allies seeking minimum wage increases that tipped workers should not be excluded. However, through direct actions, events, publications, legislative visits, town hall meetings, and much more, we have illuminated stories of hundreds of tipped workers across the country—stories of economic instability, sexual harassment, and racial discrimination. We have also exposed the slave history of the subminimum wage, as well as the rampant sexual harassment that woman workers face in the industry. In these ways, we have corrected much of the misinformation spread by the NRA and shifted public discourse on the issue.

As a result of this work, in 2014 the AFL-CIO, the nation's largest labor union umbrella, passed a resolution in support of One Fair Wage, which was followed by legislators in eight states proposing bills and ballot measures to eliminate the lower wage for tipped workers.[30] In 2015, Democratic leadership in Congress introduced the first bills in US history proposing the full elimination of the lower wage for tipped workers, and the White House announced its support for One Fair Wage as well. In 2016, both Democratic presidential candidates publicly announced their support for One Fair Wage.

In 2017, the #MeToo movement elevated the horrific experiences of sexual harassment and assault first in Hollywood and then for women in many other industries as well. Dozens of men in entertainment and politics lost their positions over incidences of sexual harassment and assault; a much smaller number of chefs and restaurateurs were also exposed. The toppling of these restaurant industry titans represented only the tip of the iceberg, but allowed us to highlight the much more pervasive issues of harassment in the restaurant industry. At the end of 2017, thanks to the #MeToo movement, Governor Cuomo responded to our efforts and announced that he would prioritize the One Fair Wage policy in New York as part of a package of anti-sexual harassment policies in 2018.

Through this campaign, we have exposed the undue influence of the NRA in every state legislature and at the federal level. Beyond all of our other work, we have launched a national campaign to expose the NRA, the corporations that hide behind the shield of the trade lobby, and the legislators who accept large financial contributions from the NRA and who consistently vote in its favor. We have created a coalition of organizations concerned about local and sustainable food, about the environment, about public health, about gender justice, about democratic practice, and about workers' rights. Together, we have released a series of reports on the hidden lobbying activities of the NRA and its member corporations. Especially in a time of grave concern about corporate contributions and tax loopholes, we are seeing that legislators are increasingly wary to associate too greatly with this powerful trade lobby, and that the NRA's influence is diminishing.

We have simultaneously built an alternative national restaurant association called RAISE (Restaurants Advancing Industry Standards in Employment), comprised of almost eight hundred restaurant owners across the country who support higher wages and better working conditions for restaurant employees, in part because they have seen the payoff of such investments, including higher productivity and profitability. We had been working with several employers around the country to eliminate the lower wage for tipped workers in their own restaurants, and many were willing to join us in pushing legislators to support One Fair Wage. When industry leader Danny Meyer decided to eliminate the subminimum wage for tipped workers in his own restaurants—and, in his case, gratuities altogether—and support One Fair Wage, several dozen restaurant companies around the nation followed suit. The *New York Times* recognized the momentum by supporting One Fair Wage in an October 2015 editorial, promptly followed by an endorsement from the *USA Today* editorial board. And many restaurant corporations have left the NRA. For example, Chipotle decided to leave the NRA and, after conversations with us, now provides paid sick days, paid family leave, and tuition reimbursements to their eighty thousand workers nationally.

Engaging in direct actions of workers to push back on the NRA, lifting up worker voices to change the public perception perpetuated by the NRA, and dividing the employer voices within the NRA all resulted in a questioning of their dominant narrative on the issue of food worker standards, and ultimately, in legislative change. Forcing this industry to pay a full minimum wage to its workers, as opposed to being the only industry in the US that demands its customers pay its workers' wages, will create a fairer balance of power, rightfully challenging a trade lobby that has wielded unbridled influence over Congress and forty-three state legislatures for almost a century.

Our successes have not gone without pushback from the NRA, of course. The NRA has set up a fully staffed organization and website to attack ROC United, and to attack me personally. They purchased three full-page ads in *USA Today* and the *Wall Street Journal*. They have urged their friends in Congress to initiate two unsuccessful congressional investigations into ROC United. Their member corporations have sued us for millions of dollars. They have targeted our university partners, engaging in academic censorship by attempting unsuccessfully to stop university professors from partnering with us. They have targeted our donors, trying to bully them into discontinuing their support for us. They have tracked my whereabouts and posted photographs of my two-year-old daughter and me on their website. They have spent hundreds of thousands of dollars on these activities, money that could have helped them engage in better business practices, namely, providing higher wages and better working conditions. Our research has shown that these improved conditions result in less employee turnover, greater employee productivity, and greater return.

Perhaps most disturbingly, the NRA has attempted to organize workers against their own wage increases. In November 2016, following a One Fair Wage victory in Maine, the NRA created "Restaurant Workers of America," an "astroturf," or fake, corporate-controlled association of both restaurant owners and workers, to promulgate the myth that tips are somehow reduced when workers receive a full minimum wage from their employers.[31] As mentioned above, the seven states that require restaurants to pay their employees the full minimum wage have the same or higher tipping averages as the forty-three states with subminimum wages for tipped workers.[32] For example, tipped workers in San Francisco, where all workers must receive the full minimum wage plus tips, receive higher tips than workers in comparable cities such as New York City or Washington, DC, from the highest tip earners to the lowest.[33] The NRA funded a campaign called "Save Our Tips" to attempt to agitate workers into opposing their own wage increases based on the misinformation that a wage increase would decrease their tips; the campaign was finally exposed on John Oliver's *Last Week Tonight* on HBO in August 2018 as a corporate-funded misinformation campaign to stop the minimum wage from being increased.[34]

These shameful attacks and purposeful misinformation have not deterred our members or our organization from continuing our pursuit of justice. They have only emboldened us.

Our hope is to join with other food system reform advocates to ultimately dismantle the undue influence of the NRA and all other major food corporations and trade lobbies. We have found that the key to winning, against the great odds of money and power, is collective, direct action of stakeholders across class, race, and issue. We must expect considerable, well-funded resistance to change from these corporate lobbies, but that should not diminish our efforts. Our experiences at ROC United prove that individuals of all backgrounds, alongside institutions, can successfully stand up to corporate power through protest, direct action, litigation, coalition development, research, public education, and much more.

Fast Food Embodied

INDUSTRIAL DIETS

Kristine Madsen and Wendi Gosliner

WHEN ANA, A SOFT-SPOKEN SIXTEEN-YEAR-OLD, first came to our pediatric obesity clinic on a cold spring morning at the behest of her family, she shared with us that she drank three or four sodas every day, which she purchased from the McDonald's next to her school. She explained that when she became sad, which happened most afternoons, soda was the only thing that made her feel better; it gave her a "pick-me-up." Ana was candid about the likelihood of successfully ceasing to drink soda. She had tried going without it, but doing so made her mood worse.

The daily soda ritual that Ana described is a pattern of behavior that is fueled by the power of the corporate food and beverage industry, and the fast-food industry specifically. Our approach in the clinic was to identify one or two behaviors that contributed most to each child's weight gain, and to help our patients address those. In Ana's case, we linked her soda consumption to her morbid obesity. As public health experts, we understand that such patterns are neither unique to patients of pediatric clinics nor simply the result of individual "poor choices." Rather, the fact that a generation of children like Ana have grown up eating ultra-processed foods that dull their ability to learn and shorten their lifespan is directly related to sustained, strategic actions by various actors, particularly the food and beverage industry.[1] This industry has engineered our environments to ensure that throughout our lifetime, we overconsume the nutrient-poor, ultra-processed, hyper-palatable foods they develop and market.

What we will here call the "industrial diet" refers to a diet rich in processed, refined, corporate-produced, mass-marketed foods that are high in fat, salt, and sugar and low in nutrient density.[2] While the industrial food system began to develop at the end of the nineteenth and into the early twentieth century, fast-food restaurants scaled the dominance of this type of diet, starting in the 1950s.[3] While foods and beverages from all types of venues comprise the industrial diet, fast food represents both the epitome and the largest purveyor of the industrial diet. Fast food is nearly ubiquitously accessible. It promotes products with multiple additives to enhance flavor and ensure a consistent taste experience wherever it is purchased. And it is served in increasingly large portion sizes at relatively affordable prices.

The US initially paved the way for massive expansion of fast-food-rich industrial diets across the globe. The number of fast-food outlets in the US increased by 85 percent between 1986 and 1996;[4] by 2016, 50 million people in the US were consuming fast food every day.[5] Fast food is steadily infiltrating global diets; between 2011 and 2016, the number of fast-food outlets increased by 30 percent globally and at least 11 countries have now surpassed the US in fast-food consumption among young people.[6]

Scientific journals have amassed considerable evidence linking changes to an industrial diet with serious health problems and significant social costs. Anthony Winson, a political economist at the University of Guelph in Ontario who coined the term "industrial diet," states: "In stark terms: The [industrial] diet is killing us."[7] The prevalence of obesity has more than tripled in the United States and doubled in seventy-three countries since 1980, contributing to four million premature deaths.[8] Frequent fast-food consumption more than doubles the risk of developing diabetes and of dying from a heart attack.[9] In addition to lives lost, these dietary changes have a high price tag for health care, with annual costs estimated at almost $400 billion for treating obesity and its complications in the US alone; global costs are expected to reach $1.2 trillion by 2025.[10]

The industrial diet represents an aspect of market failure. The low prices of fast food and ultra-processed foods do not reflect the true costs of the products. The significant health and health care costs we describe are not being borne by the corporations producing and profiting from the products; rather, they are being paid by society (negative externalities, in economic parlance). While the fast-food and food and beverage industries did not necessarily intend for the global population to become unhealthy, at a minimum they failed to give sufficient attention to the likely outcomes of cheap, ultra-processed foods becoming ubiquitously available. Even as obesity became an epidemic, the food and beverage corporations reinvested in their profitable strategies—perpetuating the health crises—while denying accountability. A critical role of our government is to intercede in such cases of market failure to ensure that there is efficiency between the costs and benefits of transactions. However, the corporate food and beverage industry uses the power the profitability to fight government intervention. They have wielded this power to maintain and feed the structures that benefit them.

As we will now describe, amassing the power to perpetuate dominance and fight government intervention is part of a three-fold strategy undergirding the corporate fast-food and beverage industry's success. First, the industry has worked to exploit human biology and psychology by engineering hyper-palatable, irresistible products. Second, fast-food and food and beverage firms flood our physical and social environments with these products while simultaneously providing multiple cues to consume them. Finally, fast-food and other food and beverage corporations have helped to push for a system that makes their products less expensive and more convenient than healthier alternatives.

"YOU CAN'T EAT JUST ONE": THE SCIENCE AND STRATEGY BEHIND HYPERPALATABILITY

As Michael Moss describes in his article "Bliss Point: The Extraordinary Science of Addictive Junk Food," the food and beverage industry has been hiring scientists and psychologists for decades to "optimize" their products to attract (and addict) more consumers.[11] Those scientists hire "flavorists" to spend long hours evaluating the texture, taste, and smell of different foods and beverages to find "the bliss point," the sensory combination that stimulates the taste buds and brain to keep us eating—and wanting more. The resultant hyperpalatable foods contain a plethora of additives to promote uniform color, texture, and flavor.[12] A McDonald's Filet-O-Fish and side of fries, a Burger King strawberry milkshake, a Wendy's Grilled Chicken Sandwich—all of these and most other fast foods owe their taste to flavorists' chemical concoctions.[13]

While numerous industrial food products are engineered for overconsumption, fast foods—mass-marketed and served in abundance—were pioneers. Beginning in the 1980s, the corporate fast-food industry began increasing portion sizes (portions are now two to five times their original size), while enhancing addictive properties to increase consumers' craving for them.[14] A partnership between McDonald's and Coca-Cola, created to enhance mutual profitability, led to "extra value meals," which can contain almost 2,000 calories—the total calories an average adult should consume in an entire day. Today, 13 percent of Americans' calories come from fast food, and more than half (58 percent) come from ultra-processed foods and beverages.[15]

Ultra-processed foods ensure that wherever you go in America—and to some degree abroad—your meal will taste exactly the same. The fast-food industry in particular, however, has engineered standardized taste, texture, and appearance of products to create familiarity—a sense of home—even in unfamiliar settings. McDonald's potato supplier, using video cameras to separate odd-sized potatoes, adds sugar to fries in the fall and leaches sugar from them in the spring to ensure total uniformity, and totally familiar French fries.[16] The standardized flavors and textures create expectations for our taste buds, influencing our taste preferences from earliest infancy through adulthood.

MASSIVE MARKETING TO ADULTS . . . AND CHILDREN

Fast-food companies make it easy for parents to feed their child, but there is a hidden cost. While fast food is convenient, inexpensive, and does not provoke arguments from the kids, these ultra-processed, standardized foods can shape the palates of children for a lifetime. The textures and complex flavors of unprocessed food are unfamiliar to children raised on industrial diets, and subsequently may become entirely undesirable. The priming of a child's palate for processed products can create lifelong fast-food consumers. Recognizing that parents may feel they are compromising their child's health when purchasing fast food for the sake of convenience, McDonald's developed strategies to win mothers over, as further described in the organizing campaign against McDonald's detailed in the next chapter.

Understanding McDonald's advertising strategy is critical to understanding the organizing campaigns that have attempted to change it. Since 1963, McDonald's has been using Ronald McDonald to capture the hearts and minds of children. And it's worked: in 2010, Ronald was as recognizable as Santa Claus.[17] In 2003, McDonald's dubbed Ronald "chief happiness officer," a not-so-subtle attempt to associate happiness with fast food.[18] These facts should hardly be surprising: Ronald is everywhere kids are. He is at birthday parties hosted at McDonald's. He is on the internet. Ronald also frequents children's hospitals, including those with McDonald's restaurants inside the hospital itself.[19]

Beyond Ronald's child-friendly character, McDonald's has created other pathways to appeal directly to children: they have been a ubiquitous sponsor of children's television programming; they created Play Places at McDonald's branches to entertain children while families eat fast food; with technology progression, children can now play games on the McWorld website and explore the virtual world, unlocking "fun" through codes on happy meals.[20] The most profitable program of all has been the McDonald's "Happy Meal," introduced in 1979, packaging a hamburger, fries, a sugary beverage, and a McDonald's cookie with a toy or prize. In 2013, Happy Meals accounted for approximately 10 percent of McDonald's sales in the US—equivalent to about $2.5 billion annually.[21] In the following chapter, Anna Lappé and Kelle Louaillier describe organizing efforts by Corporate Accountability and its allies to pressure McDonald's to adopt more responsible practices.

THE ABCS OF PRODUCT PROMOTION

In the early 1990s, the corporate food and beverage industry pursued an innovative strategy to reach children where they were: in school. Corporations like McDonald's and Pepsi funded ten-minute "educational" programs for closed-circuit school television (Channel One) in exchange for including two additional minutes of advertising. Over eight million students watched these programs every day; profit from the advertising was estimated at $30 million annually.[22] While the programs reach fewer students today, Channel One is still operational in many schools.[23] The American Association of Pediatrics notes: "School advertising also appears under the guise of educational TV: Channel One."[24] Corporate food and beverage companies also designed educational materials, including math and biology texts and nutrition guides, that included their logo.[25]

McDonald's in particular has nurtured relationships with schools, holding assemblies like "Book Time with Ronald McDonald" and "Giving Back with Ronald McDonald," described as "helping kids to give back to their school, family, friends, and community," while exposing students to Ronald's character.[26] There's also "Go Active with Ronald McDonald," promoted as a substitute for physical education classes.[27] For cash-strapped schools, these free "educational" programs can be enticing. Fast-food restaurants spend almost $5 billion each year promoting their products. McDonald's ranks first, spending about $1 billion annually to keep us coming back.

Corporate fast-food companies have not limited themselves to the interior of schools; they have also strategically sited their franchises near schools, where parents may not have control over children's eating. Ray Kroc, founder of McDonald's Corporation, wrote, "[We] spot good locations for McDonald's stores by flying over a community and looking for schools."[28] Researchers found that on average, fast-food restaurants in Chicago are located less than 0.4 miles (a five-minute walk) from schools. This is not by chance—there are three to four times as many fast-food restaurants near schools as would be expected if they were not sited with intention.[29] Research has also indicated that children whose schools are within 0.5 mile of a fast-food restaurant are more likely to be overweight than children whose schools are farther away.[30]

The onslaught doesn't stop after childhood; there is continued marketing of highly manufactured, standardized food products to adults. The corporate food and beverage industry leverages social media to create brand awareness and market directly to consumers. Of eighteen top fast-food companies, seventeen had more than one million Facebook likes in 2013, and six had more than ten million likes.[31] Industry also uses technology to analyze customers' purchases, preferences, and behaviors to fund targeted advertising for their products. For example, McDonald's uses Snapchat or GPS to identify their users' movement patterns and to focus marketing geographically to be most effective.[32]

HOW THEY WIELD THEIR POWER

We have described how fast food and ultra-processed foods hook us and create massive profits while generating multiple human and social costs (negative externalities). As we have mentioned, this type of market contradiction highlights a critical governmental responsibility: to adopt policies that can correct market inefficiencies. But the corporate food and beverage industry uses their massive power to stymie these efforts.

In 2009, when the US Congress was contemplating major legislation to improve the healthfulness of meals served to children in the National School Lunch Program and other federal food programs, food and beverage lobbying expenditures peaked at $58 million. Corporations that contributed to this lobbying included Coca-Cola, PepsiCo, McDonald's, and Yum! Brands (the parent company of KFC and Pizza Hut).[33] In recent years, the food and beverage industry has fought efforts to counter its powerful marketing forces, effectively blocking any attempts to require restaurants to post calories or to restrict toy giveaways with children's meals in at least nine states.[34] Fast-food companies partnered with Big Soda in lobbying against New York's restriction on the size of beverages sold—not surprising, given the significant profit fast-food restaurants make from selling soda.[35]

The corporate food and beverage industry also uses its substantial economic resources to reinforce its political power by contributing directly to the campaigns of members of Congress. During the 2015–2016 election cycle, food and beverage companies contributed $16 million to members of Congress, with 63 percent of the contributions going to Republicans.[36] Three of the top five food and beverage contributors to federal candidates, parties, and outside groups (e.g., PACs) were Coca-Cola ($1.4 million), the National Restaurant Association ($993,000), and McDonald's ($802,000).[37] According to the Center for Responsive Politics, in 2016 alone, food and beverage lobbying efforts totaled more than $31 million, with six of the top seven spenders being fast-food and soda companies; Coca-Cola led the pack at $7.9 million.[38]

Fast-food corporations as well as other food and beverage corporations also exert considerable influence through public relations initiatives to frame the public debate.[39] For example, companies deploy public relations campaigns that perpetuate a storyline focusing on individual behaviors and "poor choices," rather than industry practices as the cause of poor diet and obesity. Or, they may support initiatives that promote physical activity as the central solution for addressing obesity. The fact that McDonald's hands out pedometers to encourage physical activity is not in and of itself negative, but it may be misleading, considering that the average person has to walk six miles to burn off the calories in just one Big Mac.

The corporate food and beverage industry employs a variety of additional tactics to reinforce the status quo, bolstering public and political support for their products at society's expense. Some creative approaches employed include using "front groups" that sound as though they represent the interests of farmers or consumers, but are, in fact, established by industry to (1) promote their own agenda;[40] (2) associate their brands with philanthropic causes; (3) create voluntary but weak self-regulatory standards to stave off government action; (4) fight antitrust regulations that could restrict consolidation in the industry;[41] (5) fight against labor organizing in order to ensure a steady supply of cheap labor;[42] and (6) fund scientific research and scientists to shape the academic literature in the corporate interest.[43] With such vast resources and so many creative minds working to support their efforts, the corporate food and beverage industry has managed to strategically employ its resources to perpetuate its dominance.

The corporate fast-food and beverage industry designs food products to be irresistible, hyperpalatable, cheap, convenient, and generally unhealthy. They use the tremendous profits they make to structure and perpetuate a system that ensures their ongoing success. The industry lobbies public agencies and elected officials, contributes to election campaigns, supports policies favorable to their success, and aggressively fights policies and practices perceived to threaten the status quo. Corporate food and beverage industry giants use their resources to ensure that the public is confused about nutrition science and views food and nutrition issues from a perspective most favorable to the industry, all to ensure we continue to overconsume their products.

Corporate efforts have kept the US political system from adequately addressing the public harms of the industrial diet. In other countries, like Norway, Mexico, and Chile, the government has begun to recognize the significant costs of the industrial diet and has enacted policies to create greater equilibrium between the price and availability of ultra-processed, hyperpalatable foods and their cost to society. What does it take to create the type of political will necessary to overcome corporate power? Where corporate interests already capture governments, it takes sustained efforts and organizing by people committed to changing the status quo.

When people who are concerned about the health of humans and our environment come together (i.e., organize), they can create a movement that generates the political will for change. A number of examples of successful organizing have emerged in food systems. As detailed in the next chapter, the corporate fast-food industry is vulnerable to organizing efforts. The Plant Based Foods Association, established to promote policies supportive of alternatives to animal-based food products, reported annual sales of $3.5 billion in 2016, as well as faster growth than other food industries.[44]

Furthermore, millennials, who came of age as evidence about the harms of the industrial diet was exploding, are driving a healthier food revolution, leading to losses of $18 billion in market share among the top beverage and food companies in the last five years.[45] The same data sources that highlight the incredible monetary value of many food and beverage brands associated with unhealthy products (Coca-Cola, Nestlé, etc.) also suggest that these brand values have been declining in recent years due to public recognition that these products are causing obesity and diabetes. This important trend demonstrates the power and potential of collective consumer voice, particularly if that voice is part of an organizing strategy.

While the fast-food industry and other food and beverage corporations have successfully been quelling the potential for political reform, there is clearly appetite for change. The ingredients are there—shifting demand, corporate vulnerabilities, and alternative markets. Organizing and public pressure can achieve that change.

Moving a McMountain

Anna Lappé and Kelle Louaillier

IT WAS A COLD AND WINDY SPRING DAY at Hamburger University in Oak Brook, Illinois, when Hannah Robertson, a nine-year-old from a small town north of Vancouver, British Columbia, spoke truth to one of the most powerful CEOs in the world. Hannah—along with concerned parents, teachers, and community health advocates brought together by Corporate Accountability—attended McDonald's 2013 annual meeting to draw attention to the fast-food giant's outsized impact on health, and demand that the corporation end its predatory marketing to kids. Hundreds of shareholders, reporters, and financial analysts in the room and tuning in around the world waited while the microphone was lowered for Hannah. With her knees shaking, Hannah said: "There are things in life that just aren't fair ... I don't think [it's] fair when big companies try to trick kids into eating food that isn't good for them by using toys and cartoon characters." She continued: "It would be nice if you stopped trying to trick kids into wanting to eat your food all the time." She spoke to the CEO directly: "Mr. Thompson, don't you want kids to be healthy, so that they can live a long and healthy life?"[1]

Thompson, who had been briefed that the spunky girl would be speaking, replied: "First off, we don't sell junk food, Hannah."[2] The CEO's defensiveness grew as a doctor, a college student, a parent, and other health advocates also questioned him. "We are not the cause of obesity. We are not unjustly marketing to kids," Thompson replied.[3]

The story of this line of questioning and the CEO's responses swept the media: a precocious fourth grader—pigtails, black-framed glasses, ankle socks and all—challenging a Fortune 500 CEO? The media firestorm that followed was sparked by groundwork laid by Corporate Accountability, its supporters, and a global network of allies, part of an ongoing campaign to transform the fast-food industry and the behemoth at the center of it.[4]

Here, we show how ordinary people—working together to plan and build grassroots power—can shift the practices of a multi-billion-dollar transnational corporation. Through these strategies, Corporate Accountability and its allies have moved a seemingly immutable power broker, building the case that McDonald's business as usual—predatory marketing to children, a menu of unhealthy products, and unfair labor practices—is not only harmful, but a financial liability.

WHY MCDONALD'S? THE LAUNCH OF A CAMPAIGN

As described in the previous chapter, the practices and products of global food corporations are actively undermining the health and well-being of people across the planet. In 2007, Corporate Accountability organizers, members, and allies began exploring how to tackle this crisis and the unchecked power of some of the largest food corporations in the world. To develop its strategy, the team drew upon its decades-long history of challenging the most egregious abuses of global corporations, beginning in 1977 when Corporate Accountability (then known as INFACT) launched the global Nestlé boycott to compel the corporation to halt its predatory marketing of infant formula. It also drew upon the research and analysis of partner organizations, including the Rudd Center for Food Policy and Obesity and Pesticide Action Network–North America.

Through this research, it became clear that the fast-food industry—with its high-salt, high-sugar, high-calorie, and highly processed food and sugary drinks—was at the heart of the mounting crisis of diet-related disease, from heart disease and diabetes to obesity and asthma.[5] It was also clear that this industry was driving systemwide abuses, including worker exploitation (see part 4 in this volume) and inhumane treatment of animals in factory farms, among other issues. To address these impacts, Corporate Accountability decided to target the fast-food industry—and specifically, the industry leader, McDonald's.

McDonald's, the largest fast-food corporation in the world, has arguably done more to shape the food system than any other. As the world's biggest purchaser of pork, potatoes, apples, and beef, and a major purchaser of fish, lettuce, tomatoes, chicken, and pickles, McDonald's wields decisive influence over food production practices along the supply chain.[6] As one of the largest minimum wage employers, the corporation has played a decisive role in fighting federal minimum wage increases as well as other policies for low-wage worker well-being. McDonald's has also shaped the norms and policies around marketing and corporate influence over policy, pioneering predatory marketing tactics embraced across the industry, and exerting tremendous political influence, including through targeted lobbying and other political spending. By focusing on McDonald's, Corporate Accountability believed it could influence the fast-food industry as a whole and alter the landscape in which all food and beverage corporations operate.

Because McDonald's is one of the primary marketing agents and political power brokers of the dominant food system, exposing, challenging, and ultimately moving the corporation in a more socially just and ecologically sound direction would have enormous impact across the food system. Out of this analysis, Corporate Accountability developed the campaign chronicled here. Launched in 2009, the campaign was designed to shift the norms of acceptable corporate behavior and to effect lasting change in corporate practices and policies—for McDonald's, for the industry, and for the food system more broadly. The vision was to significantly reverse the corporate-driven epidemic of diet-related chronic illnesses described in the previous section. And there was another core goal: to engage everyday people in democratic social change. Here, we share seven strategies and lessons that can be applied to food justice campaigning worldwide. First stop: taking on the clown.

STRATEGY 1: EXPOSE MCDONALD'S PREDATORY MARKETING

Joe Camel was wearing oversized glasses and a brown blazer, hanging with his pal, the Marlboro Man. Dragging on cigarettes, they strolled downtown Chicago streets with a cadre of clowns holding signs that read "Time to Retire Ronald" and "Clowns for Retiring Ronald." Passers-by laughed, jumping in to take photos and sign a Retire Ronald petition to be delivered to McDonald's top executives and board members in nearby Oak Brook, Illinois.

It was May 2010 and Corporate Accountability had brought these iconic characters to the McDonald's shareholders' meeting to use humor to highlight the impact of junk food marketing icon Ronald McDonald. For nearly six decades, McDonald's had used Ronald to win hearts and minds. The idea was to challenge the "imaginative capture" that this signature character holds over children. Corporate Accountability was also asking: could we leverage this cultural currency to spark a larger public conversation about the impact of marketing on children's health?

Corporate Accountability continued to take on this brand mascot. And less than two years after Ronald and the Marlboro Man showed up at the shareholders' meeting, Corporate Accountability's reframing of Ronald was starting to be reflected in the business press: Ronald wasn't just a friendly clown any longer. He was a predatory tool in the same family as cigarette-peddling mascots. As one *Ad Age* article asked in 2012: "Is Ronald McDonald the new Joe Camel?"[7]

Ronald lost center stage at the Olympics, too, where the company had wielded the character in the past. Comparing that year's McDonald's Olympics ads to those in the past, *Chicago Business Today* noted in 2012 that they'd "gradually phased out Ronald," giving the clown a "fairly minor role" on the corporation's "biggest stage."[8] Ronald was, according to the outlet, "warming the bench this time."[9]

By 2014, McDonald's was announcing a makeover for its iconic clown, in what Corporate Accountability perceived as a sign of an embattled mascot. At that year's shareholders' meeting, the corporation's defensiveness about Ronald was on display. In response to a question about Ronald in schools from Sally Kuzemchak, a nutritionist and part of the Corporate Accountability team, then-CEO Don Thompson claimed: "We don't put Ronald out in schools."[10] (It was a claim that then-McDonald's USA president Mike Andres would contradict when he told investors later that year: "We have to get McDonald's owner-operators into schools," and called doing so the brand's "heritage.")[11]

"What do these conflicting messages about Ronald tell us?" asked Corporate Accountability's executive director, Patti Lynn. "One, the fact that McDonald's can't let him go affirms how core the clown is to this corporation's business. Two, the fact that McDonald's is trying to create distance affirms such predatory marketing to children is a growing liability."

"It wasn't overnight, either, that Corporate Accountability members and allies achieved the retirement of Joe Camel," continued Lynn. But the grassroots campaign to "send Joe Camel packing" and stop tobacco marketing to children would help pave the way for successes such as the Master Settlement Agreement (a 1998 accord between the attorneys general of forty-six states, five US territories, the District of Columbia, and the five largest tobacco corporations in the US, over the health care costs and marketing of tobacco products).[12] Adds Lynn, "With the help of Corporate Accountability's campaign, Ronald is well on his way to joining Joe in the retirement home for exploitative mascots."

STRATEGY 2: MOBILIZE THE HEALTH CARE COMMUNITY

Pediatricians, nutritionists, and other health professionals are on the frontlines of the epidemic of diet-related disease, and therefore are at the heart of Corporate Accountability's campaign. They have also been a key target of McDonald's. The corporation has long used public health officials as brand ambassadors and forged partnerships with institutions like the nation's largest association of dietitians, the Academy of Nutrition and Dietetics (AND).[13]

If Corporate Accountability was to increase pressure on McDonald's to curb marketing to kids and build upon the public discussion initiated by its Retire Ronald messaging, the engagement of the health care community was essential. To this end, the organization partnered with some of the nation's leading pediatricians, cardiologists, and children's psychologists, among others. Its first joint action was an open letter to McDonald's in May 2011 that ran in papers from New York to San Francisco. "We know the contributors to today's epidemic are manifold and a broad societal response is required," read the letter. "But marketing can no longer be ignored as a significant part of this massive problem."[14] Hundreds of health leaders called on the corporation to stop targeting children, especially as the standard-bearer for the fast-food sector. "We ask that you heed our concern and retire your marketing promotions ... from Ronald McDonald to toy giveaways."[15] To date, over three thousand health professionals and institutions worldwide have joined this call to action, amplifying the growing movement of resistance to McDonald's attempted co-optation of the health community.[16]

Corporate Accountability and its allies in health care also decided to take on McDonald's in hospitals, particularly pediatric hospitals. McDonald's stores inside hospitals are not only highly profitable, but also benefit brand perception. According to a peer-reviewed study in the medical journal *Pediatrics,* the mere presence of these stores in hospitals was linked to a "significantly increased purchase of McDonald's food by outpatients, [the] belief that the McDonald's Corporation supported the hospital financially, and [a] higher rating of the healthiness of McDonald's food."[17]

In April 2012, Corporate Accountability called on the more than two dozen US hospitals with McDonald's contracts to sever ties, on the basis of health concerns and the need for patients and visitors to have access to healthy food.[18] Since then, administrators at more than a dozen US hospitals have closed their on-site McDonald's.[19] The call has now gone global, sparking campaigns to kick McDonald's out of hospitals in Australia and the UK.[20] Allied US organizations like the Physicians Committee for Responsible Medicine have also taken up the cause, releasing a series of reports on how removing McDonald's (and other fast food) from hospitals is critical to a more healthful food environment.[21]

All of this organizing may well have played a role in the corporation cutting its ties with the world's biggest symbol of health and fitness: the Olympics. In 2017, McDonald's ended its sponsorship deal with the International Olympic Committee three years early. The corporation cited increasing cost and declining viewers, but the sustained grassroots pressure on both partners about the inappropriateness of this partnership likely played an important part in this decision as well.[22]

STRATEGY 3: PARTNER WITH THE MOST TARGETED
AND IMPACTED COMMUNITIES

"In my neighborhood there is no place to get fresh food, but there are five McDonald's," said Tanya Fields, describing the South Bronx community where she is raising her six children. Founder and executive director of the BLK ProjeK, a community-based food justice organization, Fields joined Corporate Accountability's delegation to the 2013 shareholders' meeting. A leader in the movement for food justice, Fields has seen McDonald's target her community—especially Black youth. "McDonald's is like the Nike of fast food," Fields said. "When it comes to fast-food marketing, nobody does it better. They spend a lot of money making sure they control the message, especially in the Black community."

Beyond the targeted marketing to communities of color, McDonald's also focuses on wooing moms. McDonald's has long targeted mothers like Fields. Take the 2004 "McMom" initiative offering "everything from an online newsletter . . . to individual McDonald's locations featuring 'Mom corners' and 'Mom parking.'"[23] In 2005, the corporation characterized its communications strategy as "All about the Moms," and the following year launched a "Global Moms Panel" for "guidance on such topics as balanced and active lifestyle initiatives, restaurant communications and children's well-being."[24] At that time, then-chief marketing officer Mary Dillon claimed: "We want to become the best ally we can for moms and a true partner in the well-being of families everywhere."[25] More recently, mothers who blog have become a target. As the corporation's US social media director said, mom bloggers "are key influencers for our brand . . . We need to make sure we're working with them."[26]

From the beginning of its campaign, Corporate Accountability partnered closely with those communities both most impacted by fast food and targeted marketing to children, as well as those people the corporation most tries to co-opt. With Tanya Fields and other influential mothers, including moms who blog, Corporate Accountability's campaign worked to wield their collective influence and speak up, loudly, on behalf of all children. As part of this work, Corporate Accountability launched #MomsNotLovinIt, a twist on the McDonald's tagline, "I'm Lovin' It." Beginning on Mother's Day 2013, Corporate Accountability and its community called on the corporation to end its marketing directed at kids, by bringing people together online and offline and bringing a delegation to the 2013 shareholders' meeting to drive home this message.

STRATEGY 4: UNMASK CORPORATE SPIN

Organizing health professionals and mothers to publicly challenge McDonald's in both traditional and social media were strategic steps to reveal the true face of this fast-food behemoth: an abusive corporation profiting from exploiting children and undermining parents. The next step for the campaign was to deal with another cornerstone of the corporation: exposing its exploitation of charitable activities, including Ronald McDonald House Charities (RMHC) and McTeacher's Nights, to promote its brand.

The Ronald McDonald House Charities—founded in 1984 by McDonald's—have become almost synonymous with the burger giant. While the Charities' mission and work—to support families when they're caring for a hospitalized child—are unassailable, McDonald's exploits its relationship with the institution to mute criticism of its abuses and products, and to amass sympathy that translates to brand loyalty.

What's worse, McDonald's earns this powerful association with a charity while giving very little in actual financial support (for more on corporate exploitation of charity, see part 6 of this volume). The report "Clowning Around with Charity," by public health lawyer Michele Simon, reveals that McDonald's only provides, on average, RMHC about 20 percent of its revenues.[27] Of every Happy Meal purchased, the corporation donates only one penny to the charity.[28] Meanwhile the corporation "reaps 100% of the 'branded benefit' from the charity," wrote *USA Today* on the report's findings.[29] The corporation uses the charity as an "emotionally loaded marketing vehicle," Simon explained, "while shielding itself from critics."[30] Another way McDonald's buys goodwill is with McTeacher's Nights, a so-called charitable activity for schools that offers a feel-good patina for the brand, but little back to the schools that participate.

At McTeacher's Nights, schools partner with local McDonald's stores. Teacher volunteers flip burgers, families are invited to dine out, and a small percentage of sales from the evening's event goes back to the schools. "While generously boosting sales for McDonald's," writes Simon in the report, "the return for schools can equal as little as $1 per student."[31] McDonald's uses McTeacher's Nights—much as it uses Ronald McDonald House Charities—to connect communities to its brand and foster brand loyalty.

In October 2015, Corporate Accountability and the Campaign for a Commercial-Free Childhood partnered with more than fifty local, state, and national teacher organizations in calling on McDonald's newest CEO, Steve Easterbrook, to stop McTeacher's Nights. Notably, the country's largest union, the National Education Association, representing more than three million education professionals, joined the call.[32] "Frankly, it's disrespectful for a multi-billion dollar corporation such as McDonald's to throw pennies at our schools while it uses our teachers to market its products," said Melinda Dart, vice president of the California Federation of Teachers and president of the Jefferson Elementary Federation of Teachers, both of which endorsed the call.[33] "At a time when we are working hard to help our youth adopt healthy habits, this corporation and its junk food simply have no place in our schools." The call from teachers shined the media spotlight on one of McDonald's underhanded marketing ploys, with stories on NPR's *All Things Considered,* the *Chicago Tribune* and the *Boston Globe.*[34] Just three months after McTeacher's Nights came under fire, the corporation quietly took down

McDonaldsEducates.com, one of its primary vehicles for promoting McTeacher's Nights.

While McTeacher's Nights continue around the country, some school districts have condemned and even banned them.[35] In April 2017, the Los Angeles Unified School District (LAUSD)—the second largest school district in the US—voted to end McTeacher's Nights, with the LAUSD board president arguing that McTeacher's Night "is an egregious violation of [our] policy" prohibiting "sponsorship from corporations that market, sell or produce products that may be harmful to children."[36] The California Federation of Teachers, a statewide teachers' union representing more than one hundred thousand educators, took a further step in 2018, passing a resolution rejecting McTeacher's Nights.[37] Then, the nationwide American Federation of Teachers, which represents nearly two million education professionals, passed the strongest resolution yet—opposing all junk food marketing in schools, explicitly citing McTeacher's Nights.[38] And the pressure continues as a growing number of school districts and unions pursue similar action.

STRATEGY 5: FOCUS ON STRATEGIC POLICY REFORM

In early 2010, Corporate Accountability received a call from San Francisco's Board of Supervisors. Supervisor Eric Mar had seen coverage of the Retire Ronald campaign the preceding spring and was pursuing a public health ordinance to tackle the marketing of fast food to kids, specifically the Happy Meal. Corporate Accountability was eager to add muscle to local policy.[39] In collaboration with Mar and NPLAN (now called ChangeLab Solutions), the team helped craft an ordinance that required all meals in the city sold with toy giveaways to meet strict nutrition standards. Restaurants that offered free toys with meals would have to improve the nutritional quality of the food they sold—or cut the toys. Given McDonald's offerings at the time, the Happy Meal would be out.[40]

In messaging about the policy, the coalition focused on "stories of parents that struggle every day to feed their kids, of young people dealing with the crisis of diabetes, and of the tripling of the rates of diabetes since the Happy Meal was invented just a few decades ago," explained Mar. The ordinance faced major opposition from McDonald's and the National Restaurant Association. McDonald's tried to characterize the ordinance as a "crazy San Francisco nanny state policy," Mar explained. "The industry ran full-page ads in the main dailies; there were robo-calls to San Francisco residents. McDonald's lobbyists and lawyers threatened litigation."

The coalition that Mar and Corporate Accountability organized responded to this spin with people-to-people organizing and mobilized one hundred small businesses, health professionals, and community groups to sign a full-page ad of their own.[41] "Our strength came from having parents—especially Pacific Islander, Black, Latino parents—making constant visits to supervisors," said Mar. Thanks to this powerful coalition, the dominant message about the ordinance in local media was true to what the policy, in fact, was: a commonsense public health measure to meaningfully improve the health of the city's children. All the community organizing, public testimonies, visits, phone calls, and emails paid off when the Board of Supervisors passed the Healthy Meals Incentive Ordinance with a veto-proof majority on November 2, 2010.[42] The ordinance made San Francisco the first major US city to adopt such a policy.

"Our local law had an impact on national changes," said Mar. In the wake of this policy action, McDonald's "bowed to increasing pressure from groups fighting against childhood obesity," wrote *Ad Age,* reformulating Happy Meals to include apple slices, reduce the amount of fries, and offer healthier drink choices.[43] The campaign helped spur change in other fast-food chains: in 2011, Jack in the Box—the country's fifth largest fast-food chain—announced it would discontinue toy giveaways with kids' meals.[44] That same year, Arby's did an overhaul of its kids menu, replacing fries with apple slices, cutting soda, and adding yogurt, among other changes, to make meals at least nominally healthier.[45] In July 2013, Taco Bell discontinued its toys, agreeing to phase out all kids' meals by the following year, making the corporation the first national fast-food chain to eliminate kids' meals and toys altogether.[46] And in September 2017, Panera took some of the biggest steps yet, banning sweeteners, artificial flavors, toys, unhealthy sides, and sugary drinks from their kids' menu. As Panera's chairman and CEO Ron Shaich noted in launching this initiative, "I challenge the CEOs of McDonald's, Wendy's, and Burger King to eat off of their kids' menu for a week or to re-evaluate what they're serving our children in their restaurants."[47]

Corporate Accountability sees these as signs that the campaign is changing the world around McDonald's—and forcing it to respond. These, however, are critical first steps, not ends in themselves. "'Healthier' fast-food kids' meals aren't necessarily 'healthy' for kids, nor a license to continue inundating children with marketing," said Corporate Accountability's deputy campaigns director Sriram Madhusoodanan. "Industry action constitutes progress, but isn't a substitute for binding, enforceable protections for children's health."

STRATEGY 6: CHALLENGE HEALTH ABUSES ACROSS BORDERS THROUGH POLICY AND COALITION BUILDING

Since its founding, Corporate Accountability has developed strategies that engage at different levels of governance, from cities, to states, to international institutions like the World Health Organization (WHO). This local-to-global approach is essential because the food system itself is global, with the biggest food corporations operating transnationally, constantly seeking new markets around the world. A global strategy is also key to holding accountable corporations based in the US, where the regulatory environment is industry friendly, and policies that constrain corporate power are challenging to secure. Strong policymaking by other countries can move the United States to keep up with the rest of the world. "If the corporation refuses to make systematic changes globally," said Gigi Kellett, Corporate Accountability's team lead on a variety of negotiations within the WHO, "at least it costs the corporation to differentiate its products, policies, practices, and ads in its different markets. Such added costs can be persuasive in compelling a corporation to uniformly correct a specific abuse." For a corporation like McDonald's—operating in more than one hundred countries worldwide—this observation is particularly true.[48]

Working alongside Consumers International and World Obesity, among other allies, Corporate Accountability emphasized the importance of holding transnational corporations accountable, and limiting marketing to children as a cornerstone of global obesity reduction policy. Many of these groups have joined Corporate Accountability as members of the Conflict of Interest Coalition, a network of organizations calling for stronger safeguarding of public health policymaking from manipulation by commercial interests, and in May 2010, the World Health Assembly (the decision-making body of WHO) adopted a resolution on the "marketing of foods and non-alcoholic beverages to children."[49] This groundbreaking resolution codified the global-level consensus that junk-food marketing is a significant factor in diet-related diseases, and called on governments to restrict junk-food marketing. The resolution also recommends that countries take immediate policy action at the national level, and questions the idea that voluntary regulations on marketing, like those pushed by McDonald's, are effective.

Passage of this resolution sparked local and national policies to curb junk-food marketing to children around the world. For example, over thirty countries, including many in Europe, as well as Australia, Canada, Malaysia, South Korea, and the Russian Federation, now have laws that set limits on television advertising to children.[50] In recent years, Chile, Brazil, and Mexico have all passed legislation to limit marketing to kids, in part inspired by campaigning and research conducted in the United States.[51]

To ensure global policies have teeth and actually reflect the interests of the public, Corporate Accountability has been drawing on the precedents it set with the global tobacco treaty. Currently, the food industry is considered a "stakeholder" at international and intergovernmental policymaking negotiations, and as such is engaged in both formal and informal consultations. This is a clear conflict of interest, limiting progress in reversing what is on track to become the greatest preventable health epidemic of our time. Fortunately, Corporate Accountability's history shows that change is possible. Through the campaign to challenge Big Tobacco, Corporate Accountability and its allies were successful in creating clear limits to industry influence on policymaking, codified in what is known as Article 5.3 of the WHO Framework Convention on Tobacco Control and its implementing guidelines. "Where we are today with the food industry," explains Kellett, "is where we were with the tobacco industry just before governments the world over opted to regulate it at the highest international level possible. And today countries are making enormous strides in safeguarding the health of generations to come from tobacco."

STRATEGY 7: ENGAGE SHAREHOLDERS, INVESTORS,
AND ANALYSTS

In early 2015, the Gates Foundation revealed that it had divested from three major corporations: Coca-Cola, ExxonMobil, and McDonald's.[52] This revelation represented yet another major financial and reputational blow to the corporation, signaling that public sentiment regarding the negative effects of McDonald's on health, workers, and the environment had significantly shifted since the launch of Corporate Accountability's food campaign.

"When we started this campaign in 2009, many thought McDonald's was immovable. By 2015, the corporation was spending millions to defend a brand beleaguered by grassroots campaigning," said Corporate Accountability's Patti Lynn. By 2015, *Crain's, Business Insider,* and *Forbes* all had published articles on the increasing woes of the corporation. The business press was even reporting on McDonald's financial and reputational liability of marketing to kids. Corporate Accountability's campaign raised profound questions about McDonald's business practices. In 2013, McDonald's reported slumping same-store sales, a persistent decline in millennial market share, and a drop in its share of a key demographic: families with a child under twelve.[53] By 2014, the percentage of people between nineteen and twenty-one years of age visiting McDonald's monthly in the United States had fallen nearly 13 percent over the previous three years.[54]

Analysts expressed concern that instead of reflecting on its business model and reforming it, McDonald's was throwing the "kitchen sink" at the problems: from a new office in San Francisco allowing the company to be "more plugged into the flow of ideas," to a so-called transparency campaign called "Our Food, Your Questions," from its rapid turnover of top-level executives, to its rebranding of Ronald and the Happy Meal.[55] McDonald's "kitchen sink" strategy also included stepping up its influence peddling: in 2013, its lobbyists went into overdrive, with the corporation spending close to $2.3 million in federal lobbying that year alone, with a significant focus on menu labeling.[56] From the executive turnstile and slumping sales to the shift in public attitudes toward the corporation's marketing, there were indicators aplenty that Value [the] Meal was succeeding in compelling McDonald's (and the industry at large) to shape up or decline.[57]

CONCLUSION: COURAGE IS CONTAGIOUS

"Hannah was the one who wanted to go," said Kia Robertson, Hannah's mom, when asked to explain how she and her nine-year-old found themselves at the McDonald's shareholders' meeting in 2013. "Hannah was excited to let the company know what she thought, but we were both really nervous." When mom, activist, and blogger Casey Hinds attended the corporation's shareholders' meeting with the Corporate Accountability team the following year, she, too, recalled feeling nervous, but she thought to herself: "If a nine-year-old could do it, so can I!" Courage is contagious.

As much as these seven strategies deployed by Corporate Accountability were designed to influence the corporate practices of McDonald's, they were also created to foster opportunities for everyday people to speak up for common, shared values. The campaign was meant to foster courage—and spread it. Building on lessons learned over four decades, Corporate Accountability and grassroots allies also developed these strategies to change the narrative about fast food and its marketing, and to advance game-changing global health policy.

From shareholder advocacy to media outreach to partnering with public health allies, the tactics focused on calling attention to McDonald's central role in driving an epidemic of diet-related diseases—and to push the corporation to do something real about it. Since its food campaign launched in 2009, Corporate Accountability has helped to shift the national conversation about marketing to children, helping more and more people see its predatory nature and the role such marketing plays in driving diet-related disease. The need to protect public health by creating binding, meaningful policies in the face of the actions of fast-food giants like McDonald's has also become more widely recognized.

Moreover, McDonald's fundamental business model—pushing unhealthy junk food and treating its own workers so poorly—has come squarely into question. McDonald's has been forced to a crossroads. The corporation can stubbornly attempt to market and bully its way back—whether in the courts, city halls, statehouses, Congress, or government agencies—or McDonald's can heed the dictates of the new public climate that Corporate Accountability and its many allies have fostered, and build meaningfully upon the steps it has already been forced to take. If it does not take responsibility, and fails to effect real, profound change, McDonald's—and Ronald along with it—may simply end up in the dustbin of history.

Hunger Incorporated

WHO BENEFITS FROM ANTI-HUNGER EFFORTS?

Andy Fisher

TIANNA GAINES IS a young African American woman who grew up in poverty in Philadelphia. She joined other women from a similar background in a photovoice project called "Witnesses to Hunger" to document the nature of hunger in their families and communities. Launched in 2008 by ethnographer and public health researcher Mariana Chilton, Witnesses has blossomed into a national initiative that now has substantial impacts on public policy. Witnesses to Hunger has testified in Congress, completed over two hundred interviews with the media, helped drive changes to nutrition policy in Pennsylvania, and has been featured in high-profile documentaries. Of equal importance, it has provided a role model for the anti-hunger movement, demonstrating how to effectively organize the hungry to speak for themselves. The group has also demonstrated how to advocate for policy changes needed to overcome structural preconditions.

Tianna represents a growing part of the anti-hunger sector that explores alternatives to promote public health and provide the food insecure with the skills needed to get better jobs, grow their own food, and help them build political power. Witnesses has been a transformative project, arguably bringing the most disenfranchised individuals—impoverished women of color—to the forefront of the anti-hunger movement. Unfortunately, while it represents the sector's enormous potential to address the underlying causes of hunger, Witnesses does not represent the goals or activities of a majority of the anti-hunger sector.

Witnesses and other groups like it work on the fringes of a sector that, while far from being monolithic, has largely developed operational approaches that treat the poor as clients rather than as partners of their own destiny. This top-down approach is reinforced by the sector's focus on hunger as a problem in and of itself. Hunger is a symptom of more deeply rooted issues such as poverty, racism, misogyny, a skewed economic system, and—ultimately—powerlessness. The powerful in a society are not the ones without food. Instead, it is the economically and politically marginalized that suffer from food insecurity.

Yet the anti-hunger movement in the past few decades has not focused on helping the poor to build power. Instead it has sought to *feed* the poor—through charity or federal food programs—by aligning itself with the powerful and wealthy corporate sector. While grassroots efforts that address the underlying causes of hunger are gaining credence, these efforts face intimidating barriers to change, including entrenched alliances with corporate America. This chapter explores this crossroads, explaining how the anti-hunger movement has failed to help the poor to build political and economic power. Instead, the movement has focused on constructing alliances with the corporate food industry; here, these alliances and resulting beneficiaries are highlighted.

CHARITY

Virtually all Americans encounter food charity at some point in their lives, as recipients, donors, or volunteers at a food pantry or soup kitchen. Regardless of how impressively large this system is, serving some forty-six million persons per year, it has pernicious effects on its recipients' dignity.[1] Nick Saul, longtime director of a food pantry in Toronto and coauthor of *The Stop,* calls food pantries "a slow death to the soul."[2] Waiting in long lines to receive a box of food, often in dark church basements, can be a profoundly depressing and disempowering experience. It can also be an experience that reinforces racism and classism, as poor recipients of color must rely on middle-class white volunteers to access their daily bread.[3]

Despite its best intentions, the national food banking trade association, Feeding America, further disempowers the poor through its communications. For example, a pair of 2013 public service announcements depict volunteers and staff—but not clients—as angels with wings.[4] The message is that those serving the poor are heaven sent, but the poor themselves, no matter how smiling and well dressed, are somehow less morally fit, deserving of pity.

In her book *Sweet Charity,* the authoritative volume on the charitable food sector, Jan Poppendieck contends that patrons of the emergency food system have become profoundly depoliticized. Rather than the empowered poor people of the late 1960s who marched on Washington, DC, and conducted a sit-in at the US Department of Agriculture (USDA), Poppendieck sees today's patrons as dejected objects, passively waiting in lines, their images used to raise money. In her analysis, they look more like "objects of compassion than potential allies."[5] Food banks' social service model, which all too often lacks a social change agenda, results in one of the biggest missed opportunities of the anti-hunger movement: it has not converted these tens of millions of recipients of food assistance into a powerful grassroots movement.

Even the structure of the nation's approximately two hundred food banks reflects their lack of interest in empowering the poor. Food banks are mainstream, rich, and respectable, and they intend to remain that way. One indicator of this social status can be seen in the composition of their boards of directors. The hungry are nowhere to be found on most boards. Instead, many boards consist solely of representatives of the corporations that donate food, money, and political heft to the food banks. A 2017 analysis of food bank boards indicates that 22 percent of 2,586 food bank board members work at Fortune 1000 companies or the equivalent, with Kroger, Walmart, Bank of America, and Wells Fargo the most common employers of food bank board members. Only two persons were employed by a labor union. Grassroots organizers and anti-poverty advocates are also in short supply on food bank boards, highlighting the fact that food banks tend to see themselves as permanent community institutions, appendages of the business community, with no aims to disrupt the status quo.[6]

This profile of corporate food bank leadership is an indicator of the nature of the relationship between food banks and corporate America. It is an indicator that this relationship benefits corporations perhaps as much, if not more, than it does the hungry. Through food banking, corporate America gains the following benefits:

Reduced dumping costs: Supermarkets and food processors saved $34 million per year in 2011 from reduced disposal costs associated with food donations.[7]

Tax write-offs: Corporations can deduct the full value of their philanthropic donations to charitable organizations, saving a quarter to a third of the value of the donation from their taxes. The estimated value of the food donated by companies is about $190 million per year, according to the Congressional Budget Office.[8]

Reputation building: Increasingly, the value of a company's brand is tied to public perception of corporate integrity. Corporate philanthropy plays a key role in gaining positive press and building a corporation's reputation. There are some who would argue that corporate food bank participation is as much a PR campaign as a reflection of philanthropic charity.

Profit protection: The vast majority of food banks accept large amounts of corporate food and money, but most food banks have chosen not to take a stance on inequality-related policies that affect corporate profits, such as the minimum wage, tax structure, or trade policy. Corporate philanthropy reinforces food banks' "neutral" stance on these matters.

PHILANTHROPY

Many of the nation's largest corporations have chosen anti-hunger work as a destination for their philanthropic dollars because it is a service-oriented, politically neutral approach that earns them public accolades without contradicting their financial interests. In particular, some of the nation's corporations with the worst equality reputations, such as Walmart, Monsanto, and Bank of America, have focused on funding hunger charities to heal their bruised reputations. Corporate grant-making has played a pivotal role in widening breaches between the labor, anti-hunger, and food movements, reducing their collective power. Consider the following examples.

At the same time Restaurant Opportunities Center (see part 4 in this volume) was fighting for an increase in pay for tipped workers (to 70 percent of the national minimum wage, as part of the Harkin Miller Bill of 2013), a leading national anti-hunger group, Share Our Strength (SOS), was accepting substantial donations from the opponents of this bill. Donors included Darden Restaurant Group and the National Restaurant Association. Since receiving such donations, SOS remained silent on this bill, as well as on numerous other federal, state, and local wage-raising efforts.

Similarly, Walmart has donated over $2 billion in grants and food to anti-hunger charities since 2010. These donations have been part of the company's campaign to rebuild its image as a firm that cares about the poor and to distract the public from its exploitative practices. These donations also help

Walmart gain entrance into urban markets—entrance that had previously been opposed by environmental and labor activists. At the same time that activists affiliated with the Union of Food and Commercial Workers were ferociously combating Walmart to increase its below-market wages, end abusive practices, and implement worker-friendly scheduling, these same anti-hunger groups looked the other way, particularly when they were recipients of the company's largesse. For example, the Food Research and Action Center (FRAC), the primary lobbying group on federal food programs, chose not to support the Washington, DC, City Council's bill to mandate a $12.50 starting wage at Walmart stores in the District. Instead, FRAC focused on asking Walmart to make food stamp applications available to its employees, a benefit of less impact to those in need, but one less costly to the company.

Feeding America, the trade association for the nation's food banks, has shown a penchant for entering into partnerships with corporations that produce harmful products or employ unethical practices. Sixty-eight percent of the public revenues it raised in 2016–2017 came from corporate donations and promotions.[9] The association has promoted Snickers candy bars and cheesecake from the Cheesecake Factory in the midst of a type 2 diabetes epidemic, potentially causing collateral damage to public health. Feeding America also has partnered with Monsanto (now owned by Bayer), the corporation singularly reviled by the food movement for its damage to the environment and farmer livelihoods across the globe, in the "Invest an Acre" program. This program had farmers donating the proceeds from an acre of their production to their local food bank while Archer Daniels Midland and Monsanto matched the funds.

The Ohio Association of Second Harvest Food Banks dropped out of a coalition effort to gain tougher payday loan regulations because of pressure from a corporate donor. In 2008, Rent-A-Center, a payday loan provider, complained to Feeding America (then known as America's Second Harvest) that its $500,000 contribution was being used to support legislation the company opposed. Within a few days, the association pulled its support from the coalition.[10]

Food bankers' willful blindness to the political implications of their fundraising practices extends to their sourcing of food as well. For example, Smithfield Foods regularly donates tens of thousands of pork to food banks across the country as part of its "Helping Hungry Homes" program. In Memphis, Tennessee, the CEO of the Mid-South Food Bank acknowledged

Smithfield's contribution: "Smithfield returns to us again this year as an active partner in the fight against hunger."[11] The largest pork producer in the US, Smithfield has been sued successfully three times for engaging in environmental racist practices in siting their hog factory farms next to historically marginalized communities in North Carolina. Senator Cory Booker of New Jersey called out Smithfield: "This corporation is outsourcing its pain, its costs, on to poor black people in North Carolina."[12]

Similarly, food banks have been a willing partner in the Trump administration's initiative to curry favor with farmers negatively affected by retaliatory tariffs placed on American farm products. They stand to receive $1.2 billion in "mitigation bonus commodities" of fruit, nuts, and dairy products, purchased by USDA to bolster displaced markets.[13] While food banks have strenuously fought against the Trump administration's efforts to slash food stamps, their unquestioning acceptance of these hundreds of millions of pounds of surplus food aligns their success with the president's. Once the food is distributed, food banks will tout the fact that they distributed more pounds than ever, at the same time enhancing the president's standing with his rural base and facilitating his re-election. Part of the attraction to anti-hunger work for corporate philanthropists is the framework of hunger itself. It is a sanitized rebranding of poverty, which entails a much more political and deeply rooted set of solutions. The hunger problem couches income inequality in a veil of temporary need that heralds corporate philanthropy and draws attention away from systemic causes. Hunger allows corporations to be perceived as problem solvers rather than as problem producers.

Federal Food Programs

Corporate involvement in the anti-hunger model transcends charity and philanthropy. With expenditures of roughly $80 billion, federal food programs comprise a substantial source of business for the entire food retail and manufacturing sector. The USDA purchases over $2 billion worth of food every year for schools, food banks, and other programs. Tyson held the largest contract for this program, selling more than $100 million of chicken, beef, and pork to the federal government. Schools themselves purchase another $2 billion, and one in five schools has chosen to outsource their meals programs to outside vendors, such as Aramark and Sodexo, as a way to cut costs. Protecting these programs is where the interests of the DC-based hunger lobby and the food industry dovetail.

The SNAP program (Supplemental Nutrition Assistance Program, more commonly known as food stamps) is an even bigger source of revenue for Big Food. Since its inception in the 1930s, the food stamp program initially supported the agricultural sector, but now supports a broader swath of interests, especially food processors and retailers. For example, Kraft food stamp sales comprised one-sixth of Kraft's domestic sales.[14] At Walmart, executives have acknowledged that the firm redeems an outsized share of SNAP benefits. Nationally they claim to have redeemed $13 billion, or 4 percent, of total Walmart domestic sales in 2013.[15]

To many anti-hunger groups, such as FRAC and Feeding America, the food and beverage industry is a friend. Industry sponsors their banquets, writes large checks from their foundations, and most importantly, lobbies for the passage of SNAP. In 2013, at the height of the latest Farm Bill, the food industry spent over $62 million lobbying for SNAP.[16] The anti-hunger community has made a strategic alliance with the industry to protect SNAP, demonstrating that industry can open doors that are typically closed to the more liberal-leaning groups. Through dispersing the economic benefits of this $70 billion alliance, leading strategists have sought to maximize a base of political support for SNAP.

In addition to food manufacturers, FRAC has cultivated the fast-food industry as a stakeholder in the SNAP program. For example, it supported efforts by Yum! Brands (Taco Bell, KFC, Pizza Hut) to expand a pilot project to allow homeless, disabled, and elderly SNAP participants to redeem their benefits at restaurants. FRAC staff reasoned that this program would bring the fast-food industry into the fold, creating another constituency for SNAP.[17] In her 2012 report *Food Stamps: Follow the Money,* corporate accountability advocate Michele Simon pointed out that the banking industry profits handsomely from processing SNAP transactions, adding another powerful constituency for the program.[18]

This alliance between the anti-hunger sector and the beverage and snack food industry to protect the status quo for SNAP generated controversy when this coalition advocated to allow recipients to buy soda and other unhealthy foods with SNAP benefits. Anti-hunger groups have actively courted industry groups to protect SNAP from restrictions. Ellen Vollinger, FRAC's legal/food stamp director, led the creation of the Coalition to Preserve Food Choice in SNAP, whose members include the main trade associations for the soda, candy, baking, snack food, dairy, supermarket, and high-fructose corn syrup industries.[19] Anti-hunger and industry groups lobby together on state and federal legislation related to protecting "freedom of choice" within the SNAP program. They have also developed common materials, including a joint coalition statement.[20] The anti-hunger community comes to this issue largely from a position of maintaining consumer choice, based on a belief that poor people should not suffer from paternalistic regulations, which only apply to them and not to the general public. Nonetheless, groups such as FRAC accept donations from soda companies and their trade associations, leaving themselves vulnerable to the perception of a conflict of interest.

WHO'S AT THE TABLE?

Almost all anti-hunger leaders would acknowledge the importance of increasing wages and decreasing unemployment to reduce hunger. They know that some 80 percent of SNAP households have at least one working individual.[21] They also know that wages and related benefits comprise 70 percent of the income of the bottom fifth of non-elderly American households.[22] They know that the relative value of the minimum wage has shrunk considerably below its 1968 peak, which would be worth $18.30 per hour in 2015 if it had kept pace with productivity.[23]

Yet very few anti-hunger groups dedicate significant time and resources to raising wages. Their policy platforms have typically not called for wage increases, and few of their policy advocacy resources are dedicated to this end. Few anti-hunger groups have joined with striking fast-food workers to demand a $15 minimum wage, for example, or supported ballot initiatives in cities and states around the country for the same goal. Instead, they have focused almost exclusively on strengthening federal food programs as a tool for redistributing public resources to the poor. They have been modestly successful in this realm, having protected and grown these programs through an age of neoliberal austerity. Nonetheless, federal food programs cannot by themselves solve the hunger problem. An exclusive focus on them ignores some of the other key roles of the government in ensuring the right to food, specifically around setting the conditions under which labor operates. Over the past few decades, labor has experienced numerous policy setbacks that have weakened their hand. As candidates from both the Republican and Democratic Parties have accurately noted, the loss of well-paying manufacturing jobs has hollowed out many communities in the Rustbelt and beyond.

Moreover, the anti-hunger community's virtually exclusive focus on strengthening the safety net has left them vulnerable. Persistently high caseloads for SNAP in recent years, despite the recovering economy, have raised great opposition to the program, providing ammunition to the right that the program fosters government dependency. Federal food programs become seen as the primary, if not only, defense against hunger, instead of part of a broader strategy that focuses on income inequality and poverty reduction. After all, SNAP does not build the wealth and skills people need to get off government assistance in the first place. Many households remain on SNAP for long periods of time, with a median time frame of eight years, according to one USDA study.[24] By design, safety net programs cannot solve what has become a persistent and ongoing problem of underemployment and unemployment.

It was not always this way. Throughout the 1960s, 1970s, and into the 1980s, the poor were at the forefront of anti-poverty and anti-hunger work. The 1964 Economic Opportunity Act created a national network of community action agencies (CAAs) across the country to fight the war on poverty. Federal regulations mandated that CAA boards of directors include one-third poor people, to foster their leadership and gain their perspectives. Even into the 1980s, the National Anti-Hunger Coalition, led by impoverished women of color, dramatically shaped the federal anti-hunger policy agenda.

In spite of this progressive legacy, anti-hunger groups today remain isolated from the progressive community, such as those involved in labor and trade issues. The potential for social change would be astounding if they could mobilize even a small fraction of the tens of millions of poor people with whom they work on a daily basis toward a broader agenda to reduce income inequality. What is holding back this alliance-building?

On one level, anti-hunger groups' reliance on corporate donors and a bipartisan support base has meant that they must advocate only within a "nutrition safety zone"—a set of programs on which there exists general consensus that threatens neither the ideology nor the economic interests of their base of support. At a minimum, finding funding for nutrition program advocacy is arguably much easier than getting money for community organizing, especially from corporate sources.

On another level, it is the absence of the participation of the poor themselves in the leadership of anti-hunger groups that influences their policy agenda. Most anti-hunger groups are not membership oriented, and, as noted, few of the board members of food banks come from the ranks of the hungry. In other words, most anti-hunger groups are not held accountable to those they serve.

Some observers believe that as a result, the anti-hunger leadership prioritizes strategies, such as an overwhelming emphasis on federal food aid, that do not fully account for the self-articulated needs and desires of the poor. It would be difficult indeed to find a survey in which the impoverished said their highest priority was to improve the food stamp program. Instead, they typically want safer communities, better jobs, better schools for their kids, and higher wages. Most poor participants wish to escape federal food programs such as SNAP, even if they are necessary.

As New York anti-hunger leader Joel Berg states, "It is darn hard to organize among individuals whose top goal is to no longer be a part of the group being organized."[25] It is also exceedingly difficult to organize people around solutions that are not their priorities. Effective community organizing requires listening to people explaining their needs and desires, and then building a campaign around that goal. The lack of participation of low-income individuals at the forefront of the anti-hunger movement is both a symptom and a cause of a top-down, insider strategy that focuses on feeding the poor and not empowering them. This approach may solve today's hunger, but not tomorrow's, merely kicking the can down the road and into the future. Food charity is the solution of an industry that chooses to perpetuate itself (in a self-congratulatory fashion), rather than work itself out of business.

Still, the potential to do anti-hunger work differently exists. In addition to Witnesses, the organization described at the start of this chapter, Freedom 90 and the Alameda County Community Food Bank provide two additional examples of how anti-hunger organizations can address the root causes of hunger in a transformative way. These examples, and the example provided by the United Food and Commercial Workers in the next chapter, prove that a different way of addressing hunger is not only possible, but also entirely necessary.

Across the province of Ontario, Canada, "church ladies" running food pantries have decided to get serious and organize. They have declared that they do not want to keep feeding people indefinitely, but instead want the government to preemptively reduce the incidence of poverty. With the help of an experienced labor organizer, they've formed a union, Freedom 90, a parody of the Freedom 55 financial planning advertisements that promise the good life to Canadians who work hard and invest their savings wisely, so they can retire by fifty-five. Tongue in cheek, these activists demand to be able to retire by the time they are ninety. They argue that poverty has been rebranded as hunger to mask its cause: inadequate incomes due to low wages, stagnant welfare rates, and increasingly part-time employment. They see food banks as a means for the government to avoid its commitment to citizens' right to food, and as a means to minimize taxes on the middle and upper classes. Freedom 90 members believe that organizing will pressure labor markets to raise wages and increase social assistance rates by "put[ting] food in the budget." Moreover, Freedom 90 has made strides in bridging the divide between food bank volunteers and clients, fostering an understanding that they share the common goal of wanting social justice, rather than charity.

ALAMEDA COUNTY COMMUNITY FOOD BANK

In Oakland, recipients of food boxes from the Alameda County Community Food Bank have organized themselves into a community-based advisory committee that drives the food bank's policy agenda. They advocate on policies that affect the bottom line of low-income persons in Alameda County, such as minimum wage, housing subsidies, childcare, and even bus passes. Their efforts have played a key role in the food bank, leveraging its considerable power to advocate for policies that would normally be considered unrealistic.

Through their narrow agenda and alliances with corporate America, the anti-hunger community has kept food insecurity at bay, but has not significantly reduced its prevalence. Food insecurity rates have ebbed and flowed since the USDA started tracking it in the 1990s, but in relative terms, have not been reduced. Unfortunately, this approach has resulted in collateral damage on multiple levels. It has resulted in missed opportunities to improve the health of the poor, who suffer from higher levels of diet-related diseases such as type 2 diabetes. Through the ubiquity of the emergency food system, it has communicated to the poor that they are not capable of feeding themselves, while mis-educating the public that the solution to hunger is food, not political and economic power. It has reinforced an oligopolistic food system, dependent upon the cheap labor of workers and farmers.

This hunger industrial complex has divided prospective coalitions, diminishing the ability to effectively address income inequality and poverty in a more systematic fashion. The anti-hunger sector remains largely aloof from, if not at odds with, its potential allies in the public health, food systems, and labor sectors. Anti-hunger advocates find themselves between a rock (the knowledge that their strategies are incomplete to resolve the hunger problem) and a hard place (the nation's political realities). There seems not to exist an immediate out to this uncomfortable position, so the hunger movement remains in a holding pattern, waiting for the political winds to change direction.

At this crossroads, the anti-hunger sector will need to decide its path. Will the sector continue to ignore the degradation of its "clients," continuing down the hunger management path, in which feeding people through charity and food programs is seen as the solution? Or have times changed sufficiently such that the sector can more fully address income inequality without jeopardizing its hard-fought gains in food aid, and so choose the path of income equality, in which building collective power for social and economic justice is the primary strategy?

Progress over Poverty through Political Power

Jim Araby

ANTI-HUNGER ACTIVISTS TODAY FACE multiple dilemmas: as political power, wealth, and influence become concentrated among fewer people, and frequently in the hands of corporations, influencing decision makers through traditional forms of protest and progress has become more challenging. Yet even though the anti-hunger sector in the United States has become increasingly dominated by corporate power—or what Andy Fisher has described as "hunger incorporated"—organizations that nimbly adapt to changing conditions can create lasting, positive change. Activists, academics, organizers, and elected officials can tackle issues of poverty, hunger, and corporate influence. To do so, it is important that they focus on impacting the organizational structures of the US food system, while also creating relevant change in local communities.

In the same way that many anti-hunger organizations face multiple dilemmas, the United Food and Commercial Workers (UFCW) Union and its membership are also experiencing an evolutionary change. This is a shift that advocacy and membership-driven organizations must also undertake as the dynamics of the culture and economy evolve. Both nationally and regionally, UFCW leadership recognizes that in order for the union to remain relevant, we must adapt our organizational strategy to address the large-scale consolidation of the food industry.

The union still fights hard to win and maintain strong bargaining positions with food employers. Yet union leaders also recognize that in order to win, and to maintain the high standards achieved through decades of struggle, our efforts must extend beyond the traditional bargaining table. UFCW must reach out to communities, immigrant rights' groups, and food advocacy groups to foster credibility with people most hurt by dramatic changes in the economy and the food system. UFCW has come to realize that, in order to win progress for workers, we must complement targeted anti-hunger efforts by engaging in broader, intersectional solidarity strategies as well, with a wider array of actors that also care about poverty, hunger, and justice in the food system.

To implement these strategies, UFCW's recent efforts in California include building bridges with unlikely allies. These alliances allow UFCW to exercise its political power in new ways, widening its sociopolitical vision to wield greater influence within the California food supply chain. Throughout this process, the union has helped win broad increases in wages, workplace protections, and paid sick days. We recognize that at a fundamental, structural level, addressing hunger means addressing subminimal wages and helping workers obtain critical workplace protections. UFCW continues to fight to increase the level of engagement of its members and community allies and partners.

INITIAL ANALYSIS

In late 2012, the union leadership recognized a key factor: the UFCW operates in a core area of the California economy. As such, opportunities to participate in significant public policy debates on behalf of UFCW members were clear. Following this recognition, the UFCW began strategizing about how to tackle issues that were affecting the union's main industry, including the negative effects of part-time work and large employers' use of legal loopholes to avoid providing employee health care coverage. For example, in 2012 alone, more than seven million eligible Californians lacked health insurance at some point during the year.

Many employers, particularly in the non-union sector, were shifting their part-time employees onto the California Medical Assistance Program, a Medicaid program known as "Medi-Cal," shifting the financial burden onto the taxpayer. In effect, the taxpayers of California were subsidizing unscrupulous employers while also allowing non-union companies to operate at a comparative cost advantage. Many UFCW strategies dovetailed with federal efforts to expand health care coverage through the Affordable Care Act.

One key, analytical point of departure was the understanding that the UFCW plays a pivotal role in the private-sector economy. As the largest private-sector union in California, and in a state with growing union density, the UFCW's ability to leverage its position in a crucial area of the economy had been underutilized. Additionally, the UFCW needed to better understand the changing nature of the food supply chain—the ways in which food is produced, processed, shipped, marketed, and sold. This demanded research and outreach.

Toward that end, in early 2013, the UFCW Western States Council engaged the Food Labor Research Center at the University of California, Berkeley, the Food Chain Workers Alliance, and UC Davis professor Chris Benner to undertake a study of our workers and our industry. *Shelved,* the resulting study released in June 2014, contained industry and government data, as well as information gleaned from close to one thousand worker surveys and twenty in-depth interviews with workers and employers throughout the state.[1]

This comprehensive study of the industry found that while the California food retail industry had thrived, a low-cost non-union business model had encouraged significant downward pressure on wages and working conditions. Low-cost and low-skill operations such as Walmart and Target, along with non-union "natural" and gourmet food stores and "ethnic markets" like El Super, have pushed workers into poverty and onto the public tax rolls. Startlingly, this study found that 36 percent of California food retail workers use some form of public assistance, at a cost of $662 million to state taxpayers. With regard to hunger, the report found that nearly one-third of all California food retail workers (29.3 percent) faced low or very-low food security.

The study also found that unionized workers, due to low-wage competition, have seen their wage rates decline by 16.7 percent in the last decade, resulting in even some unionized food retail workers facing food insecurity. While a "union advantage" for wages and working conditions still holds, the unionization rate among grocery store workers has declined by almost one-quarter during the last decade. This is due mainly to the growth of general merchandise stores that sell food. While some of the major union stores pursued dubious financial strategies such as share buy-backs, debt repayments, and dividend increases, more thoughtful approaches emphasized investment in employees, productivity, and capital improvements. Union density also fell because of larger economic forces, including consolidation of unionized employers, which resulted in the closing of many union stores. Large competitors such as Target and Walmart also had positional advantages due to their ability to use economies of scale with both perishable and nonperishable goods.

The implications of the report guided the council leadership and broader political community. Policy recommendations based upon the *Shelved* report included raising wages for food retail workers by expanding collective bargaining agreements and raising state and city minimum wage levels. This was part of a campaign for legislation to reduce incentives for "low-road" employers to provide substandard wages, benefits, and reliance on part-time workers. (Low-road employers are those who provide exploitative wages and working conditions, and/or violate workers' rights, while "high-road" employers strive to provide livable wages and working conditions to their employees.) Additionally, the recommendations in the report aimed to create a level playing field for unionized employers by linking any government subsidy, such as tax breaks, zoning assistance or Cal Fresh Works Fund loans, to the provision of quality full-time jobs with livable wages and benefits.

The purpose of the report was to compile key economic information about our industry in order to provide an empirical foundation for our public policy initiatives. Moreover, the process of creating the report was an indication that UFCW was willing to look honestly at its sociopolitical situation and the challenges we faced. Some of *Shelved*'s grim economic data also encouraged us to reach out to community and food justice organizations. For example, with regard to food security and hunger, it became clear that neither the union nor other food justice groups such as anti-hunger groups could tackle the issue alone and without broader analysis of the root causes of increased poverty and food insecurity in one of the state's largest employment sectors. The report showed the interconnections between declining wages, poverty and food insecurity, access to health care, and worker voice and control over worker schedules and lives. For example, one key factor causing poverty for food industry workers is the limited access to full-time work. Part-time workers require lower income investments and fewer health care benefits, and for that reason, many large employers try to limit the number of full-time employees. We realized we needed to work on this broad set of issues with a broad set of groups. These are groups we felt we had a moral obligation to ally with, as well as a political imperative to join. In sum, we committed ourselves to facing the rapidly changing world around us.

2013 LEGISLATION: ORGANIZATIONAL POSITIONING AND STRATEGIZING FOR POLITICAL POWER

Even before *Shelved* was published, the UFCW had some sense of the situation, and began to work on legislation to address some of the issues ultimately raised in the report. In February 2013, Los Angeles Democratic Assembly member Jimmy Gomez introduced the UFCW-sponsored bill AB 880. This bill, entitled the Fair Share Health Care Law, would require large employers with Medi-Cal–enrolled employees to pay a premium to a trust fund that would provide reimbursements to California health care providers. We knew, even before the report was published, that employers who were increasingly moving in the direction of low-wage, part-time jobs were contributing to the overall decline in wages and increase in food insecurity among workers in our sector and statewide. Requiring these employers to pay for their employees' use of publicly funded health care would be a disincentive to move in this low-wage direction.

Initiating the legislation established a number of important markers for the UFCW in California. Taking this legislative initiative sent a message to the political world that the UFCW in California was ready to take political leadership, rather than follow the lead of others. This new approach captured the attention of statewide labor leadership, as well as the business community and other institutional players in Sacramento, the state capital.

Organizationally, the UFCW understood that solidifying the union's presence in California would be a major component of legislative battles. UFCW recognized that building communities and alliances requires a common ethic and common goals, as well as a clear oppositional target. By taking the initiative, the union defied tradition and expectations, tested political allies, and challenged its own organizational capacity.

Context is key in understanding this fight. It is important to note that in 2012, the Democrats in the legislature had achieved a two-thirds supermajority, giving them the power to initiate and pass tax bills and override potential gubernatorial vetoes. That kind of power is rare in legislative bodies, offering unprecedented opportunities as well as potential contradictions.

As the proposed Fair Share Health Care Law was introduced, the UFCW mobilized its membership for an intense battle. The union engaged rank-and-file members through direct mail, educational programs, and ongoing lobbying as the bill made its way through the legislative process. One of our primary goals was to create internal organizational unity, as well as to increase the political knowledge and skills of the UFCW membership. The union's belief was that if it engaged UFCW members with clearly defined vital issues, they would respond with enthusiasm. That is precisely what happened.

In late March of 2013, the bill was double referred to the Health and Revenue and Tax Committees of the Assembly. ("Double referring" occurs when legislation is referred to two committees rather than a single committee for review.) As several special elections were taking place concurrently, a concrete two-thirds majority was never solidified. Yet the UFCW and its allies at the State Federation of Labor held lobby days in February, March, and April, actively urging union members to garner the support needed to bring the bill to the floor for a vote.

By mid-May, this work had paid off. The UFCW had forty-eight dependable votes, and we subsequently pushed for the bill to be brought to the floor. The bill passed out of the Assembly Rules and Assembly Health Committee in April, and out of the Appropriations Committee in May. Then, AB 880 was finally brought to the floor of the Assembly at the end of June 2013, the last day to vote bills out of the house of origin. Unfortunately, three Democrats voted against the bill and five abstained, preventing it from moving to the Senate.

LESSONS LEARNED

The defeat of AB 880 was nevertheless in many ways a victory. The legislative battle bolstered the UFCW's organizational capacity and taught us several political lessons. First, we recognized that we cannot assume the automatic support of all Democrats, even those who previously supported the union. We saw the need to recognize our assumptions, holding one another accountable to interrogate them. Second, we learned that personalizing political efforts is necessary, as lobbying "Assembly members" as abstract entities is neither possible nor effective. By personalizing members' requests for support, our organizers entered into a personal relationship with individual legislative members, creating mutual responsibilities and obligations. Although personalizing can also be polarizing, we contend that it is necessary for effective organizing. We believe the tension this process creates often de-escalates with victory. Third, we have learned that members of union organizations are the most effective spokespeople. A lobbyist can develop strategy and provide key information, but union members are the core embodiments of policies, experiencing struggle firsthand. Fourth, even if opponents have more money, union members can overcome this advantage through great personal dedication: steadfast loyalty is the union's ultimate advantage. Fifth, in democratic societies, power and justice should take place in the public—as opposed to the private, corporate—sphere. By asserting power in the public sphere, the UFCW expresses its members' determination to be recognized. Sixth, achieving justice often requires conflict, but that conflict can also serve to clarify obstacles. In many instances, self-definition is born of opposition. By questioning our organizational past, by opposing entrenched interests, and even by opposing some previous political allies, the UFCW Western States Council began to redefine itself, and it gave birth to a qualitatively different organization. Finally, we believe that power is wasted unless it is utilized to achieve our political aims. Although there are times when demonstrating restraint in the exercise of power is a strategic necessity (numerous US foreign policy examples come to mind), there are also moments when the refusal to utilize power means lost opportunities. Political caution at a moment of great economic crisis is irresponsible.

BUILDING COMMUNITY SUPPORT: CONNECTING THE FOOD CHAIN

One of the union's initial efforts at expanding our outreach to community organizations was to hire a staff person to work with the Jobs with Justice (JWJ) organization in San Francisco. JWJ is an alliance of labor, community, faith-based, and student organizations that fights for workers in their communities and workplaces.

Some of their priority campaigns included the successful Fight for $15, which helped raise the minimum wage in San Francisco, as well as the *Retail Workers Bill of Rights,* passed in November 2014. The latter promoted full-time work, predictable schedules, and job security for tens of thousands of retail, restaurant, custodial, and security workers. The UFCW Western States Council hired organizer Michelle Lim to work full time on solidifying UFCW's relationship with JWJ, helping to build a strategic alliance that would have long-term benefits for both UFCW members and JWJ organizers. This work in San Francisco is a model for key partnerships in other cities; it builds community support for the UFCW and leads to organizing opportunities in the non-union sector.

Such research and community outreach are also an initial investment in connecting the union analytically and organizationally with other links in the complex and changing food chain in California. The council determined that it needed to be acutely aware of and actively engaged with workers in the producing, logistics, transportation, storage, marketing and global dimensions of the food system.

2014 LEGISLATIVE VICTORIES

As the 2014 legislative session began, the UFCW was prepared to initiate a number of bills that could politically "move the ball down the field." These bills were chosen based on a number of criteria, namely: Would the bill be helpful to UFCW members and the unionized sector of the industry? Would the bill have a reasonable possibility of passage and signature by the governor? Were there opportunities to build effective coalitions around the bills that would also increase long-term political relationships and capacity? Was there a larger "public good" derived from the bills that would garner favorable public opinion and potential allies? The UFCW initiated and promoted two bills that fit those criteria: AB 1792 and AB 1522.

AB 1792 was an offshoot of the previous year's tax bill (AB 880). Rather than fighting the retail industry, the UFCW decided to take a smaller but significant step. AB 1792 called for a report from the largest five hundred employers in California that would show how many of their employees were using Medi-Cal. This bill was also an outcome of *Shelved,* the study described above.

Our clear intent was to provide the data that could substantiate the existence of a major public policy scandal: the use of public tax dollars to avoid providing adequate health care for workers. The bill required the State Department of Health Care Services to annually inform the Employment Development Department of the names and social security numbers of all recipients of the Medi-Cal program, and to determine the attendant costs of state and federally funded benefits provided by the Medi-Cal program.

AB 1792 sailed through the Assembly and the Senate with bipartisan support and was signed by Governor Brown on September 30, 2014. UFCW demonstrated, through the passage of AB 1792, the ability of the union to assert unilateral power while at the same time entering into strategic alliances that added to UFCW knowledge and enhanced our reputation. The union also tested the organizing principle that the "action is in the reaction": reactions to group initiatives are as important as the initial action, as these dynamics help clarify subsequent strategies.

By remaining disciplined and exercising strength when necessary, and compromising when the time was right, the union demonstrated a beneficial mix of risk and political maturity. UFCW's organization had local knowledge of the political terrain, important allies, and the passion necessary for sustained commitment.

Governor Brown also signed AB 1522, the paid sick days bill. UFCW once again demonstrated the ability to skillfully maneuver through a difficult political process. In this case, because the governor did not want home care workers covered in the bill, it was opposed by the Service Employees International Union (SEIU) and the American Federation of State, County and Municipal Employees (AFSCME), both major political players in Sacramento.

UFCW's strategy was to remain supportive of the bill because it knew it would help 4.5 million workers obtain three mandated sick days, which would provide a minimum of decency for those suffering from illness. UFCW partnered with the state building and construction trades unions, as well as many other community partners and allies, to push the bill forward. Though employers and other major organizations opposed the bill, it passed, and Governor Brown signed it.

2015 LEGISLATIVE ACTION

In February 2015, the UFCW Western States Council kicked off its legislative agenda by bringing local members and leadership to Sacramento to lobby its bills. These included bills on fair scheduling, worker retention, and raising the minimum wage—all issues that, as mentioned above, *Shelved* connected to addressing poverty and food security for low-wage workers.

The Fair Scheduling Bill would require at least five days' advance notice on work schedules; with this bill, no caregiver would miss their child's doctor's appointment, meetings with teachers, or other important family obligations due to the chaotic scheduling practices of retailers. However, the Fair Scheduling Bill failed to get out of committee in the Assembly. The opposition, mainly the California Retail Association, the California Grocers' Association, and large individual retailers like Walmart, successfully lobbied legislators to kill this bill.

In the wake of hostile corporate takeovers, mergers designed only for stockholders or corporate executives, and other irresponsible business practices, the UFCW is also sponsoring the Grocery Worker Retention Bill. Authored by Assembly member Lorena Gonzalez from San Diego and coauthored by Senator Connie Leyva, this bill would require any new employer that purchases an existing grocery store to retain its current workers for at least ninety days. It is the union's belief that the expertise, productivity, and commitment of UFCW union workers provide clear competitive advantages for any business.

UFCW has also joined with a broad-based, statewide coalition to significantly raise the minimum wage in California and to index that increase to the cost of living. California is one of the most expensive places to live in the country. No family that is working full time should live in poverty, but that is exactly what is happening to tens of thousands of hardworking people. Raising and indexing the minimum wage would provide hope and decency for every worker.

UFCW members approached meetings with legislators with the respect their offices deserved, while also maintaining an understanding of our own standing as workers, voters, and proud representatives of our fellow union members. UFCW members' efforts did not go unnoticed; as a result of their dedication and commitment, Governor Brown signed both the Grocery Worker Retention bill and the $15 per hour minimum wage bill in 2015.

POLITICS AND INDEPENDENT ACTION

At the same time that the Western States Council was taking the initiative legislatively, UFCW shifted its overall approach to political engagement. In the past, UFCW tended to participate in political campaigns by following the leads of state and local labor federations. While generally this is an effective approach, the union has also determined that acting independently can be in its best interests.

To that end, the Western States Council created a 527-organization political committee that has the ability to run independent expenditure campaigns. Independent action also allows UFCW to craft its own messages, tailored to its members' interests.

The other reason for pursuing independent political action is the understanding that UFCW is challenging the social structure that locks people and institutions in place. There are times when an organization, in order to be effective, has to break away from predictable strategies. Predictability can foster vulnerability. UFCW has now explicitly stated that it will choreograph its own public actions. The UFCW council also believes that this new stance encourages a sense of organizational identity and membership loyalty.

THE NATURE OF POWER

One of the most famous dictums about power, attributed to Lord Dahlberg-Acton in 1887, is "Power corrupts; absolute power corrupts absolutely." Dahlberg-Acton was referring to the behavior of popes and kings when he articulated this axiom—the kind of inaccessible and unaccountable power that was unilateral, domineering, and opaque. But as US civil rights leader Bayard Rustin pointed out in his famous 1965 essay, "From Protest to Politics," the absence of power also corrupts.[2] Powerlessness leaves people and organizations vulnerable, directionless, and depressed.

In other words, if we do not exercise power, then someone else will. In the past, UFCW let other organizations shape its political orientation and fate. The problem UFCW was facing was not that it was without close friends and allies, but that it did not recognize its own potential for gathering and utilizing power. As the great organizer Fred Ross explained, "Organizing is providing people with the opportunity to become aware of their own capabilities and potential." The leaders of the Western States Council have since embraced that message.

UFCW's successes over the past three years in the state legislature have made the industry take notice. Two major industry lobbyist associations, California Retailers and California Grocers, have hired more lobbyists and have extended their outreach to non-affiliated businesses. Additionally, industries within the food system are continuing to consolidate into larger corporate entities.

While these two factors may give UFCW's opposition access to greater resources, they also present opportunities for union strengthening. First, corporate consolidation could potentially make these organizations more bureaucratic and less responsive. Second, UFCW can leverage the outcomes of further concentration of power by arguing that these companies can afford positive change, since their bottom-line costs will be minimal.

Ultimately, the success of the UFCW-affiliated organizations will rely on people who support it, the accuracy and relevance of its research, and its ability to effectively communicate its message about who it is and what it stands for.

"BLUE STATE" EXCEPTIONALISM?

The success of UFCW begs the question, "Can this only happen in 'blue' states?" This question is an important one and must be asked if we are to pursue larger fights around social and economic inequality. A brief history of California and its politics shows that while the fights listed above are more likely to take place in blue state, the only reason unions, community groups, and progressive elected officials exist in California is because organizations and leaders there decided to fight for the issues outlined above.

In 1994, California and its politics were much different than they are today. The city of Los Angeles was still dealing with the aftershocks of the L.A. uprising in 1992, Republican Pete Wilson was governor, the City of Los Angeles was led by Republican Richard Riordan, Democrats only held a slim majority in the state legislature, and California passed an anti-immigrant ballot proposition (Proposition 187) that restricted state services to immigrants and undocumented workers.

Proposition 187 became the catalyst by which many progressive groups previously operating in silos recognized that much more had to be done. Unions, community groups, and foundations began to work more closely together and invest in strategies that developed capacity at the local and state levels. Key leaders built a vision to get candidates elected into legislative office who shared the values of the majority of Californians, and strategic investments were made in cities like Los Angeles to change the power structure. Leaders like Miguel Contreras, from the Los Angeles County Labor Federation, and Anthony Thigpenn, a longtime community activist and leader in the city of Los Angeles, organized their constituencies to engage in political activism. Unions such as SEIU, AFSCME, UNITE HERE, and the California Nurses Association began to invest in union-organizing campaigns that grew their memberships. Unions then turned around and talked to those new members about why politics mattered and mobilized workers across California to begin to think about a new vision for the state.

Within four years of the passage of Proposition 187, the City of Los Angeles had elected its first Latino Democratic mayor, Antonio Villaragosa, and the state had elected Democrat Gray Davis to the governorship. Progressive policies were enacted at both the state and local levels throughout the late 1990s and early 2000s, and while progressives suffered a defeat in 2003 with the recall of Gray Davis and the election of Republican governor Arnold Schwarzenegger, progressives expanded their hold on local power, winning in places like Orange County, San Diego, and Sacramento.

Yet clearly the story did not end with the election of mayoral and gubernatorial candidates who supported progressive policies during their campaigns. The key lesson is not simply to invest in organizing and infrastructure to get some candidates elected, but to then continue to demonstrate intersectional power to pressure those elected—regardless of party—to actually follow through and pass policies that work to uplift millions out of poverty.

The story of California becoming—and *remaining*—a blue state is not one of destiny, but one of politics, organizing, and persistence. It is a story of wealthy individuals and foundations, community organizations, elected officials, and unions working together to fight for a broader vision of progress in the country's largest state. While California remains a blue "wall" of resistance to the national tide of conservatism, the struggle for power and equity remains.

In order for other states to replicate what California has become, they need to make smart investments in organizing, be persistent in their engagement, and make a coordinated effort across communities.

A NEW TRADITION

Creating a new tradition may seem like an oxymoron; how can tradition be new? But in the forward-thinking movement of the UFCW, the foundations of change grow out of the past. Creating something new is grounded in the resources of traditions, yet anticipates something unique. We can create our own future, even under economic and political conditions not of our choosing.

PART SEVEN

Trade

CALL TO ACTION—
THE CORPORATE STOCK IN TRADE

Raj Patel and Maywa Montenegro de Wit

COLLECTIVE RESPONSE—
FOOD SOVEREIGNTY IN JAPAN AND BEYOND

Ayumi Kinezuka and Maywa Montenegro de Wit

The Corporate Stock in Trade

Raj Patel and Maywa Montenegro de Wit

IN SEPTEMBER 2003, the World Trade Organization met in Cancún to seal a round of tariff reductions and other trade-related rules nearly four years after the failures of the Seattle negotiations, and two years after the resuscitation of the US-led multilateral trade agenda in Doha. At the Mexico meeting, countries of the Global South were pressed to concede the agricultural subsidies that, in part, had prompted their walkout four years before. The EU and US delegations were in no mood to let up the pressure. Social movements, building on tactics developed outside earlier negotiations of the WTO, the World Bank, the Free Trade Agreement of the Americas, and Multilateral Agreement on Investment in the 1990s, stationed themselves at the perimeter of the Ministerial Conference. Among them was La Vía Campesina, an international federation of two hundred million farmers, peasants, and landless and agricultural workers from around the world. A number of delegations at the protest were from South Korea, home of industrial giants like Samsung and Hyundai and of vigorous and militant peasant movements like the Korean Peasant League and the Korean Peasant Association.[1] Also present were members of the Korea Advanced Farmers Federation, at one time led by fifty-five-year-old Lee Kyung Hae, whose forty-acre experimental and teaching farm had been sold in foreclosure four years before. On Wednesday September 10, Lee scaled the barricades around the trade negotiation wearing a sign saying "WTO! Kills. FARMERS." He flipped open a rusty Swiss Army knife, stabbed himself in the heart, and died minutes later.

In the days following Lee's death, a new chant spread through the front-lines of the protest, one that recognized that while he may have hailed from South Korea, his tragedy was one that mattered internationally: "Lee, hermano, te has hecho mexicano." Lee, brother, you have become Mexican.

It's not hard to understand this international solidarity, to see how Mexican campesinos were able to see in Lee's death the fall of a comrade. Under the World Trade Organization, farmers had been made to compete against one another, leaving only those with access to land, capital, and occasional state support able to survive the downward pressure on income. Lee was not the first, and has hardly been the last, to die disputing the merits of an economic policy that had dispossessed him. But even as peasants immolate themselves and governments struggle over agricultural trade issues, prevailing common sense holds that free trade is good.

The problem with this conventional wisdom is not only that it is contravened by decades of evidence, from Mexico to Malawi, Tokyo to Ohio. It is also that the ideas of free trade are a cornerstone of today's international capitalist food system but are seldom scrutinized publicly. Asking why it's wrong gives us purchase on such central questions as these: who owns what, who does what, who gets what, and what do they do with their wealth? To see who profits from international trade in the food system is to glimpse the levers of control on the buying and selling of goods, at what scale this exchange occurs, and where (or to whom) value is flowing as a result. Because it involves such socially central questions, we need to peel back the technocratic language around trade to show how it masks some profound political decisions.

Here, we make three main arguments: the first is that the dynamics of modern "free trade" have less to do with rational economic thought than with how nation-states and later corporations have positioned themselves as global hegemons, using trade barriers to nurture domestic agricultural industry and finance, and then collapsing those barriers to take advantage of global markets and prevent others from doing the same. Second is that economic arguments are made to suit prevailing hegemonic politics, and "free trade" has been particularly effective in serving capitalist interests, as seen in the rise of agrofood multinational corporations with unprecedented market power and control. Third is that free trade, like every instrument of hegemony, requires active and ongoing justification. With evidence mounting of trade liberalization's ill effects, it takes a potent mix of naturalization, obfuscation, and reimagined histories to keep the conventional wisdom running.

To tell this story, this chapter unfolds through history, theory, politics, and practice. We first revisit how trade has evolved in the past 150 years, using the lens of food regimes. We then examine a fundamental tenet of liberal trade theory, asking how it holds up under political and historical scrutiny. Next, we look more closely at modern trade institutions, including the North

American Free Trade Agreement (NAFTA) and the World Trade Organization, to illustrate how agrofood corporations justify, utilize, and expand "free trade" under the guise of both consumer choice/value and national interests. We look at specific practices initiated under NAFTA and expanded under the WTO to explore how agriculture is permeated in areas from extrajudicial tribunals to intellectual property on seeds. In the following chapter, we return to the frontlines—in a real and metaphorical sense. Whether outside WTO Ministerials, in classrooms, around meeting tables, or on farms worldwide, people are designing and enacting alternatives to free trade. Through the story of the Nouminren farmers' movement in Japan, we introduce food sovereignty as a theory and practice that counters the concentration of power and wealth enabled by liberalized trade, therein reclaiming peoples' rights to determine by and for whom their food systems work.

A BRIEF HISTORY OF ORGANIZING TRADE

During the last great wave of colonial expansion (1870–1914), world food trade was largely structured by and around the British Empire. Tropical crops such as sugar, tea, coffee, bananas, and rubber flowed into Britain's borders from her colonies, including India, Ceylon, Barbados, and the Bahamas, while temperate crops like wheat came in from fledgling states like Canada and the US. The repeal of the British Corn Laws in the 1840s was critical in setting the stage. In a move heavily favored by the class of industrial capitalists, this repeal lowered barriers to "free trade," enabling imports of raw materials and cheapening the price of food for wage workers. This first era of globalization, then, brought slave-grown plantation crops, factory workers, and free trade rules to fuel the Industrial Revolution.

By the end of the Second World War, the US had emerged as the new hegemonic power in the world food system. From the 1940s through the 1970s, Cold War political alliances largely defined the boundaries of trade, and US agriculture strengthened significantly under farm supports and protectionist policies, reversing the previous era's "free trade" scheme. Tariffs and subsidies—alongside technological revolutions in crop and animal breeding, mechanization, and chemicals—helped generate a historically unprecedented food surplus. This period was characterized by the US developing ways to continue overproduction by developing ways of disposing of the fruits of its overproduction. Those included food stamps, school lunch programs, and foreign food aid. Underwritten by Public Law 480, food aid became particularly effective in facilitating the postwar "development project," in which political classes in countries of the Global South were persuaded that the trajectory of the US and other settler states was "universally desirable and universally achievable."[2]

The legacies of this era were shrinking Global South rural populations, the creation of dependency on cheap foreign food imports, the transformation of agricultural systems in the Global South for export crops destined for the Global North, and opening up space for future markets. Another legacy was the emergence of northern agricultural corporations, including input corporations—makers of those Green Revolution pesticides, fertilizers, and farm machinery—and food industries specializing in oils, sugars, and many processed, "durable" foods. But the growth of such agrofood corporations also brought about new tensions. Once strengthened by protectionist trade policy, the larger firms started seeing tariffs as a hindrance on their ability to penetrate foreign markets. The accelerating growth in power, influence, and control of global food sourcing, processes, and sales was starting to push back against the mercantile limits of the postwar order, from which it had benefited earlier.[3]

From the early 1970s until the present, the food system has been structured less by a particular country than by transnational agrofood corporations. Ushered in by a series of crises in the Nixon era, this period dovetails with the broader "globalization project" that has predominated since the collapse of Bretton Woods, the dissolution of the gold-backed dollar, and the rise of neoliberalism worldwide. Writing in 1993, Harriet Friedmann remained agnostic about which trends would predominate in food systems, but she saw clearly the developments under way.[4] Export agriculture from southern countries was an explicit aim of Structural Adjustment Policies imposed by International Monetary Fund creditors. Industry was shifting to "food" over agriculture, bringing about a new class of workers in food processing and services. There was a new convergence of year-round global sourcing, homogenous production conditions, and standardized global diets. Twenty years later, we can add the heightened fungibility of grain, meat, and biofuel markets, the growing influence of the retail sector (the "supermarket revolution"), highly mobile and migratory labor forces, and oligopsony control by a few powerful agrofood firms.[5]

The role of the World Trade Organization as international arbiter of "free trade" has been central to these sweeping changes. Previously known at the Global Agreement on Tariffs and Trade (or GATT), this body emerged when international efforts to create the "World Food Board" foundered in the 1940s due to US opposition. Implicated in what Friedmann calls a program for "private global regulation," the WTO restricts the rights of sovereign states to regulate food and agriculture. Instead, she suggests, "agro-food corporations are the major agents attempting to regulate agro-food conditions, that is, to organize stable conditions of production and consumption which allow them to plan investment, sourcing of agricultural raw materials, and marketing."[6]

Importantly, the ascendancy of private global regulation does not mean a diminished power of the state. As David Goodman and Michael Watts point out, the conventional view of neoliberal food regimes are ones defined by the global circuits of capital and the undermining of state autonomy.[7] But, they suggest, "while it would be wrong-headed to deny the extent to which agriculture has been deregulated in the last decade . . . the pace and direction of liberalisation remains uneven and underdetermined. . . . *The state continues to play a central role* in domestic restructuring and negotiation a competitive global environment" (emphasis added). Many scholars have subsequently argued that even neoliberals never honestly believed that state institutions would wither away. Indeed, the technologies of neoliberal governance, including information technology, genetics/genomics, and transportation innovations, among others, have expanded the apparatus of the state in ways that not even the "fairy tale" crafters themselves anticipated.[8]

Both the state and private capital, we assume, figure deeply in processes of globalization that form the underlying ethos for the current food order—one Phillip McMichael has explicitly dubbed the "corporate food regime." Insofar as food systems have long been inscribed by trade relations, from colonial time until the present, trade is at the very heart of this neoliberal-era order. But it is a particular kind of trade—organized by states on behalf of agrofood monopolies, adjudicated in part by lobbyists in proceedings where trade agreements are hammered out beyond democratic view—that defines this contemporary period. As McMichael argues:

> Within the terms of the corporate food regime, neo-liberal policies (particularly liberalization and financial deregulation) have encouraged agribusiness consolidation, including strategic alliances between agribusiness, the chemical industry and biotechnology. Most importantly, dismantling national marketing boards, eliminating small farmer subsidies and rural credit, and liberalizing trade and investment relations have accelerated de-peasantization and legitimized a wholesale conversion of the global South into a "world farm."[9]

For peasant leaders José Bové and François Dufour, a signpost of the corporate regime is easy to see: corporations can now source "food from nowhere" to supply affluent markets anywhere.[10]

Perhaps no case better illustrates this than Mexico under NAFTA, in which consolidation of agribusiness is conditioning a permanent food crisis associated with the neoliberal era. Despite earlier agrarian crises—triggered by the dismantling of the Mexican national food system in the 1980s, when the Mexican Constitution was reformed to allow the dismantling of the *eijido* system and foreign investment in farmland—campesinos have tenaciously clung to their farmland, often by resorting to off-farm work and family remittances from the US.[11] In 1994, NAFTA blew the lid off of an already unstable arrangement by institutionalizing liberalized trade in corn. Mexico's dependence on food imports has soared in the past twenty-five years, with 46 percent of basic grains now imported, mainly from the US.[12]

If food crisis is endemic to this global food regime—producing new dispossession of land, casualizations of work, displacement of people into informal economies where need will never register as purchasing power—then why does free trade persist?[13] If NAFTA is so obviously corrosive, then why are the US, Mexico, and Canada renegotiating it, as we speak? In short, the answer is power, politics, and the entrenchment of institutions that serve elite interests. But there is also a subtler ingredient: something needed to smooth the surface, to naturalize things, to make it seem like the status quo is necessary, normal, and should not be disturbed. This something is the magical thinking of comparative advantage, the economic theory at the heart of free trade.

THE MAGICAL THINKING OF COMPARATIVE ADVANTAGE

Understanding and appreciating comparative advantage provides an induction into an august circle. Think of comparative advantage as a kind of intellectual hazing ritual. It's so important, the economics profession even has some lore around it, the appreciation of which is a prerequisite to the entry to the fraternity of economists.[14] In a key essay, Paul Samuelson, winner of the first Nobel Memorial Prize in Economics in 1970, recalls a brainstorming session in which noted thinkers were brought together to "cross-fertilize" their ideas.[15] It didn't go well. Stanislaw Ulam, the noted mathematician, challenged Samuelson: "Name me one proposition in all of the social sciences which is both true and non-trivial." Samuelson didn't have the answer with him, but a few years later his response was this: "Comparative advantage." He wrote: "That it is logically true need not be argued before a mathematician; that it is not trivial is attested by the thousands of important and intelligent men who have never been able to grasp the doctrine for themselves or to believe it after it was explained to them."[16]

Explaining comparative advantage is straightforward—here's the World Trade Organization's attempt:

> Suppose country A is better than country B at making automobiles, and country B is better than country A at making bread. It is obvious (the academics would say "trivial") that both would benefit if A specialized in automobiles, B specialized in bread and they traded their products. That is a case of **absolute advantage.**
>
> But what if a country is bad at making everything? Will trade drive all producers out of business? The answer, according to [David] Ricardo, is no. The reason is the principle of **comparative advantage.**
>
> It says countries A and B still stand to benefit from trading with each other even if A is better than B at making everything. If A is much more superior at making automobiles and only slightly superior at making bread, then A should still invest resources in what it does best—producing automobiles— and export the product to B. B should still invest in what it does best— making bread—and export that product to A, even if it is not as efficient as A. Both would still benefit from the trade. A country does not have to be best at anything to gain from trade. That is comparative advantage.
>
> The theory dates back to classical economist David Ricardo. It is one of the most widely accepted among economists. It is also one of the most misunderstood among non-economists because it is confused with absolute advantage.
>
> It is often claimed, for example, that some countries have no comparative advantage in anything. That is virtually impossible.
>
> Think about it . . .[17]

The ellipsis at the end of this explanation assumes that if you don't get it the first time, a few more attempts to wrap your head around the arithmetic of comparative advantage will ultimately leave you convinced. The question persists, then: Why do any number of important and intelligent men, in Samuelson's words, not grasp or believe the theory? Why can't they grasp that trade barriers are straitjackets, mistakenly donned in the belief that they're bulletproof vests? That removing the jacket offers freedom, a means for markets in both countries to allocate resources more efficiently? The potted history of free trade is often told from Ricardo's forging of it, the early British adaptation of it, and its creeping victories against the tide of protection, with a disastrous deviation in the interwar years, until the General Agreement on Tariffs and Trade in 1947 restored the world back to its course en route to the World Trade Organization, with fewer and fewer people failing to understand its bounties.[18]

LIBERATING AGRICULTURE
FROM TRADE LIBERALIZATION?

Defenders of free trade will often contrast the "pro-people" rhetoric of trade sceptics with the logic of comparative advantage. Compared with the situation before trade, allowing specialization and the free flow of goods means that there are more goods, and the prices are lower. When the pie is bigger, the slices are cheaper, and more people get to eat it. That's better for *all* consumers. In other words, defenders of free trade argue that the real beneficiaries of trade skepticism aren't "the people." When you prevent trade, you're really just putting money in the hands of a small cabal of producers, who in turn steal more money from consumers through higher prices. There's an egalitarian kernel within this narrative that is important to take seriously: rather than tie money up in the hands of a few producers, free trade supposedly expands the circulation of goods, lowers prices, and therefore distributes consumption more evenly.

Yet this egalitarian argument in favor of trade founders in the real world. In part, this is because while consumer gains across an economy may be substantial, individual consumers see relatively little gain—it is usually the capitalists further up the supply chain who benefit the most from lower input costs, more biddable legal protections, more precarious workers, and governments keen to attract their attentions. Agriculture provides cheaper food to consumers at an extraordinary cost to climate, ecosystems, and those consumers' own health. It also pits small farmers not only against their larger and wealthier compatriots, but against other smallholders across the planet.

Historically, the problem of—as Samuelson puts it—intelligent men failing to understand trade liberalization has been explained by Filipino sociologist and activist Walden Bello. He writes that "the problem is very basic: while seemingly compelling in theory, there is very little empirical evidence that radically liberalized regimes in trade, finance, and investment actually bring about net benefits globally."[19]

Instead, as Peter Rosset points out, the argument of comparative advantage is *itself* an engine for transforming society. Countries have comparative advantages relative to one another because of their different resource endowments, different mineral wealth, soil fertility, and the like, but also different degrees of worker wages, environmental standards, and price distortions like subsidies or monopoly pressure. For some countries, the comparative "advantage . . . may be nothing more than a lower-paid, more exploited workforce."[20] "Cheap goods" in countries A and B are far more easily explained by capitalism's quest for cheap nature, money, work, care, food, energy, and lives, by country A's colonization of country B, than it is by any God-given difference between two places.[21] Trade agreements help an elite bloc of capitalists in countries A and B maintain hegemonic power and, as we'll see, when that dominance wavers, economists can be asked to offer new supporting theories. Indeed, the current crises in trade agreements can be understood not as a sudden collective failure to understand Samuelson, but as an outcome of a longer history to which Samuelson was oblivious.

TRADE IN THE NATIONAL INTEREST

A certain history has attached to the founding of free trade, one in which first Britain, and then the rest of the world, gradually came to understand the supposed wisdom of free trade in the nineteenth century, lost faith in the early and aberrant twentieth century, then returned to full wisdom with the collapse of the Soviet Union and the creation of the World Trade Organization. The trouble with this story is that it's not quite what happened.[22] The dynamics of modern free trade have less to do with the creep of the Enlightenment and more to do with how the United Kingdom and then United States were able to position themselves as global superpowers, establishing an order favorable to private industry and finance. They then endure by "kicking away the ladder" of national economic protection—to use Ha-Joon Chang's phrase—to prevent others' use of similar policies. This pattern is captured nicely in a quote by Ulysses S. Grant:

> For centuries England has relied on protection, has carried it to extremes and has obtained satisfactory results from it. There is no doubt that it is to this system that it owes its present strength. After two centuries, England has found it convenient to adopt free trade because it thinks that protection can no longer offer it anything. Very well then, Gentlemen, my knowledge of our country leads me to believe that within 200 years, when America has gotten out of protection all that it can offer, it too will adopt free trade.[23]

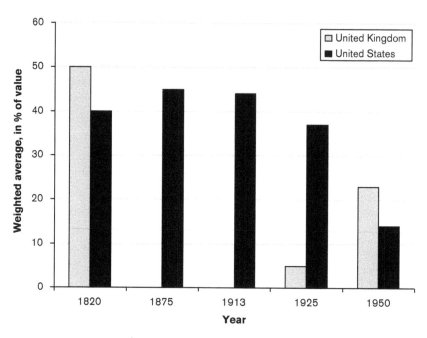

FIGURE 4. Average tariff rates on manufactured products for the UK and US. Credit: Paul Bairoch. Source: Paul Bairoch, *Economics and World History: Myths and Paradoxes* (Brighton: Wheastheaf, 1993).

It's a sentiment that certainly seems borne out by the evidence. As figure 4 shows, the UK zeroed tariffs on industrial goods throughout the late nineteenth and early twentieth centuries, a time when its industries were the planet's most efficient. With the decline in relative British industrial power, barriers crept up, at the same time as increasingly efficient US industries and corporations won concessions for lower tariff barriers. Following suit, most countries have developed formidable industrial capacity behind tariff walls. A bloc of large-enough companies can urge a nation to drop those barriers once the profits from international trade outweigh the benefits of domestic protection. The central—and surely unoriginal—argument of our chapter is that economic arguments are made to suit prevailing hegemonic politics. To be clear, hegemony isn't simply a matter of corporate rule. It's the complex interactions of the capitalist state, civil society institutions, the private sector, and household spheres that, working together, subordinate the interests of subaltern groups (read: poor, nonwhite, non-citizen, etc.) to those of the elites. To the extent that free trade has been useful, it has been to serve and stabilize the hegemonic bloc that commissioned the idea.

Those commissioners are now deeply embroiled in renegotiating NAFTA, the trade agreement that has perhaps taught us most about the specific tropes and false promises of mixing food and free trade. The reason for the renegotiation is precisely a crisis in the hegemony of free trade. The theory that free trade was universally beneficial was always fragile. In the protests in Seattle, that theory was vulnerable to critiques from the left that decried the environmental and worker injustices created by international free trade. In more recent politics, the assertion that free trade is universally beneficial has been vulnerable to the argument from the right that foreign firms steal jobs from American workers.

NAFTA: TEMPLATE FOR THE WORLD

The 1994 free trade agreement between the US, Mexico, and Canada was "in many ways... the model trade agreement," suggests Rosset.[24] NAFTA set the mold for the Central American Free Trade Agreement (CAFTA), the Transatlantic Trade and Investment Partnership (TTIP), the Comprehensive Economic and Trade Agreement (CETA), the Trans-Pacific Partnership (TPP), and dozens of others. One of the innovative features of the new generation of free trade agreements signaled by NAFTA was that signatory nations allowed themselves to be bound by the rulings of a supranational court constituted by the trade agreement. NAFTA was the first to include corporate arbitration panels, giving private corporations the power to sue national governments. Beyond implementing run-of-the-mill policies like tariffs and import quotas, this trilateral agreement carved out a wider berth for hegemonic control, including issues only indirectly related to trade like investments and competition between foreign and domestic firms.

Food and agriculture were central to promises made by NAFTA advocates from the start. During debates that unfolded in the early 1990s, US farmers and ranchers were promised prosperity from unrestricted trade. The USDA circulated a factsheet at the time, showing growers that they could expect boons from coming "higher agricultural export prices." President Clinton stumped memorably for NAFTA, tethering trade to immigration: "By raising the incomes of Mexicans, which this [NAFTA] will do, they'll be able to buy more of our products and there will be much less pressure on them to come to this country in the form of illegal immigration."[25]

This was, to say the least, disingenuous. Research by Maria Narayani Lasala-Blanco, among others, indicates that US NAFTA negotiators knew that if agricultural tariff barriers between Mexico and the US were lowered, the effect on Mexico's peasant economy would be apocalyptic.[26] US farm subsidies allowed US exports to be sold at levels below the cost of production in Mexico. Against such competition, Mexican peasants would be wiped out. That's why US negotiators hadn't thought to include agriculture when expanding the US-Canada trade agreement to Mexico. When NAFTA first started, the US didn't put agriculture on the table. Mexico did. The Mexican government argued that the improving effects of competition would leave behind a competitive farming sector, with those backward peasants unable to compete urged by the "invisible hand" to the cities, where they would provide a labor force that would, surely, be taken up by any low-cost industry that wanted to relocate there from the US. Thus, the argument ran, would Mexico transform itself from a developing to a developed country. In order for that to happen, the peasantry needed to be staked. The US accepted the sacrifice.

Nearly twenty-five years on, NAFTA's record provides its own rebuttal. In a 2009 paper—"Agricultural Dumping under NAFTA"—Timothy Wise and coauthors found that, after 1994, US grain exports to Mexico increased dramatically: upward of 400 percent, 500 percent, even 600 percent increases in corn, soybeans, wheat, cotton, and meat, all basic dietary items for Mexico.[27] Running these surpluses below the costs of production, what came to be known as "dumping" characterized the first twelve years of NAFTA. During this time, corn prices fell precipitously (50 percent between 1990 and 2003) and tortilla prices in Mexico tripled.[28] An estimated 5.3 million Mexicans left family farms. Rural poverty went up to 55 percent, and many left farming to look for work. According to Mexico's 2007 national census, of those who left farming households, 3 million found some work in seasonal export farm labor, while the remaining 2.3 million left agriculture altogether.[29] Many of these migrants crossed into the US—rather contrary to Clintonian visions.

Correlation, of course, is not causation. Such trends nevertheless show that NAFTA did not align with touted windfalls for US and Mexican farmers. Its impacts almost invariably fell hardest on farmers with small landholdings. From 1993 through 2012, the US lost nearly 22 percent of small-scale farmers, and 5 percent of mid-sized farmers. Farmland ownership consolidated accordingly, with large-scale farms increasing in number by roughly 107 percent.[30] Cheaper corn and soy prices enabled by free trade (and also by the Farm Bill) had knock-on effects for the meat industry. Concentrated Animal Feeding Operations (CAFOs) have expanded dramatically in poultry and hog production, coinciding with the demise of independent animal producers in the US. Mexican producers, meanwhile, counted some successes in winter fruits and vegetables. But while strawberries and tomatoes generated some rural jobs, these tended to be in the industrialized sector, where labor needs were light relative to the peasant systems displaced.

It is worth asking, then, who won what? In a recent policy brief, the Institute for Agriculture and Trade Policy (IATP) puts some names to the principal beneficiaries: "The top 10 companies exporting foodstuffs from the U.S. to Mexico include grain companies Bartlett Grain, ADM, Cargill and CHS, as well as meat companies such as Tyson Foods and JBS, according to Panjiva, a trade data company. The top 10 companies shipping north include Driscoll's, a berry grower; Grupo Viz, a Mexican meat supplier; Mondelez, the U.S. snacks company; and Mission Produce, an avocado producer."[31] Here, NAFTA reveals much about the links between corporate concentration in the food system and free trade. Since 1994, agribusiness market share has dramatically concentrated in nearly all sectors, including seeds, fertilizer, meat, and crop production.[32] Policy analysts attribute these trends to many things, but the role of free trade cannot be overemphasized. "One of the major consequences of NAFTA," writes William Heffernan, "was the consolidation and restructuring of the agri-food system on the continent."[33]

EXPANDING FREE TRADE TO THE GLOBAL LEVEL

Just as NAFTA came into force in 1994, another trade regime—this one at the world level—was striving to modernize "free trade" in the age of globalization. Formerly known as the General Agreement on Tariffs and Trade, the World Trade Organization was established on January 1, 1995, with 123 nations already signed on. Like NAFTA, the WTO approached agriculture with zeal, and with similar caveats for industrial farmers in the US and EU. While the rest of the world's farmers were pushed toward free market competition, US and EU farmers were shielded. The WTO's Agreement on Agriculture was one set of rules and exemptions that policed this trade, but the WTO also imposed agricultural policy through intellectual property rules, government procurement policies, sanitary and phytosanitary guidelines, and investment rules that formed the broader political economy context for agriculture. The intellectual property (IP) provisos of its Trade Related Intellectual Property Rights (TRIPS) agreement necessitated that every country develop a way to manage intellectual property—a provision demanded by Disney and pharmaceutical companies, but beneficial to seed oligopolies too.

TRIPs required countries to provide basic minimum IP rights through patenting, plant breeders' rights, or an "effective *sui generis* system." Geographical indicators for food also came into focus, as the WTO moved to disallow country-of-origin labels that give additional value to farmers in the marketplace. State procurement policies similarly met with WTO nettles. Communities around the world endeavoring to grow locally, organically, and agroecologically often use government purchases to buoy their efforts; farm-to-school programs, for example, incentivize purchasing from local farmers. But these have been directly undercut by WTO arbitrations against the "local," specifically by claims that "providing preferential treatment for domestic goods, services and suppliers discriminates against foreign suppliers and therefore acts as a trade barrier in this sector."

Another key instrument of the WTO, first road-tested under NAFTA, are provisions that grant foreign corporations the power to sue national governments. Formally called "investor-state dispute settlement," or ISDS, this mechanism goes far beyond traditional trade issues, granting foreign investors new rights to own and control land and natural resources, to establish or acquire local firms, and to operate them at an advantage over domestic enterprises. If corporations believe that domestic policy contravenes their trade pact privileges—for example, by favoring local companies or contravening "expected future profits"—they are empowered to sue states for damages. Importantly, these ISDS cases are litigated outside any domestic legal system, in tribunals where corporate lawyer panels may award large amounts of public money to corporations for revenue they might have earned but for the challenged measures.[34]

Sugar disputes illustrate how these investor-state settlements can trammel over public interest. In 2003 Corn Products International, a US agribusiness that produces high-fructose corn syrup (HFCS), challenged the Mexican government for infringing on its rights. At issue was a government tax that Mexico was levying on beverages sweetened with HFCS—a sweetener linked to obesity—but not on those sweetened with cane sugar. Corn Products International argued that Mexico's HFCS tax violated the country's obligation under NAFTA to provide foreign investors with "national treatment." For its part, Mexico argued that the tax was a legitimate counter to US refusals to open American markets to Mexican cane sugar, as stipulated by

NAFTA. It also said that the tax helped safeguard hundreds of thousands of Mexican jobs in the cane sugar industry.

The ISDS tribunal found the agribusiness giant's case more convincing and awarded the company $58.4 million in damages. Soon after, the US multinational Archer Daniels Midland lodged a very similar case with the tribunals, and was awarded $37 million.[35] Then in 2004, Cargill, the largest privately held corporation in the US, rounded out the sugar wars with an even broader challenge to the Mexican government. High-fructose corn syrup, Cargill argued, should be allowed into Mexico not only under "national treatment" obligations, but under a whole raft of claims, including "most favored nation treatment," "expropriation," and "fair and equitable treatment and performance standards." The tribunal again ruled in the corporation's favor, awarding Cargill a sum of $77.3 million—the largest award to that point granted by ISDS under a US free trade agreement.[36]

In part due to such sugar wars, the Mexican diet has been transformed over the last two decades, bringing soaring rates of obesity. Consumption of beans has dropped by half, and fruit and vegetables by nearly one-third. In their place, Mexican consumers now see a cornucopia of HFC-sweetened beverages and processed foods. "Even in the most remote villages," according to the *Guardian,* "little stores sell packaged biscuits, pastries, doughnuts and cakes, and sodas and non-carbonated sweetened drinks. When you're hungry, you can buy a Gansito snack cake and a soda for about a dollar. It's fast and cheap and delicious."[37]

The sweep of the WTO's purview over the food system—from trade liberalization to intellectual property to corporate tribunals—was the reason for the La Vía Campesina slogan "Not agriculture out of the WTO, but the WTO out of agriculture." Simply excising the WTO's Agreement on Agriculture would have struck just one of the many charters against peasants within the WTO apparatus; much better would be to remove the apparatus from all the practices of agriculture it now affects.

La Vía Campesina's battle continues, as we show below. Meanwhile the consequences of a globalization that drives inequality, worker insecurity, and environmental evisceration, and yet presents trade and internationalism as signs of the national interest, have made themselves increasingly clear. Today, the "globalist" architects of multilateral trade agreements find themselves not irrelevant exactly, but making deals on a bilateral rather than multilateral basis. It's not that the fiction of a national interest has abated, nor have capitalist demands for low-wage work, cheap resources, markets, concessions, and exemptions become any less acute. But as the social and environmental costs of free trade have become more visible, and as critics have grown in their voice and power, trade proponents are confronting new challenges trying to shore up the legitimacy of free trade. For the first time in decades, the crises of neoliberalism have tipped the scales; we are seeing a sizable rebalancing of power between globalization and the blocs of proponents and opponents of this kind of hegemony.

MULTIPLE TRAJECTORIES OF TRADE ALTERNATIVES

One trend in seeking to defend the global economic order can be found in reformist tactics. Former chief economist for the World Bank Larry Summers speaks of a "responsible nationalism" to soften the hard edges of globalism: "countries are expected to pursue their citizens' economic welfare as a primary objective but where their ability to harm the interests of citizens elsewhere is circumscribed."[38] Still another trend, more central to agriculture, can be found in paternalistic ideas of "fair trade" as a remedy for poverty in the Global South. Fair trade promises better pay for producers via short value chains and premiums for coffee, bananas, chocolate, and other tasty crops. But there is scant evidence so far that fair-trade labels do much to provide equity or sustainability.[39] What's more, the whole system takes for granted that Latin America, the Caribbean, and other parts of the Global South ought to task themselves in perpetuity with growing our bananas. It doesn't force us to confront how these countries became a US fruit bowl.

Rejecting either of these globalist solutions, both right-wing and left-wing populisms have gathered momentum. One face of this countermovement can be seen in the rise of Trump (US), Le Pen (France), Johnson (UK), Kaczyński (Poland), Babiš (Czech Republic), Modi (India), Erdogan (Turkey), Duterte (Philippines), and other politicians of the "alt-right." Rising to prominence not in spite of, but because of rank displays of nativism, misogyny, bigotry, and xenophobia, their response to globalism can be seen in taking back control from "dangerous and threatening crowds."[40] Proposals include building border walls between the US and Mexico or at the peripheries of the EU; Islamophobic travel restrictions; and blaming wage depression and unemployment (often the upshots of free trade agreements) on a mass of unfairly advantaged Others—be they Mexicans, Muslims, Blacks, Syrians, or Surinamese. The racist thinking that shaped some resistance to the TPP and

NAFTA within the United States was exemplified by Trump's populist appeals. For even if Trump was never honest about ditching free trade, the social power he stirred up in the Heartland was real. Invoking the abominations of outsourced jobs, rural depression, and lost wages, he tapped in to neoliberal dysfunction and hitched the outrage to authoritarian rule.

Yet not all critics of free trade agreements are nativists. In July 2018, Manuel López Obrador, known to most Mexicans as simply "AMLO," won Mexico's presidential election by a comfortable margin. He campaigned on a vow not unlike US president Donald Trump's—to "make rural Mexico great again"—but his impetus had very different roots. Reviving a twenty-first-century manifesto for agrarianism based on Mexican revolutionary Emiliano Zapata's original 1911 Plan de Ayala, AMLO committed to promoting self-sufficiency in key crops by 2024. He pushed back against the fortified NAFTA eagerly sought by his predecessor and by Donald Trump. He made explicit calls for "food sovereignty."

Similarly, when La Vía Campesina formed three decades ago, it was to reject globalization without resorting to tired calls about blood and soil and country first. By providing a vision for food sovereignty based on international solidarity, equality, dignity, and human rights, LVC quickly became the planet's largest organized opposition to free trade. To be sure, LVC has not been immune to the recent chauvinist trends; latent nationalisms have metastasized into Islamophobia seeded by organizations like the Bharatiya Kisan Union (BKU) in India. But as the exigencies of neoliberal crisis have deepened the need to draw a bright line between two rejections of free trade—one based on right-wing atomism and hatred, another based on interdependence and solidarity—food sovereignty movements have strengthened their analyses and deepened their resolve. In particular, by embracing anti-racist, anti-patriarchal, and anti-colonial precepts, they fortify the division between authoritarian rejections of free trade and progressive ones, as these are lines that chauvinists will not cross.

Still, ambitious inclusive visions of equity are not enough. Just as free trade moves from magical thinking into shaping reality through networks of Cargills, Nestlés, and Bayer-Monsantos, through Washington, DC, Wall Street, the World Bank, and the WTO, so too do alternative ideas require actions by organized communities. It is now to farmers in Japan who are undertaking such activities that we turn.

Food Sovereignty in Japan and Beyond

Ayumi Kinezuka and Maywa Montenegro de Wit

FROM TOYOTA TO MITSUBISHI, TOSHIBA TO SONY, Japan is known for its high-tech industry. We, the people of Japan, are also renowned for our food—sushi, teriyaki, and edamame are household words, even in the US— but how many people think of the rice, soybean, and wheat farmers who grow the key ingredients?

We are here to tell you Japanese farmers do indeed exist. In fact, farming makes up an essential part of our unique culture and traditions, which are highly dependent upon local environments unique to our small island country. Most of Japan belongs to a mild and humid climatic zone, but from north to south, the islands also vary greatly in rainfall, temperature, and soil. Over time, Japanese farmers have developed various farming cultures specific to local regions, each of which is based on complex geographical conditions and climates with four distinct seasons.

Unfortunately, during the post–World War II economic boom in Japan, our agriculture faced a great decline. Alongside many developing countries at the time, we received massive imports of surplus US wheat, and new trade policies created dependencies on imported industrial foods. Since the 1980s, neoliberal trade policies have forced small- and medium-scale farmers to compete with large-scale farmers, and have accelerated the import of agricultural products. Even rice, our country's main staple, has not been safe from competition with foreign rice imports. The government points to high GDP numbers as shining evidence of the success of free trade policy. But the darker side is shown in other numbers. Today's food sufficiency rate—a measure of national autonomy in food supply—is dismally low: Japan only grows 38 percent of the food it consumes, while the US grows closer to 80 percent. Now more dependent on imports, Japan is experiencing the erosion of regionally specific traditional cultures, an uptick in health problems linked to imported processed food, and widening income disparities in a country renowned for a strong middle class. Young people from farming communities don't see opportunities at home, so they are moving to urban areas, causing a situation in which there is a lack of agricultural successors in most rural villages. Hourly income of rice farmers has dropped as low as 256 yen (about USD $2.25), which is about one-third of the minimum wage in the country. In sum, Japanese family farming is in crisis—in large part because of an agricultural ministry that promotes free trade policies as "national progress."

One of us (Ayumi) is part of *Nouminren,* a Japanese agrarian movement that is fighting back against these interconnected trends. Nouminren, which means "Family Farmers Movement," was founded in 1989 to promote the autonomous development of Japanese agriculture and make farmers' livelihoods more stable. Importantly, we seek to unite the often-disconnected interest groups in the Japanese food system. Working with Shokkenren (National Coalition of Workers, Farmers, and Consumers for Safe Food and Health), we seek to revitalize the country's agriculture and build solidarity in establishing food sovereignty. Shokkenren was established in 1990 and is comprised of various groups, including farmers, workers, consumers, medical workers, teachers, and small- and medium-sized wholesalers; these groups are often seen as separate "links" in a "food chain." Together, our groups see the possibility of deep connections between various peoples who work in agriculture, food safety, and health. These cross-sectoral alliances represent a strategy for overcoming the crisis in agriculture—in Japan and beyond.

One of our first projects as an organization was to establish the Food Research Lab, an independent food analysis center to address food safety. "Food safety?" you ask. "How does this relate to free trade?" Food safety is indeed one of the biggest issues that Japanese consumers now face.[1] Our liberalized trade system brings enormous amounts of imported agricultural products that reach Japanese ports every day; inspection stations are understaffed and monitoring systems are far from adequate. As a result, food contamination proliferates. For example, residue tests show high amounts of chemicals in spinach, while food poisoning has been caused by methamidophos (a pesticide sold in the US as "Monitor") in frozen processed dumplings, and by expired meat used in fast-food hamburgers.[2] To make matters worse, these incidents are not just limited to items from abroad. Japanese companies, retail chains, and even famous hotels have been caught with contaminated food and products with fraudulent claims of origin. As corporations have increasingly gained control of our agrofood and trade system, the government's regulatory capacities have failed to keep pace.[3]

PEOPLE-CENTERED SCIENCE

Japan joined the WTO in 1996. Many people, including farmers and consumers, feared further degradation of food safety with rising volumes of imports. In response, Nouminren decided to act by building the Food Research Lab, which would collect and provide scientific data on agricultural products. What is special about this laboratory, built in 1996, is that it relies solely on collective, crowdsourced contributions of farmers and consumers; its research develops free from pressures by companies or governments. The lab has assembled data by testing chemical residues in items ranging from school lunch bread, to Chinese herbal medicines, to chopsticks. Our citizen science has had measurable successes: as a result of high chemical loads found in frozen spinach from China, a national food sanitation law was revised and the government introduced something called the "Positive List" system, which in general prohibits the sale of food products containing an excess of health-damaging chemical residues.

The activities of the Food Research Lab have continued to expand, as we have obtained new equipment and tools. In the late 1990s we acquired the ability to analyze genetically modified organisms, and in 2003, to assay heavy metals. In 2011, soon after the nuclear meltdown in Fukushima, we obtained a sodium iodide scintillation detector and a germanium semiconductor detector to measure radioactivity. The lab now functions to inspect many toxicological aspects of imported agricultural products, including radiation, chemical residues, and genetic and metal contamination. In terms of GMOs, the lab closely monitors the growth of wild canola near shipping ports. Japan imports GM canola seeds for oil, and these transgenic seeds can escape shipping containers and take root nearby. Indeed, many samples of wild canola have tested positive for transgenic material. Through these and other actions, Nouminren has succeeded in pressuring the national government to tighten its surveillance and safety measures on imported products, as well as in warning local canola growers of the dangers of genetic contamination.

But even while we have celebrated these successes, government deregulation is relentless. New threats have come in the guise of the Trans-Pacific Partnership (TPP) and the Regional Comprehensive Economic Partnership

(RCEP), two international free trade agreements that Japan is aggressively promoting. For the past five years, to prepare for passage of the TPP, Japanese officials have been carrying out "agricultural reform," restructuring national agriculture to be more globally competitive. This restructuring has further exacerbated existing inequities in agriculture that have been created over several decades, when the ruling Liberal Democratic Party took measures to give more favorable treatment to agribusiness.

A good illustration of these cozy relations between corporations and the state is Keidanren, a business federation composed of about 1,350 Japanese companies, 109 industrial associations, and 47 regional economic groups. The former chairperson of Keidanren—also chairman of Sumimoto Chemical Co. Ltd.—lobbied strongly for passage of the TPP and promoted policies to allow GMOs into the country, with the chemical tie-ins and intellectual property rights of Monsanto. Under pressure from Keidanren and its constituent firms, the government in recent years has been removing trade restrictions, abolishing protections for small food retailers, and changing agrarian policy to allow corporate access to farmland. As a result, Japan has witnessed a major decline in the price of farm products, aging of its farming population, and expansion of abandoned farmland to as much as 398,000 hectares in total (about the size of Rhode Island).

Nouminren rejects these trends, which are turning the soils and agrarian knowledge of Japan into simply an island of extractive possibility for business. This corporate-friendly approach, ushered in and enabled by free trade pacts like TPP, will adversely affect not just farmers but all the people of our country.

As mentioned previously, Shokkenren was founded to provide solutions that link farmers, consumers, workers, and wholesalers. We see this as a critical part of building a stronger movement to oppose the power of neoliberalism. Our work is also premised on the idea of people-centered science. Our experiences have shown us that in the hands of the privileged and powerful, science—whether it be atomic physics or genetic engineering—is often conducted with little concern for human and planetary welfare. But the Food Research Lab, we like to say, "is constituted by and working for people." To this end, both collection and publication of data are public, with the lab working to gather and disseminate information in many ways, such as through websites and newspaper stories.

Politically, this work has led to some interesting developments. For years we have been combining our lab research with on-the-ground policy advocacy. Through our own newspapers and magazines, we have criticized national farm policy, demanding suspension of current "agricultural reform" efforts. We have called for more funding and government resources to restore biodiverse agriculture, and to shore up our sinking food sufficiency rate. These campaigns have started to shift popular thinking in the country, where (thanks to the government's excellent propaganda) many people, especially in cities, assume that "free trade" is the natural progression of Japan's economic development. Greater citizen awareness, in turn, puts more pressure on state officials to respond to our political demands. Specifically, we are asking that the government first remove agriculture from the TPP and other trade agreements to allow the import control of agricultural products. Second, we seek the establishment of a price guarantee system at the level of Europe and the US based on the production costs of major crops. And finally, we seek support for a base of family farming, taking measures to secure diverse successors of farming.

Unfortunately, as this book goes to press, the fate of the TPP remains unknown. As the preceding chapter suggests, civil society movements in countries across Asia, the US, and Latin America are struggling fiercely against the passage of the TPP. Here in Japan, in 2013, roughly four thousand farmers from across the country staged a protest in Tokyo over signs that Prime Minister Abe was about to sign onto the TPP alongside the US and other nations.[4] By 2016, the tides had turned, and TPP had become a political hot potato in the US elections. Opposition to TPP on the Republican side helped usher in President Trump—who quickly withdrew the US from the trade pact. Many people assumed the TPP was dead, but Japan is now at the center of efforts to revive it. In September 2017, at a meeting of the eleven remaining TPP countries, Kazuhisa Shibuya, our government's spokesman on the TPP, told reporters: "I would like to once again emphasize the crucial importance of establishing . . . a free, multilateral trade system based upon high-standard rules in the Asia-Pacific, which really fits the 21st century."[5] Shibuya insisted that he will even try to get the US to join the TPP.

FOOD MOVEMENTS AT A CROSSROADS

These shifts in tides between globalization and nationalism put us at a new crossroads. In the US, Trump-style populist rhetoric promises a return to nationalist policies, which may be better for farmers domestically and abroad—but is tinged with racist and isolationist sentiments.[6] In Japan (and for transnational corporations based in the US and beyond), the globalized pathway appears to have no race, no borders, no problems with mixing all foods and peoples together. But it inevitably crushes local cultures, economies, heritages, and worldviews unless they provide the profits required by big business.

The concept of food sovereignty suggests there is another pathway. Nouminren joined the international peasant movement, La Vía Campesina, in 2005, after working for several years at the national level. Throughout this text, I have used the word "food sufficiency," meaning "the extent to which a country can satisfy its food needs from its own domestic production."[7] But food sovereignty goes far beyond this concept, asking how food is produced, by whom, and according to whose decision-making and rights. As defined by La Vía Campesina, "Food sovereignty is the right of peoples, communities and countries to define their own agricultural, labor, fishing, food and land policies, which are ecologically, socially, economically and culturally appropriate to their particular circumstances."[8]

According to this philosophy, food sovereignty combines concepts of *territorial sovereignty,* which is a holistic notion of the land as a whole, including not just arable land, but the cultures and ecosystems with which farmlands are interconnected, and *people's sovereignty,* which gives people the rights to determine their own food and agricultural policies.[9]

The history of food sovereignty is deeply tied to trade. The first instances of "soberanía alimentaria" can be traced back to a 1980s Mexican government program responding to the country's growing dependency on foreign capital and imported basic foods.[10] In the 1990s, as the Global Agreement on Trade and Tariffs (now the WTO) moved to incorporate agriculture into global trade negotiations, leaders of peasant-based organizations around the world pushed back. At a 1996 meeting in Tlaxcala, Mexico, organized as La Vía Campesina, activists presented "food sovereignty" in sharp defiance of GATT trade strategies that treated food like so much surplus, dumping excess grain across foreign borders and undermining peasant livelihoods globally.[11]

Today, La Vía Campesina continues to invoke food sovereignty as a radical alternative to communities' widespread loss of control over food markets, environments, land, and rural cultures. Importantly, food sovereignty does not deny trade. Rather, it promotes the establishment and practice of trade policy for the sustainable production of safe, healthy, and earth-friendly food. International trade, moreover, should not be given prominence over trade among communities and districts within a country. Trade policy can be used to support, rather than undermine, smallholders who produce food for local consumption using sustainable practices. This means limiting global trade to certain conditions, such as a period of unstable food production in a certain region or season, trade of particular products grown only in certain regions of the world, or trade of goods with special quality. However, trade policies at all levels must respect the people's right to food sovereignty and decision-making power.

Nouminren is now seeking to develop a model of food sovereignty that is appropriate to Japanese contexts. For example, in an effort to counteract corporate control of food and agriculture, the direct marketing system known as *sanchoku* or *teikei,* was built upon existing networks between producers and consumers. Under this system, suitable crops are selected to grow in particular environments to produce safe farm products with less dependence on agrochemicals. Direct shops, local produce sections at supermarkets, school lunch programs, processed farm products, and farm-to-table restaurants are some of the many activities supported by Nouminren farmers. In many of these cases, women play a major role in creating diversity within the program, which further contributes to the region's sustainable production and revitalization.

Indeed, the issue of gender equity is still a big challenge for Nouminren, just as it is for many other organizations in Japan and around the world. Often, the problems Japanese women face on a day-to-day basis are considered too personal or insignificant to be brought into the public sphere. Many women bear the burdens of both farmwork and domestic work, frequently combined with care for family elders. Moreover, both physical and mental domestic violence is invisible—"behind the closed door," as women do not, or cannot, speak out. To help counter these trends, Nouminren women have created their own division within the organization. Ensuring a safe place for female farmers to meet and discuss their concerns, the Nouminren women's division emphasizes the importance of building spaces of solidarity between women—where they can speak out freely about their personal and domestic issues—and educational trainings that put the violations women suffer in a larger social framework. Rural women have long distanced themselves from political issues, often hiding behind the excuse of lack of time. But in offering more solidarity, and more influence in politics, Nouminren women hold up the idea of *making* time—or rather, being in time—for social reform through collective action.

This issue of solidarity brings us back to some recent questions surrounding nationalism and sovereignty. President Trump has been much in the international news for promoting "sovereignty" lately. At the UN, he appeared at the podium invoking sovereignty more than twenty-one times, using it to invoke American exceptionalism. "I will always put America first," President Trump said. "Just like you, as the leaders of your countries, will always and should always put your countries first."[12] In Trump-world, the idea is that the US can invoke the sovereignties that it likes and denounce those it doesn't like. It comes from a narrow domestic prism in which some countries and their peoples become "evil" or "terrorists," and others become "good guys." It allows for the selective imposition of US policies, and intervention in democratic processes in countries whose leaders are summarily denounced as "dictators." It even—very terrifyingly for those of us in Japan—leads to saber-rattling of the sort recently seen on the peninsula, where to protect US sovereignty, Trump said, "we will have no choice but to totally destroy North Korea."

This is not the sovereignty supported or invoked by La Vía Campesina, nor the sovereignty that makes sense for Nouminren and its family farmers. Confronting the toxicity of nationalism and patriarchy can even begin in our own ranks, as La Vía Campesina is showing with the 2017 Euskal Declaration, which emerged from their VII International Conference in Basque Country, and states: "Patriarchy is an enemy of our movement. The feminist character of La Vía Campesina strengthens our unity and commitment to the struggle, with equality and gender equity."[13] So, while it would be tempting to say that we support simply the "opposite" of Trump's sovereignty—which mixes individualism, racism, nationalism, and American exceptionalism—the truth is, food sovereignty is far more complicated than that. As I mentioned earlier, Nouminren was founded in the late 1980s to promote an "autonomous" farming movement. We *do* seek independence from corporations, as well as freedom from nation-states that would like to squeeze out not just Japanese smallholders, but Japanese agricultural activities altogether.[14] We seek to restore our nation's relative self-sufficiency and independence in agriculture. These goals are autonomous insofar as they reject the culture of dependency fostered by long histories of imperialism, foreign development projects, and free trade.

At the same time, we seek solidarity with allies who share a common vision of human rights, environmental rights, peace, and democracy. So, autonomy does not mean isolationism or autarky for us. It means fighting against oppressive relationships while also nurturing egalitarian ties to one another and to the Earth. We can reject the extractive relationships with corporations and government elites—abroad and at home—that exploit our country, impoverish our farmers, and make our eaters sick. We can simultaneously practice independence from those who do not share equitably while expressing *inter*dependence with those who do. These values draw in part from the idea of "the time being," which comes from Zen master Dogen Zenji, who wrote nearly eight hundred years ago in a book entitled *Shobogenzo:*

> Do not think that time simply flies away. Do not understand "flying" as the only function of time. If time simply flew away, a separation would exist between you and time. So if you understand time as only passing, then you do not understand the time being. To grasp this truly, every being that exists in the entire world is linked together as moments in time, and at the same time they exist as individual moments of time. Because all moments are the time being, they are your time being.

For many Japanese, time and memory are profoundly important to a sense of being. Each of us is a *time being*. So too is nature. A gingko tree, as described by Japanese American author Ruth Ozeki, is a time being: "Leaves are shaped like little green fans, and in the autumn they turn bright yellow and fall off and cover the ground, painting everything pure golden."[15] And whales are time beings, with lifespans of more than a century, who survive and live and presumably have long memories.

Agriculture itself is a time being. The farmer connects her morning times and night times, her work times and resting times, to the rhythms of nature: animal and crop life cycles, rainfall patterns, seasons with their own peculiar times of lightness and dark, cold and warmth. Some of these seem permanent, but in many ways the whole world is fleeting, because all things—including bees and crops and microbes and rice and mountains, and even you and me—are just "flowing through for the time being."[16]

This means that social movements—and even corporations—are time beings too. Corporations survive by generating wealth from time—the laboring time of their workers. Movements survive by effecting change in dominant systems, sometimes rapidly and sometimes over long periods of struggle. Whatever we do now should keep these different paces and processes in mind. Our Food Research Lab will not upend the colossal power of Monsanto-Bayer or the WTO overnight. But we would be foolish to mistake speed with movement, as Dogen Zenji might say. Nouminren stands in solidarity with time beings around the world who envision another way of doing things: growing food in harmony with ecosystems, sharing the rights and responsibilities associated with keeping food systems safe, and trading not in order to achieve power over others, but to share the fruits of our labor and land.

Conclusion

STAND UP, BITE BACK

Saru Jayaraman and Kathryn De Master

TARGETING CORPORATE INFLUENCE in the food system—given its breadth, scope, and diversity—entails implementing an extraordinarily diverse array of strategies, from traditional organizing efforts to new and emerging forms of collective action.

Traditional organizing efforts include ways that food workers, organized by a myriad of organizations—from Restaurant Opportunities Centers United to the Fight for $15 to OUR Walmart to the Coalition of Immokalee Workers—are confronting corporate power through direct actions, litigation, research and communications efforts, and policy advocacy. Many of the stories in this book describe traditional organizing efforts.

To pass a statewide ban on fracking in New York, for example, Food and Water Watch was part of a large coalition of organizations that organized hundreds of thousands of residents of New York State to attend "community meetings, public hearings, film screenings, rallies, and protest marches." They also submitted hundreds of thousands of public comments, wrote letters to editors, called elected officials, and more. Corporate Accountability similarly has worked with organizations of affected individuals alongside health experts, good government groups, and corporate watchdog organizations to directly confront McDonald's in shareholder meetings, in the media, and with legislative policy efforts. And finally, the United Food and Commercial Workers Union organized their own members alongside other community and labor organizations in California to win several landmark bills that address poverty and food insecurity, demonstrating the greatest political power of any food justice organization in this book.

All of these efforts involve the key element of community organizing and social movement activity as defined by the vast literature on social movements—mobilizing a base of directly affected individuals to engage in contentious direct action, including protests that target those with power over their lives for concrete improvements in the food system and in people's lives.[1]

In addition to traditional organizing campaigns, some of the efforts described in this book have utilized new and emerging forms of collective action that do not directly fit traditional models for community organizing. Farmers organizing through the Organic Seed Alliance and the Open Source Seed Initiative, for example, are acting collectively to resist corporate control of seeds through public plant breeding and noncorporatized seed production. This represents an emerging form of organized collective resistance. Similarly, the Pesticide Action Network's (PAN) Drift Catcher program represents an innovative model of community-based participatory action research. PAN supports communities that are engaged in citizen science, employing the Drift Catcher monitoring device to collect data on pesticide drift. PAN then analyzes the data and assists community members who use this data to press for pesticide policy change by sharing it with the media and in public fora. In Japan, a collective response to the corporate-driven injustices of current trade regimes includes ways that farmers have worked to build community around principles of food sovereignty.

All of these forms of collective action are essential. Farmer-driven seed production and community-driven research and citizen science are critical foundations for balancing the power between corporations and people. The groups engaged in traditional organizing described in the book also rely on participatory research and alternative means of production as elements of a campaign. For Corporate Accountability, exposing information on McDonald's predatory marketing, health impacts, and undue government influence have all been critical to building the foundation for mobilization. But more change is needed. Kiki Hubbard of the Organic Seed Alliance, for example, argues that greater public outcry is ultimately needed, including direct action to fight for greater antitrust regulation in the seed industry. Some of this is already happening—Hubbard notes that several hundred people have attended antitrust hearings and eighteen thousand people have submitted public comments on the need for greater antitrust regulation— but far more is necessary to push back on the powerful corporate forces that control antitrust regulation at present. And since PAN focuses more on community-driven data collection than on training communities to organize and mobilize with that data, many communities could use greater support for direct organizing to use the data collected by the innovative Drift Catcher program to advocate for policy change. Even the groups engaged in traditional organizing profiled in this book would say that more support for organizing—more mobilization of affected peoples to engage in direct action to confront corporate power—is needed for them to win as well. Regardless of the form of work currently undertaken, it is clear that more collective direct action by affected peoples is needed on every issue in the food system.

Ultimately, the only way to change the power imbalance between people and corporations is for the largest number of people possible to directly demand that change. No amount of data alone will be as threatening to a corporation as large groups of people who are directly affected by that corporation's actions taking that science to the corporation's doors, or to elected officials who are being influenced by corporations, and demanding change. As Wenonah Hauter and Seth Gladstone note in their piece on winning the fracking ban in New York, the most important element in that campaign were the hundreds of people who "came out at every possible opportunity to Governor Cuomo's public and private events in an attempt to engage directly with the governor and make their opposition to fracking known to him. He simply could not appear in public without encountering dozens, hundreds, or even thousands of loud, animated 'fractivists' holding ban-fracking signs and shouting ban-fracking chants."

Although conscientious consumer behavior might succeed at getting a corporation to shift its marketing or products, this will not fundamentally alter the power that corporation has over our democracy. For example, while Walmart has added an "Organics" section as a result of perceived consumer demand, the corporation benefits from this niche market while further diluting the concept. To change the way in which Walmart pays its workers, or treats farmers in its supply chain, or to demand equal voice between people and corporations in defining organics, will require far more than consumers shopping differently. It will require Walmart workers, consumers, and the general public to mobilize in a myriad of ways to demand change, since, in the immortal words of Frederick Douglass, "Power concedes nothing without a demand."

The diverse campaigns described in this book largely adhere to core social movement organizing principles: they involve or directly inform collective efforts by the people who are the most affected, and they engage in direct, contentious action that targets corporate powers to win concrete, transformative change in people's lives. However, given the complexity and diversity of food issues, we realize that simply providing examples of campaigns that follow these principles will not be sufficient to inspire more such activity across the food system. Far more organizing is necessary to win a greater balance of power between people and corporations. For this reason, we are offering, in tandem with this book and in partnership with the Midwest Academy, a new Community Organizing Training Program, offered to all those interested in food justice. In this conclusion, we provide some of the key practical tools and skills that will be offered through this new training program.

Community organizing, as defined here, is not new. For centuries, oppressed peoples have engaged in collective action all over the world. Over the last century, theoreticians such as Paolo Frere, Saul Alinsky, and more recently, Marshall Ganz and Theda Skocpol, have codified this collective action into widely respected skills and tools used by both the left and the right ends of the political spectrum. Schools and institutes such as the Highlander Academy and the Midwest Academy have been providing training on this definition of collective action for decades. However, with notable exceptions, this highly effective and well-established community organizing practice and social movement activity has been largely absent from most food justice work. It is time for food justice work to utilize the tools and skills of this trade.

We review the principles of community organizing and social movement activity here:

First, we argue that effective community organizing involves collective action by those who are most affected. It requires people—often those with limited means—being willing to stand up, have their voices heard, and take risks by collectively pushing back against powerful elites. An individual writing, speaking, or advocating *on behalf* of many others may be doing laudable work, but we argue that this is not community organizing. Similarly, advocates engaged in coalition efforts to change policy or reform regulations, without bases of people actually engaging in collective direct action themselves, are also not engaged in community organizing. We argue that collective action by people who are the most affected by corporate actions is the way to counterbalance the power of corporate elites. Advocates acting independently, without bases of people willing to act, will lack the collective authority needed to combat corporate power successfully over time.

Second, successful community organizing requires direct and often contentious action targeting those in power. By this definition, laudable initiatives that train young people to grow urban gardens, or teach consumers how to eat and shop differently, or partner with corporations to improve their sustainability practices, are not engaged in community organizing activities. None of these activities directly confront and combat corporate power. As the many examples in this book highlight, directly contending with powerful corporate elites is necessary to achieve transformative structural change, rather than marginal shifts in practices.

Third, community organizing aims to win transformative, concrete, and measurable improvements in the lives of people. Higher wages and better workplace benefits, for example, represent such a tangible improvement. Achieving seed sovereignty for small-scale farmers is a concrete benefit. Protecting a state's drinking water from fracking pollutants is also a measurable and significant achievement. These changes are most often won through legislative policy change, or sometimes through corporate policy change, driven by community organizing. Achieving concrete improvements is only transformative and lasting when codified in policy change. Books, training centers, schools, and academic fields have been built around this specific definition of organizing. This school of thought provides concrete strategies and actions that advocates, activists, scholars, and communities can employ to address corporate power over our food system.

Ultimately, an organizing vision for a new food democracy must include a diverse coalition of affected peoples targeting corporate power collectively, with a unified set of demands. Some of this activity is already beginning to take shape, but much more is needed, sustained over longer periods of time, to achieve transformative change. For this reason, as we have worked to document the success stories in this book, we have simultaneously collaborated with the Midwest Academy and Food and Water Watch to create and launch a new organizing training program specifically for advocates interested in food systems change. We seek to increase the amount of organizing happening to combat the undue influence of corporations, and fight for equity, sustainability, and collective prosperity.

The skills and tools offered here, and in greater depth by the Midwest Academy and other organizing training programs, are essential to combat corporate control of our food system. Judy Hertz, executive director of the Midwest Academy, offers us some the basic elements of that training program in "Afterword: Taking Action to Create Change." We hope these elements will serve as an inspiration to join us in spreading organizing skills and resources among the many organizations and activists who seek to change the food system.

Fundamentally, the reason that corporations control so much of our food system is their unbridled, unregulated, unchecked power over our democracy. To balance this unbridled power requires the collective power of affected people demanding that their voices be heard. Considering the drastic climate change on the horizon, combined with widespread environmental pollution, public health crises, and the greatest levels of income inequality in the US since the Gilded Age, we have no choice but to act. Indeed, the question cannot be *whether* we act, but *how* we deploy community organizing resources and skills to power a food rebellion and *bite back*.

Afterword

TAKING ACTION TO CREATE CHANGE

Judy Hertz

BY THIS POINT, YOU WILL HAVE REALIZED that we need to change the underlying structures of our food system in order to bring about the changes we are seeking. We are pitting ourselves against serious corporate power structures and the public policies that support them.

The stories in this book illustrate some of the issue campaigns that organizations have conducted to fight for change—organized efforts to change particular public or corporate policies.

Are you ready to take action?

You may have read this far in the book and become a bit daunted by the task. Individual, local actions—while useful—are usually not enough by themselves to change the behavior of large corporations.

Here, you will find a system for analyzing power and putting together an effective issue campaign.

We know that if we all work together, we can create a better food system, because people just like us have brought about similar transformations.

The next time you are sitting in a coffee shop, or a college classroom, at the airport or the Department of Motor Vehicles, take a look around. Is the air filled with smoke? Are half the people in the room smoking cigarettes?

No, they are not. Second-hand smoke causes cancer, and we have clean indoor air laws in the United States that prohibit smoking indoors in most public places. The lives of millions of people have been saved because they were not forced to breathe second-hand smoke, which is a known carcinogen.

This didn't just happen. We all owe a huge debt of thanks to the community organizers and public health workers and the organizations they work for that fought for years to get these laws passed. They achieved heroic victories, but they started out just the way we are, and did years of strategic issue campaigns to change public and corporate policies.

These organizers used some of the tools discussed here.

THE MIDWEST ACADEMY STRATEGY CHART: A TOOL FOR ANALYSIS

At the Midwest Academy, we teach organizers a tool called the *strategy chart,* which helps to put all the pieces of an issue campaign together. The chart takes you through a series of questions that form a deeper analysis of the power you will need to win the change you are seeking.

As you can see from the strategy chart diagram in figure 5, there are five columns:

Column 1, Goals, helps you define what you want to win.

Column 2, Organizational Considerations, helps you assess your own power and that of your organization, and think about how you are going to build it.

Column 3, Constituency and Allies, gives you a place to make a list of people and organizations you need to recruit, because they have some power to move the decision-makers.

Column 3, Decision-Maker, is the place to start the analysis of what it will take to get the person in power to say yes to you.

Column 5, Tactics, is a list of the ways that you are going to show off your power (what you have in columns 2 and 3) to the decision-maker. Tactics include all the actions you typically think of community organizations doing—from writing letters and making phone calls to big public meetings and sit-ins.

As you read this chapter, we hope that you will see why tactics only make sense once you have done the rest of the strategy chart analysis. That is how you will determine what is it going to take to get the person with the authority (a corporate CEO or a number of legislative representatives, for example) to make the decision that you want.

Goals	Organizational Considerations	Constituency and Allies	Decision-Maker	Tactics
Long-term What you really want. Example: Fair and livable wages for all workers in state! **Intermediate** What you are trying to win now. Example: $15 state minimum-wage law. **Short-term** A step to the intermediate goal. Example: Get Rep. Smith to vote yes. *Goals are always concrete improvements in people's lives!*	**What resources can you put in now?** • Number of people? • Social media lists? • How much time? • Meeting space, copiers, etc.? • Money? *Use numbers. Be specific!* **How will you build your organization?** • How many new members? • Money to raise? • New leaders? • Public recognition *How much? How many? Be specific!* **Internal problems?** • How to solve/reduce.	**Who cares about the issue?** • Whose problem is it most directly? • What power do they have over the decision-maker? • Who else will be an ally on this issue? • How are they organized; where can you find them? • What risks are they taking? What might they gain? *How many? Be specific!* **Opponents?** What will opponents do? Can you divide them or reduce their influence?	**The person who has the power to give you what you want** • Elected or appointed or corporate? • Do you have electoral or consumer power? • Analyze your potential power over them very concretely so that you can use it strategically! • Are there real consequences for the decision-maker if they say no? *Always a person with a name, not an institution!*	**How you will show power to the decision-maker so s/he will say yes to the goals?** **1. Show power directly to the decision-maker** • Letter writing • Petitions • Phone calling • Social media tactics • Group visits to decision-makers • Media events • Rallies • Actions • Public forums • Strategic civil disobedience • Be creative! **2. Public education and organization building** • Teach-ins • Media events, etc. • Social media • Rallies/banners

© Midwest Academy 2018   www.midwestacademy.com   312-427-2304

FIGURE 5. The Midwest Academy Strategy Chart. Source: Midwest Academy.

A WORD ABOUT POWER

Before we start the strategy chart, let's step back for a moment and think about why decision-makers make the decisions that they do.

It would be nice to think that they carefully evaluate the facts, and make a rational choice.

We would also like to think that decision-makers listen to the stories and experiences of their constituents, customers, and workers.

And, of course, there are many good elected officials and corporate executives who do just that.

If you can win by presenting facts and telling stories, please do so.

Unfortunately, most of the world is far more complicated. For example, even though the vast majority of scientists agree that human activity is causing global warming, we are nowhere near taking the action as a country that is needed to slow the process.

Moving away from fossil fuels would cost oil company executives their jobs; would cost shareholders their investment; and would cost oil workers their source of employment. Oil companies have given donations to many elected officials to win their support.

Of course, in the longer term, there are plenty of jobs in green energy, and profits, too. But it can be difficult to get these decision-makers to think about the long term, which is much more unknown and insecure than the present.

This makes it difficult for CEOs and elected officials to hear the facts about global warming, and to see the stories they are told as more than individual sad cases.

The same is true in the food industry. The changes we are asking for—living wage jobs, food without dangerous additives, viable family farms—are structural changes that would harm the short-term profits and diminish the power of multinational corporations.

So we must be prepared to analyze and build real power within our campaigns for change, and not just expect the food industry and elected officials to be persuaded that we are right.

Being right is not enough.

The Midwest Academy strategy chart is about building real power to fight for change, when we are up against serious power on the other side.

COLUMN 1: GOALS

What Do You Want to Win? Problems versus Issues

When we first start thinking about something that makes us mad, we are often thinking about a problem—a broad area of concern.

Children eating too much sugar in their diets is a problem. Pesticides making agricultural workers sick, killing beneficial insects and butterflies, and poisoning our food is a problem.

In order to tackle any of these problems, we generally need to break them down into smaller issues. An *issue is the solution or partial solution* that we might work for, small and specific enough that we can write a public or corporate policy to address it.

Clear labeling of food packages so that mothers can easily see how much sugar is in their children's cereal is an issue. Ending the subminimum wage for tipped workers, either locally or nationally, is an issue.

You know you've turned a problem into an issue when you can name the person or people who have the power to pass a law or policy to make it happen: the secretary of the US Department of Agriculture can require better food labeling, and members of your state legislature or Congress can vote for a higher minimum wage.

Now, any problem area will have many possible issues that could address it. To reduce sugar in kids' diets, we could improve food labels; limit the amount of added sugar that is permitted; tax the sales of sugared drinks; regulate school lunches; and many more possibilities.

So your first step generally is to make a long list of possible solutions to the problem before you start to consider which issue is the best one to start with.

It is important to remember that even when the problem—childhood obesity and diabetes, in our example—is slapping you in the face, you still have to choose your best approach, which solution to work for first. The most obvious solution is not always the best choice.

Choosing which issue to work on is a combination of art and science. You are looking for something that you can win, and that you can build a group of enthusiastic activists around—hopefully, an organization!

Here are some questions to help you get started.

Is there momentum right now around a particular issue that you can build on? If the wind is in your sails because this issue has just been won in five other localities, that can be a good reason to take on an issue.

Are there other people who want to work on this issue with you? Is there an organization to support or help build? Having an enthusiastic group to work with is important.

Which issues match your overall capacity? If you want to end lower wages for tipped workers, do you have the resources to address this at the national level? Or is your organization more local, in which case you may be looking at a city ordinance?

Can you name the decision-maker? What do you know about them? Would they support or oppose you? If oppose, why and how much? What would it take to get them to say yes?

How much power are you going up against, and do you have enough power on your side to get the decision-maker to yes? Are you just asking for more information to be made available? Are you directly cutting corporate profits?

Moving from a problem to an issue is the beginning of strategic analysis. Of course, you will have both long-term and more immediate goals, and it is very important to keep both in mind.

Your long-term goal might be dignity and a living wage for food service workers. Your intermediate goal could be ending the tipped minimum wage in your state. The short-term goal could be getting a particular state representative to vote yes.

Before you totally settle on your issue, you will want to review the rest of your strategy chart. The five columns work together. How large an issue you can win will obviously be impacted by how much power you have (columns 2 and 3) in relation to the power of the decision-maker (column 4). So, you will be going back and forth as you do the chart.

COLUMN 2: ORGANIZATIONAL CONSIDERATIONS

The Overall Importance of Organizations

The media just loves it when one angry mom single-handedly defeats a big corporation. She's a hero and a saint, and a great representation of all that is right with America.

However, that's not usually how change happens.

Big corporations have enormous public relations and marketing budgets. They have staffs of lobbyists and fleets of attorneys. They have massive lobbying budgets and advertising that reaches millions of people, with a message that may be totally misleading.

As organizers and activists, we will never be able to match the amount of money that corporations spend. But we need to match and surpass their ability to reach large numbers of people and get them to take organized and strategic action.

Sometimes, this happens spontaneously. The news reports that something bad happened, there's negative publicity, people are angry and speak out, and a change gets made. This is most likely when the fix is easy, not too expensive, and doesn't require structural changes to the way food is produced.

More frequently, there's a great deal of tsk-tsking, and then everything just keeps going along the way it was.

Making real policy changes almost always requires long-term persistence, a significant activist presence in multiple locations, and growing numbers of people speaking up. For that, you generally need organizational infrastructure.

Whether you have an organization or not, column 2 asks you to list your current resources. How many people do you have? Are they hard-core activist leaders, or people you can call on now and then to write a letter or make a phone call?

How much money do you have? Can you afford to print flyers? Can you pay for a website? Is there money for buses to the state capital, if that's what you need? What else will you need to spend money on?

Do you have a public presence—a Facebook page with lots of followers, a big email list, phone lists, regular media coverage?

Organizations can build a presence, and create lists and develop leadership, especially if they are systematic about it. Ideally, working in an organization, as opposed to just an informal group, provides the structure to persist and grow that is needed if we are going to restructure a whole sector of our economy.

The best organizations plan for continual growth, so that each new round of issue work helps create more activists, with more reach in more places. This is more likely to happen if you plan for it in advance.

It is best to be very honest as you think about your current and future resources! Lack of clarity here can lead to burning out your staff and volunteers by expecting them to do more than is humanly possible.

COLUMN 3: CONSTITUENCY AND ALLIES

You and Who Else: How Much Power Can You Build?

Now it is time to make as long a list as you can of who shares your concern about the change you are trying to make.

Who is directly impacted by this problem, or will benefit from your proposed solution?

Who may not be directly impacted, but cares about the people who are?

Your aim is to make a big list of potential supporters, and then start to talk to them, and see who can be recruited to take action.

Of course, you are not just looking for anybody. A key question to answer first is, who does the decision-maker care about, and why? As you consider this question, you will be back and forth with your analysis in column 4. We'll say more about that in the next section.

If you can find people wholesale rather than retail, it will help you grow your effort bigger, faster. By wholesale, we mean already organized somehow.

Imagine standing on a street corner looking for parents of young children who eat sugared cereal. Now imagine that you can address a PTA meeting at your local elementary school. That is what we mean by retail versus wholesale.

At the PTA, if you are lucky, you can build a relationship with the president, and recruit her for your effort. Then when you need people to write letters, for example, you can ask her to have PTA members from her school write letters at the monthly meeting.

Other places to find people already organized into groups include religious congregations, labor unions, civic associations, professional organizations and social service agencies. The list is only limited by your imagination.

Expanding your constituencies and allies is the key to building real power. Remember, we are doing this organizing because we have realized that being right is not enough. We need to be able to make a credible electoral challenge or a believable profit-cutting threat, or show someone that their current path will damage their reputation in a meaningful way. To do this on a large scale, we have to go beyond the usual band of committed activists and demonstrate that a significant number of people are very concerned.

COLUMN 4: DECISION-MAKER

Who Needs to Say Yes, and What Will It Take to Get There?

For any change that you are trying to make, you need to know who has the ultimate power to say yes and make it happen.

Does it require a new law? Then you are looking at a legislative body of some kind—local, state, or national. Issue campaigns are won by changing the votes of individual representatives, so it is important to name names. Find the representatives who are most likely to support you. They can help identify the ones who will be most opposed, and those who are potentially moveable. This last group, the swing votes, are the people you will need to develop strategy charts and issue campaigns around.

Are you working to change a corporate policy? Then you are ultimately targeting the CEO.

You may start with a friendly conversation, to determine whether this person is someone who will be persuaded by facts and reason, and stories about the negative impact of the status quo.

You may get information from, and build a relationship with, people at a lower level—department heads and legislative assistants.

But remember that these people are hired to carry out the wishes of their boss. Often, the biggest wish of their boss is that people like you never come near them! Don't let yourself be stalled endlessly by people whose main job is to keep you busy and away from the boss. They may do this rudely, or with a show of kindness, but be prepared to note when slowdown tactics are being used against you, and don't be afraid to go right to the person with the actual power to say yes.

If you don't get to yes merely with a reasonable ask, you will need to do a full power analysis.

The key question is, what is the relationship of your power to the power of the decision-maker? By "your power," we mean you and your organization and all the constituents and allies you can recruit (column 3).

If the decision-maker is elected, can you organize voters in their district to vote them out of office? A credible threat to do just that has opened the minds of many elected officials. Of course, you can also frame this positively, if it makes sense in the situation: you will make clear what a champion they are if they do the right thing, and it will help them electorally.

If the decision-maker is a corporate CEO, can you organize enough customers to cut the company's profits significantly? You may make it clear that you believe their actions are despicable, but as long as they can continue to make a profit, they aren't likely to change. Framed more positively, what is the advantage to their bottom line if they do change?

Both corporate CEOs and elected officials are often looking toward their next, higher position. Can you create the kind of public awareness that will make them appear to be a bad choice for higher office or a different corporation? Or make them appear to be the hero of the hour, and an excellent choice for promotion?

Perhaps this sounds unkind or even rude to you. If so, please take a moment to contemplate how rude it is for millions of American children to get diabetes because their diets include so much added sugar. Or how impolite it is that waitstaff must often accept sexual harassment from customers in order to earn enough money to support themselves and their families. Or that farmworkers are routinely exposed to dangerous chemicals in the fields.

Challenging the status quo almost always seems rude to someone who is being asked to make a significant change. But the status quo itself is causing great hardship to many people, whose main failing is that they don't have enough money to buy their way out of their current situation.

We've been trained to shake our heads sadly at the inevitability of suffering for many people, or even to believe that it is somehow their own fault. But heaven forbid that we would fail to say please and thank you! Let's broaden our definition of what is rude and unacceptable.

This is a good place to note that all of the activities we are discussing here can be carried out politely, if you so choose. We differentiate between power and tone. If you have a very large number of voters who are prepared to switch to a different candidate, you do not have to shout at the incumbent when you ask her to change her position on a particular piece of legislation. You only need to calmly let her know exactly what your request is, and how many people are prepared to act with you.

Shouting rarely makes you more persuasive. Shouting is tone; the numbers of people who will vote or purchase differently is power.

However, sometimes people are very angry because they feel they have been taken advantage of, and they want to say so loudly and clearly when they have the opportunity. Sometimes, it is useful to be satiric or mocking. Tone is something that you need to discuss as a group, and make a choice about. The people who are taking action together should feel comfortable with the tone that is chosen. Just remember that tone is not the same as power.

Decision-makers would always prefer that you be polite. They would also always rather meet with only one or two people. They would prefer that you not present power. Remember, they are trying to keep you from winning.

Power analysis sounds complicated, and we're not going to tell you it's simple. But it is also not rocket science. You can find the facts that you need if you dig around. The internet is a terrific resource. You can also talk to people who have experience in the area.

Here are some of the kinds of questions you want to answer.

For an elected official:

What were the results of the last few elections? Is the person getting more or less popular?

Who lives in the official's district? How are these people impacted by the problem you are trying to change? Are some of them already members of your organization? Who can you recruit?

How has the person voted on similar issues in the past? What is the person's voting record? What have they said publicly that can be used— promises or goals stated?

For a corporate CEO:

Do they sell their products or services to the general public, or to other businesses? You will have much more chance of success if they sell to the public. What is your relationship (or what can you build) with the people who buy from this corporation?

Is this a profitable sector? Is it competitive? If margins are thin, or there is competition for market share, the CEO may be more vulnerable. For example, when customers rebelled against Bank of America's effort to impose a $5 monthly ATM fee, the corporation reacted quickly because banking is very competitive, there is very little brand loyalty (it doesn't matter to me if my money is in Chase Bank instead of Bank of America), and they did not want to lose market share.

Is there significant brand loyalty? If you can hurt their reputation, will it matter to their bottom line? Think how much more difficult it would be to get people to change from McDonald's to Burger King, than from Bank of America to Chase.

Do they have a reputation for being ecologically concerned, or treating their workers well? They will want to keep this good image, and that makes them vulnerable.

For all kinds of decision-makers, what are their personal vulnerabilities?

Is there a scandal brewing, and therefore any bad publicity will be multiplied? (You may not even need to mention the scandal; the decision-maker may just be more motivated.)

Do they have ambition for higher office, or to run a bigger corporation—and therefore if you make them look like they aren't doing a good job where they are, it may hurt them?

In general, what you are looking for in your analysis is the answer to the question, What is it that we can do that will be seen as so bad by the decision-maker that they will change their position on this issue in order to get us to stop? Or more positively, what incentive can we give them to agree with us?

Always try to look at the question from the decision-maker's particular point of view. Look at how are they actually evaluating what you are doing, not how would you be feeling if you were them. Try to avoid wishful thinking or imagining that you will win merely by persuading them that you are right.

COLUMN 5: TACTICS

What the Constituents and Allies Do to the Decision-Maker to Get Them to Say Yes

Tactics are what most people associate with organizing: letters, phone calls, office visits, picketing, town hall meetings, sit-ins, and so on.

The analysis in the first four columns of the strategy chart should enable you to design much more effective tactics, because you will have answered some key questions.

What will it take to get the decision-maker to say yes? Can we threaten their reelection or their profits? Can we threaten them with regulation that would be worse than just saying yes to us now? Can we make them look like heroes and boost their chance to get that new job they are hoping for?

Who needs to be carrying out the tactics so that the decision-maker will take us seriously?

All too often, we approach an elected official with people who do not even live in their district, or people who live in their district but would never, ever consider voting for them, even if they do what we are asking. Thus, we pose no real threat to the politician, and we are basically trying to persuade them with facts and stories.

Similarly, we may approach a corporation with requests, but not be able to disrupt the status quo of their profits. Yes, we're annoying, but usually we go away after a while.

Digging in on the power analysis requires some serious work up front, but it enables us to be taken seriously when we mobilize our constituents to communicate their wishes to the decision-makers.

Which tactics you choose is less important than the substance of the power (number of voters, number of potential customers, etc.) that is shown through the tactic.

Everything you have heard about handwritten letters being better than form letters is true. Addresses are essential so that elected officials can tell that the people who are communicating are in their district. Similarly, people who are customers should say so. The numbers that you have to amass depend on what has happened before: a thousand people is often insignificant in Chicago, but even twenty-five is a big number in Pierre, South Dakota. A multinational corporation may be less worried about a boycott in the US if their profits are large overseas.

The best tactics show power directly, and are fun—or at least satisfying—for the people who are carrying them out, but surprising to the decision-makers. A national organization once sent delegations to take over dozens of local mortgage offices, and to ask the managers to fax a letter to corporate headquarters. Imagine being the CEO's thoughts as letters flowed in from across the country!

HOW TO FIND OUT MORE

Obviously, we've just scratched the surface here.

The Midwest Academy has a book, *Organizing for Social Change,* which provides more information, available through many booksellers. The Midwest Academy also has a five-day training for organizers. See our website at www.midwestacademy.com for dates, location, and costs.

And now, the Midwest Academy is partnering with the authors of this book and the UC Berkeley Food Institute to bring organizing training to food justice efforts. First, we will be jointly offering a five-day training for leaders of food justice organizations to learn how to pivot their organizations and engage in real base-building and targeted organizing campaigns. Second, we will be offering training to young people interested in organizing to change the food system, to create a pipeline of new organizers that can help shift the balance of power. People have built collective power and resisted the most powerful opponents for centuries. With organizing training, we can collectively overcome the challenges outlined in this book—and many more that confront the food system—both for our own health and well-being and for that of future generations.

ACKNOWLEDGMENTS

SARU JAYARAMAN

Thank you to my colleagues at the Goldman School of Public Policy and at the Restaurant Opportunities Centers (ROC) United, without whom nothing would be possible. I'd especially like to thank researchers and assistants Diana Liu, Teofilo Reyes, Veronica Avila, Celine Chen, and Bryan Trujillo for their help on this book.

Many thanks to the Berkeley Food Institute and, in particular, to Bob Epstein, for his vision and support of this work.

Our gratitude to the authors in this book, and in particular Judy Hertz and the Midwest Academy for sharing their organizing brilliance.

And last but not least, thank you to Zachary, Akeela, and Lina, and my parents and sisters for being such a constant source of love and support.

KATHRYN DE MASTER

Thank you to the many people who made this book possible: the authors, the organizers, and the many people fighting back tirelessly against corporate power in the food system. Many thanks to the Berkeley Food Institute for organizing the faculty seminars out of which this collaborative book project emerged. Thank you for deft and committed research and editorial contributions from several anonymous assistants and editors. Thank you to the amazing staff at Corporate Accountability. Thanks especially to the staff at UC Press for your guidance and patience throughout the process. Thank you for the incredible inspiration and encouragement from colleagues and students at UW Madison, Brown University, and UC Berkeley's Department of Environmental Science, Policy, and Management—especially the many students of "Sustenance and Sustainability" who are working today to create a more just agrofood system. Finally, thank you most especially to my family and dear friends for your love and support.

NOTES

INTRODUCTION

1. George Monbiot, "Taming Corporate Power: The Key Political Issue of Our Age," *Guardian*, December 8, 2014, www.theguardian.com/commentisfree/2014/dec/08/taming-corporate-power-key-political-issue-alternative.

2. David Korten, *When Corporations Rule the World* (Sterling, VA: Kumerian Press, 1995).

3. Since 1886 the federal courts have extended the certain rights and constitutional protections under the Fourteenth Amendment to the Constitution to "Corporate Persons." See, among other cases, First National Bank of Boston v. Bellotti, 435 U.S. 765 (1978), Santa Clara County v. Southern Pacific Railroad Company, 118 U.S. 394 (1886), and Citizens United v. Federal Election Commission 558 U.S. 310 (2010), described in Alex Park, "10 Supreme Court Rulings—Before Hobby Lobby—That Turned Corporations into People," *Mother Jones,* July 10, 2014, www.motherjones.com/politics/2014/07/how-supreme-court-turned-corporations-people-200-year-saga/.

4. Citizens United.

5. Philip H. Howard, *Concentration and Power in the Food System: Who Controls What We Eat?*, (New York: Bloomsbury, 2016); see also Wenonah Hauter, *Foodopoly: The Battle over the Future of Food and Farming in America* (New York: New Press, 2012).

6. Howard, *Concentration and Power in the Food System;* Hauter, *Foodopoly.*

7. See William Heffernan, "Concentration of Ownership and Control in Agriculture," in *Hungry for Profit: The Agribusiness Threat to Farmers, Food, and the Environment,* ed. Fred Magdoff, John Bellamy Foster, and Frederick H. Buttel, 61–75 (New York: Monthly Review Press, 2000), and William Heffernan, with Mary Hendrickson and Robert Gronski, *Consolidation in the Food and Agriculture System* (report to National Farmers Union, Columbia: University of Missouri, February 5, 1999).

8. Howard, *Concentration and Power in the Food System;* see also Hauter, *Foodopoly.*

9. Hauter, *Foodopoly.*

10. Howard, *Concentration and Power in the Food System;* see also Hauter, *Foodopoly.*

11. Christopher Leonard, *The Meat Racket: The Secret Takeover of America's Food Business* (New York: Simon and Schuster, 2014.

12. Mary Hendrickson and William Heffernan, *Concentration of Agricultural Markets* (Columbia: Department of Rural Sociology, University of Missouri, 2005).

13. Berne Declaration, *Agropology: A Handful of Corporations Control World Food Production* (Zurich: EcoNexus, September 2013), www.econexus.info/sites/econexus/files/Agropoly_Econexus_BerneDeclaration_wide-format.pdf.

14. Hauter, *Foodopoly.*

15. https://sjinsights.net/2014/09/29/new-research-sheds-light-on-daily-ad-exposures/.

16. Jack Ralph Kloppenburg Jr., "Planetary Patriots or Sophisticated Scoundrels?" *Biotechnology and Development Monitor* 16 (September 1993): 24.

17. Jane L. Collins, *Threads: Gender, Labor, and Power in the Global Apparel Industry* (Chicago: University of Chicago Press, 2003).

18. For recent examples, see Alison Hope Alkon and Julie Guthman, *The New Food Activism: Opposition, Cooperation, and Collective Action* (Oakland: University of California Press, 2017), and Joshua Sbicca, *Food Justice Now! Deepening the Roots of Social Struggle* (Minneapolis: University of Minnesota Press, 2018).

19. See, for example, Julie Guthman, *Agrarian Dreams: The Paradox of Organic Farming in California* (Berkeley: University of California Press, 2004), and Philip H. Howard, "Organic Industry Structure: Acquisitions and Alliances, Top 100 Food Producers in North America" (poster, Michigan State University, January 2016), https://msu.edu/~howardp/OrganicJan16.pdf.

20. See Sidney G. Tarrow, *Power in Movement: Social Movements and Contentious Politics,* 3rd ed. (New York: Cambridge University Press, 2011).

HOW CORPORATIONS CONTROL OUR SEEDS

1. Cary Fowler and Patrick R. Mooney, *Shattering: Food, Politics, and the Loss of Genetic Diversity* (Tucson: University of Arizona Press, 1990); Helena Paul and Ricarda Steinbrecher, *Hungry Corporations: Transnational Biotech Companies Colonise the Food Chain* (London: Zed Books, 2003).

2. ETC Group, *Putting the Cartel before the Horse . . . and Farm, Seeds, Soil and Peasants Etc.: Who Will Control the Agricultural Inputs?* (Montreal, September 4, 2013), 1–40, www.etcgroup.org/putting_the_cartel_before_the_horse_2013.

3. Richard B. Du Boff and Edward S. Herman, "Mergers, Concentration, and the Erosion of Democracy," *Monthly Review,* May 1, 2001, http://monthlyreview.org/2001/05/01/mergers-concentration-and-the-erosion-of-democracy/.

4. ETC Group, *Breaking Bad: Big Ag Mega-Mergers in Play* (Montreal, December 15, 2015), 1–20, www.etcgroup.org/content/breaking-bad-big-ag-mega-mergers-play.

5. Richard C. Lewontin, "The Maturing of Capitalist Agriculture: Farmer as Proletarian," in *Hungry for Profit: The Agribusiness Threat to Farmers, Food, and the Environment,* ed. Fred Magdoff, John Bellamy Foster, and Frederick H. Buttel (New York: Monthly Review Press, 2000), 93–106.

6. Irene Musselli Moretti, *Tracking the Trend Towards Market Concentration: The Case of the Agricultural Input Industry* (Geneva: United Nations Conference on Trade and Development, April 20, 2006), 1–60, http://unctad.org/en/docs/ditccom200516_en.pdf.

7. Jonathan Nitzan and Shimshon Bichler, *Capital as Power: A Study of Order and Creorder* (London: Routledge, 2009).

8. William Heffernan, with Mary Hendrickson and Robert Gronski, *Consolidation in the Food and Agriculture System* (report to National Farmers Union, Columbia: University of Missouri, February 5, 1999), 1–19, www.foodcircles.missouri.edu/whstudy.pdf.

9. Philip H. Howard, "Visualizing Consolidation in the Global Seed Industry: 1996–2008," *Sustainability* 1, no. 4 (December 8, 2009): 1266–87, doi:10.3390/su1041266.

10. Pam Smith, "The Business of Seed," AgWeb—The Home Page of Agriculture, July 29, 2011, accessed June 29, 2012, www.agweb.com/article/the_business_of_seed/.

11. Food and Agricultural Policy Research Institute, University of Missouri (FAPRI-MU), *U.S. Baseline Briefing Book: Projections for Agricultural and Biofuel Markets* (Columbia, MO: FAPRI-MU, March 2016), 1–56, www.fapri.missouri.edu/wp-content/uploads/2016/03/FAPRI-MU-Report-02-16.pdf.

12. Patrick Winters, "Syngenta to Buy Biotech Seedmaker Devgen for $523 Million," *Bloomberg,* September 21, 2012, www.bloomberg.com/news/articles/2012-09-21/syngenta-agrees-to-buy-biotech-rival-devgen-for-523-million-1-.

13. ETC Group, *Putting the Cartel before the Horse,* 1–40.

14. ETC Group, *Gene Giants Seek "Philanthrogopoly"* (Montreal, March 7, 2013), 1–17, www.etcgroup.org/content/gene-giants-seek-philanthrogopoly.

15. Mark Schapiro, "Seeds of Disaster," *Mother Jones* 7, no. 10, (December 1982), 12.

16. Michael S. Carolan, "Saving Seeds, Saving Culture: A Case Study of a Heritage Seed Bank," *Society and Natural Resources* 20, no. 8 (July 19, 2007): 739–50, https://doi.org/10.1080/08941920601091345.

17. Matthew Dillon, "Monsanto Buys Seminis," *New Farm,* February 22, 2005, http://newfarm.rodaleinstitute.org/features/2005/0205/seminisbuy/.

18. Schapiro, "Seeds of Disaster," 13.

19. Kristina Hubbard, *Out of Hand: Farmers Face the Consequences of a Consolidated Seed Industry* (report for the Farmer to Farmer Campaign on Genetic Engineering, Washington, DC: National Family Farm Coalition, December 2009), 1–56, www.farmertofarmercampaign.com/Out%20of%20Hand.FullReport.pdf.

20. Michael E. Gray, "Relevance of Traditional Integrated Pest Management (IPM) Strategies for Commercial Corn Producers in a Transgenic Agroecosystem: A Bygone Era?" *Journal of Agricultural and Food Chemistry* 59, no. 11 (June 8, 2011): 5852–58, https://doi.org/10.1021/jf102673s.

21. Sara Schafer, "Behind the Seed Scene," AgWeb—The Home Page of Agriculture, July 27, 2012, accessed August 16, 2016, www.agweb.com/article/behind_the_seed_scene/.

22. Walter Adams and James W. Brock, *The Bigness Complex: Industry, Labor, and Government in the American Economy,* 2nd ed. (Stanford, CA: Stanford Economics and Finance, 2004).

23. Rachel Schurman and William A. Munro, *Fighting for the Future of Food: Activists versus Agribusiness in the Struggle over Biotechnology* (Minneapolis: University of Minnesota Press, 2010).

24. Schurman and Munro, *Fighting for the Future.*

25. Paul A. Stitt, *Fighting the Food Giants* (Manitowoc, WI: Natural Press, 1980).

26. Karen McMahon, "Mycogen Purchases Cargill Seed," *Farm Industry News,* February 1, 2001, http://farmindustrynews.com/mycogen-purchases-cargill-seed.

27. Stefano Padulosi, Judith Thompson, and Per Rudebjer, *Fighting Poverty, Hunger and Malnutrition with Neglected and Underutilized Species (NUS): Needs, Challenges and the Way Forward* (Rome: Bioversity International, 2013), www.bioversityinternational.org/e-library/publications/detail/fighting-poverty-hunger-and-malnutrition-with-neglected-and-underutilized-species-nus-needs-challenges-and-the-way-forward/.

28. Leland L. Glenna et al., "Intellectual Property, Scientific Independence, and the Efficacy and Environmental Impacts of Genetically Engineered Crops: Intellectual Property, Scientific Independence," *Rural Sociology* 80, no. 2 (June 2015): 147–72, https://doi.org/10.1111/ruso.12062.

29. Emily Dupraz, "Monsanto and the Per Se Illegal Rule for Bundled Discounts" (SSRN Scholarly Paper, Rochester, NY: Social Science Research Network, April 1, 2012), 1–36, http://papers.ssrn.com/abstract=2032615.

30. Ben A. Woodcock et al., "Impacts of Neonicotinoid Use on Long-Term Population Changes in Wild Bees in England," *Nature Communications* 7 (August 16, 2016): 1–8, https://doi.org/10.1038/ncomms12459.

31. Dave Goulson, "Review: An Overview of the Environmental Risks Posed by Neonicotinoid Insecticides," *Journal of Applied Ecology* 50, no. 4 (August 2013): 977–87, https://doi.org/10.1111/1365-2664.12111; Sarah Stevens and Peter Jenkins, *Heavy Costs: Weighing the Value of Neonicotinoid Insects in Agriculture* (Washington, DC: Center for Food Safety, March 2014), 1–20, www.centerforfoodsafety.org/files/neonic-efficacy_digital_29226.pdf.

32. Jack Ralph Kloppenburg Jr., *First the Seed: The Political Economy of Plant Biotechnology, 1492–2000,* 2nd ed. (Madison: University of Wisconsin Press, 2004), http://hdl.handle.net/2027/heb.06255.

33. Jack Ralph Kloppenburg Jr., "Re-Purposing the Master's Tools: The Open Source Seed Initiative and the Struggle for Seed Sovereignty," *Journal of Peasant*

Studies 41, no. 6 (November 2, 2014): 1225–46, https://doi.org/10.1080/03066150.2013.875897.

34. Debbie Barker, Bill Freese, and George Kimbrell, *Seed Giants vs. U.S. Farmers* (Washington, DC: Center for Food Safety, 2013), 1–46, www.centerforfoodsafety.org/reports/1770/seed-giants-vs-us-farmers#.

35. Andy Meek, "Down and Out in Covington," *Memphis Daily News,* June 22, 2006, www.memphisdailynews.com/editorial/Article.aspx?id=30496.

36. Matthew Dillon, "Organic Vegetable Farmers–WARNING–You May Be Engaging in Contract Agreements with Monsanto," *Seed Broadcast Blog,* March 16, 2010, http://blog.seedalliance.org/2010/03/16/organic-vegetable-farmers-warning-you-may-be-engaging-in-contract-agreements-with-monsanto/.

37. Rebekah Fraser, "Seed Research: Seed Cleaning Takes a Bath," *Growing Magazine,* 2009, www.growingmagazine.com/article-3671.aspx.

38. Michael Mascarenhas and Lawrence Busch, "Seeds of Change: Intellectual Property Rights, Genetically Modified Soybeans and Seed Saving in the United States," *Sociologia Ruralis* 46, no. 2 (April 2006): 122–38, https://doi.org/10.1111/j.1467-9523.2006.00406.x.

39. Martin Gilens, *Affluence and Influence: Economic Inequality and Political Power in America* (Princeton: Princeton University Press, 2012); Larry M. Bartels, *Unequal Democracy: The Political Economy of the New Gilded Age* (Princeton: Princeton University Press, 2009); Kay Lehman Schlozman, Sidney Verba, and Henry E. Brady, *The Unheavenly Chorus: Unequal Political Voice and the Broken Promise of American Democracy* (Princeton: Princeton University Press, 2012).

40. Philip H. Howard, "Transnational Corporations," in *Achieving Sustainability: Visions, Principles and Practices,* ed. Debra Rowe (Detroit: Macmillan, 2014), 737–42.

41. Philip H. Howard, "Too Big to Ale? Globalization and Consolidation in the Beer Industry," in *The Geography of Beer: Regions, Environment, and Society,* ed. Mark W. Patterson and Nancy Hoast Pullen (New York: Springer, 2014), 155–65.

42. US Department of Justice, *Competition and Agriculture: Voices from the Workshops on Agriculture and Antitrust Enforcement in Our 21st Century Economy and Thoughts on the Way Forward* (Washington, DC, 2012).

43. Tom Philpott, "DOJ Mysteriously Quits Monsanto Antitrust Investigation," *Mother Jones,* December 1, 2012, www.motherjones.com/tom-philpott/2012/11/dojs-monsantoseed-industry-investigation-ends-thud.

44. Chuck Neubauer, "Monsanto Chief Accuses Rival DuPont of Deceit," *Washington Times,* August 18, 2009, www.washingtontimes.com/news/2009/aug/18/monsanto-chief-accuses-rival-dupont of deceit/, "Antitrust Probe of Monsanto May Turn on Anti-Stacking Provisions," *Corporate Crime Reporter,* May 10, 2010, www.corporatecrimereporter.com/monsanto051010.htm.

45. Daryl Lim, "Self-Replicating Technologies and the Challenge for the Patent and Antitrust Laws," *Cardozo Arts and Entertainment Law Journal* 32, no. 1 (2013): 131–223.

46. David Pitt, "DuPont Wins Fight for South African Seed Company," *Associated Press,* July 31, 2013, www.stltoday.com/business/local/dupont-wins-fight-for-south-african-seed-company/article_7dfca80c-a480-5a56-9b42-16a21d52bfaf.html.

47. James Matson, Minli Tang, and Sarah Wynn, "Intellectual Property and Market Power in the Seed Industry: The Shifting Foundation of Our Food System" (SSRN Scholarly Paper, Rochester, NY: Social Science Research Network, September 1, 2012), 1–38, http://papers.ssrn.com/abstract=2153098.

48. Philip H. Howard, "Intellectual Property and Consolidation in the Food System," *Crop Science* 55, no. 6 (2015): 2489–95.

49. Philip Pardey et al., "The Evolving Landscape of Plant Varietal Rights in the United States, 1930–2008," *Nature Biotechnology* 31, no. 1 (2013): 25.

50. Philip H. Howard, *Concentration and Power in the Food System: Who Controls What We Eat?* (New York: Bloomsbury Academic, 2016), 111.

51. GRAIN, "New Mega-Treaty in the Pipeline: What Does RCEP Mean for Farmers' Seeds in Asia?" *Against the Grain,* March 7, 2016, www.grain.org/article /entries/5405-new-mega-treaty-in-the-pipeline-what-does-rcep-mean-for-farmers-seeds-in-asia.

TAKING BACK OUR SEEDS

1. William Tracy and Michael Sligh, eds., *Proceedings of the 2014 Summit on Seeds & Breeds for 21st Century Agriculture* (Pittsboro, NC: Rural Advancement Foundation International, 2014).

2. Attorneys General of Montana, Iowa, Maine, Maryland, Mississippi, New Hampshire, New Mexico, Ohio, Oklahoma, Oregon, South Dakota, Tennessee, Vermont, and West Virginia. Comments regarding Competition in the Agriculture Industry, 2010, submitted to the US Departments of Justice and Agriculture on March 11, 2010.

3. Bowman v. Monsanto Company, No. 11–796 (U.S. May 13, 2013).

4. Jim Myers, personal communication, November 26, 2013.

5. Robert Barham and David Joynt, Heat tolerant broccoli, US Patent 6,784,345, filed June 22, 2001, and issued August 31, 2004.

6. Lisa Hamilton, "Linux for Lettuce," *VQR,* May 14, 2014.

7. Tracy and Sligh, *Proceedings,* 1.

8. Tracy and Sligh, *Proceedings,* 53.

9. Food and Water Watch, *Public Research, Private Gain* (Washington, DC: Food and Water Watch, 2012), 6.

10. Food and Water Watch, *Public Research,* 1.

11. Andrew Pollack, "Crop Scientists Say Biotechnology Seed Companies Are Thwarting Research," *New York Times,* February 19, 2009.

12. Leland Glenna, "The Purpose-Driven University: The Role of University Research in the Era of Science Commercialization," Agriculture, Food and Human Values Society 2017 Presidential Address (Clinton, SC: AFHVS, 2017).

13. Bhaven N. Sampat, "Patenting and U.S. Academic Research in the 20th Century: The World before and after Bayh-Dole," *Research Policy* 35, no. 6 (June 2006): 776.

14. William F. Tracy et al., *Intellectual Property Rights and Public Plant Breeding: Recommendations, and Proceedings of a Conference on Best Practices for Intellectual Property Protection of Publicly Developed Plant Germplasm*, Raleigh, NC, August 12–13, 2016, iv–x.

15. Matthew Dillon, "Monsanto Buys Seminis," *New Farm*, February 22, 2005, http://newfarm.rodaleinstitute.org/features/2005/0205/seminisbuy/.

16. Kristina Hubbard and Jared Zystro, *State of Organic Seed, 2016* (Port Townsend, WA: Organic Seed Alliance, 2016), 30.

17. Hubbard and Zystro, *State of Organic Seed*, 16.

18. New America, "America's Monopoly Problem: What Should the Next President Do About It?" Capitol Visitors Center, June 29, 2016, Washington, DC.

PESTICIDE PURVEYORS AND CORPORATE POWER

Brief sections of this chapter were previously published in the following works by the author: *Pesticide Drift and the Pursuit of Environmental Justice* (Cambridge: MIT Press, 2011); "Abandoned Bodies and Spaces of Sacrifice: Pesticide Drift Activism and the Contestation of Neoliberal Environmental Politics in California," *Geoforum* 39, no. 3 (2008): 1197–1214; "'Accidents' and Invisibilities: Scaled Discourse and the Naturalization of Regulatory Neglect in California's Pesticide Drift Conflict," *Political Geography* 25, no. 5 (2006): 506–29.

1. Jill Lindsey Harrison, *Pesticide Drift and the Pursuit of Environmental Justice* (Cambridge: MIT Press, 2011).

2. Susan Kegley, Anne Katten, and Marion Moses, *Secondhand Pesticides: Airborne Pesticide Drift in California* (San Francisco: Pesticide Action Network, 2003); Michael O'Malley, "Pesticides," in *Current Occupational and Environmental Medicine*, 5th ed., ed. Joseph LaDou and Robert Harrison (New York: Lange Medical Books, 2014), 573–616.

3. Harrison, *Pesticide Drift*, 25–49.

4. Carol Dansereau, "MITC in Our Air: Air Monitoring Results, Poisoning Cases, and the Need for Action to Protect Workers and Families" (Farm Worker Pesticide Project, 2009), www.fwpp.org; California Department of Pesticide Regulation (DPR), *Pesticide Air Monitoring Results Conducted by the Air Resources Board, 1986–2000* (Sacramento: California Department of Pesticide Regulation, 2002); Kegley, Katten, and Moses, "Secondhand Pesticides," 22–41; K. Mills and S.E. Kegley, *Air Monitoring for Chlorpyrifos in Lindsay, California: June–July 2004 and July–August 2005* (technical report, Pesticide Action Network, 2006), accessed May 15, 2019, www.pesticideresearch.com/site/docs/Lindsay-CP_7_18_06.pdf; Karl Tupper et al., *Air Monitoring for Pesticides in Hastings, Florida, December 6–14, 2006* (technical report, Pesticide Action Network, 2007), accessed May 15, 2019,

www.pesticideresearch.com/site/docs/DriftCatcher/HastingsFL02_19_08wc.pdf; Karl Tupper et al., *Air Monitoring in Hastings, Florida, October 1–December 6, 2007* (technical report, Pesticide Action Network, 2008), accessed May 15, 2019, www .pesticideresearch.com/site/docs/DriftCatcher/FL-TechReport9–22–08-finalSM .pdf.

5. Joe Thornton, *Pandora's Poison: Chlorine, Health, and a New Environmental Strategy* (Cambridge: MIT Press: 2000), 30–31.

6. US Department of Agriculture, Agricultural Marketing Service, *Pesticide Data Program Annual Summary, Calendar Year 2015* (Washington, DC, 2015), ix; see also Ryan E. Galt, "Scaling Up Political Ecology: The Case of Illegal Pesticides on Fresh Vegetables Imported into the United States, 1996–2006," *Annals of the Association of American Geographers* 100, no. 2 (2010): 327–55.

7. Phil Brown, *Toxic Exposures: Contested Illnesses and the Environmental Health Movement* (New York: Columbia University Press, 2007); Harrison, *Pesticide Drift*, 41–46; Mary O'Brien, *Making Better Environmental Decisions: An Alternative to Risk Assessment* (Cambridge: MIT Press, 2000).

8. Ryan E. Galt, "Overlap of US FDA Residue Tests and Pesticides Used on Imported Vegetables: Empirical Findings and Policy Recommendations," *Food Policy* 34 (2009).

9. Donald Atwood and Claire Paisley-Jones, *Pesticides Industry Sales and Usage: 2008–2012 Market Estimates* (Washington, DC: US Environmental Protection Agency, Office of Chemical Safety and Pollution Prevention, Office of Pesticide Programs, Biological and Economic Analysis Division, 2017), 9, www.epa.gov/sites /production/files/2017–01/documents/pesticides-industry-sales-usage-2016_0.pdf; see also David Pimentel and Lois Levitan, "Pesticides: Amounts Applied and Amounts Reaching Pests," *Bioscience* 36 (1986): 86–91.

10. Jim Hightower, *Hard Tomatoes, Hard Times* (Cambridge: Schenkman, 1973); Steven Stoll, *The Fruits of Natural Advantage: Making the Industrial Countryside in California* (Berkeley: University of California Press, 1998).

11. Christopher Bosso, *Pesticides and Politics: The Life Cycle of a Public Issue* (Pittsburgh: University of Pittsburgh Press, 1987), 28.

12. Mary O'Brien, *Environmental Decisions;* see also Carolyn Raffensperger and Joel Tickner, eds., *Protecting Public Health and the Environment: Implementing the Precautionary Principle* (Washington, DC: Island Press, 1999); see also Thornton, *Pandora's Poison,* and Kerry H. Whiteside, *Precautionary Politics: Principle and Practice in Confronting Environmental Risk.* (Cambridge: MIT Press, 2006).

13. Jill Lindsey Harrison and Sarah E. Lloyd, "Illegality at Work: Deportability and the Productive New Era of Immigration Enforcement," *Antipode* 44, no. 2 (2012): 365–85.

14. Edmund Russell, *War and Nature: Fighting Humans and Insects with Chemicals from World War I to Silent Spring* (Cambridge: Cambridge University Press, 2001).

15. Russell, *War and Nature.*

16. ETC Group, *Breaking Bad: Big Ag Mega-Mergers in Play* (Montreal, December 15 2015), 12, www.etcgroup.org/content/breaking-bad-big-ag-mega-mergers-play.

17. ETC Group, *Breaking Bad*, 4.

18. International Panel of Experts on Sustainable Food Systems and Pat Mooney, *Too Big to Feed: Exploring the Impacts of Mega-Mergers, Consolidation, Concentration of Power in the Agri-Food Sector* (Brussels: IPES-Food, October 2017), 23, accessed October 17, 2017, www.ipes-food.org/_img/upload/files/Concentration_FullReport.pdf.

19. Jim Panousis, "Ag's Largest Advertisers," *AgriMarketing* 46, no. 6 (2008): 33.

20. Michael Bell, *Farming for Us All: Practical Agriculture and the Cultivation of Sustainability* (University Park: Pennsylvania State University Press, 2004); see also Michael Carolan, "Do You See What I See? Epistemic Barriers to Sustainable Agriculture," *Rural Sociology* 71, no. 2 (2006): 232–60; see also Jessie K. Luna, "Getting out of the Dirt: Racialized Modernity and Environmental Inequality in the Cotton Sector of Burkina Faso," *Environmental Sociology* 4, no. 2 (November 2017): 221–34, https://doi.org/10.1080/23251042.2017.1396657.

21. Rajeev Patel, Robert J. Torres, and Peter Rosset, "Genetic Engineering in Agriculture and Corporate Engineering in Public Debate: Risk, Public Relations, and Public Debate over Genetically Modified Crops," *International Journal of Occupational and Environmental Health* 11, no. 4 (2005).

22. Margaret Kroma and Cornelia Butler Flora, "Greening Pesticides: A Historical Analysis of the Social Construction of Farm Chemical Advertisements," *Agriculture and Human Values* 20, no. 1 (2003).

23. CropLife America, "Our Values," accessed October 17, 2017, www.croplifeamerica.org/our-values/.

24. CropLife America, "Our Values."

25. Zev Ross, *Toxic Fraud: Deceptive Advertising by Pest Control Companies in California* (Californians for Pesticide Reform and California Public Interest Research Group, 1998), http://pesticidereform.org/article.php?id=13.

26. Patel, Torres, and Rosset, "Genetic Engineering."

27. Bayer AG, "Feeding a Growing World Population," Bayer Crop Science UK, 2007, accessed November 28, 2017, https://cropscience.bayer.co.uk/tools-and-services/stewardship-food-and-environment/producing-more-using-less/feeding-a-growing-world-population/.

28. Mark Winne, *Closing the Food Gap: Resetting the Table in the Land of Plenty* (Boston: Beacon, 2008).

29. John P. Reganold and Jonathan M. Wachter, "Organic Agriculture in the Twenty-First Century," *Nature Plants* 2 (February 2016): 1–8.

30. Carl Pray and Keith Fuglie, "Agricultural Research by the Private Sector," *Annual Review of Resource Economics* 7 (October 2015): 399–424.

31. Valerio Gennaro and Lorenzo Tomatis, "Business Bias: How Epidemiologic Studies May Underestimate or Fail to Detect Increased Risks of Cancer and Other

Diseases," *International Journal of Occupational and Environmental Health* 11, no. 4 (July 2013): 356–59, https://doi.org/10.1179/oeh.2005.11.4.356.

32. Carey Gillam, "New 'Monsanto Papers' Add to Questions of Regulatory Collusion, Scientific Mischief," *Huffington Post,* August 1, 2017, www.huffingtonpost.com/entry/newly-released-monsanto-papers-add-to-questions-of_us_597fc800e4bod187a5968fbf.

33. Center for Media Democracy, "Dennis Avery," CMD, 2017, accessed October 17, 2017, www.sourcewatch.org/index.php/Dennis_Avery; Sheldon Rampton and John Stauber, *Trust Us, We're Experts! How Industry Manipulates Science and Gambles with Your Future* (New York: Jeremy P. Tarcher, 2002).

34. Dennis T. Avery, *Saving the Planet with Pesticides and Plastic,* 2nd ed. (Indianapolis: Hudson Institute, 2000).

35. Sheldon Krimsky, *Science in the Private Interest: Has the Lure of Profits Corrupted Biomedical Research?* (Lanham, MD: Rowman and Littlefield, 2003); see also Jennifer Washburn, *University Inc: The Corporate Corruption of Higher Education* (New York: Basic Books, 2005).

36. Rachel Aviv, "A Valuable Reputation," *New Yorker,* February 10, 2014, www.newyorker.com/magazine/2014/02/10/a-valuable-reputation; see also Tyrone B. Hayes, "There Is No Denying This: Defusing the Confusion about Atrazine," *BioScience* 54, no. 12 (2004): 1138–49, https://doi.org/10.1641/0006–3568(2004)054[1138:TINDTD]2.0.CO;2; Clare Howard, "Pest Control: Syngenta's Secret Campaign to Discredit Atrazine's Critics," *100 Reporters,* June 17, 2013, https://100r.org/2013/06/pest-control-syngentas-secret-campaign-to-discredit-atrazines-critics/.

37. Daniel Lee Kleinman, *Impure Cultures: University Biology and the World of Commerce* (Madison: University of Wisconsin Press, 2003), 44.

38. Bodil Als-Nielsen et al., "Association of Funding and Conclusions in Randomized Drug Trials: A Reflection of Treatment Effect or Adverse Events?," *Journal of the American Medical Association* 290, no. 7 (August 2003): 921–28, https://doi.org/10.1001/jama.290.7.921.

39. Daniel Faber, *Capitalizing on Environmental Injustice: The Polluter-Industrial Complex in the Age of Globalization* (Lanham, MD: Rowman and Littlefield, 2008); Pesticide Action Network, "Undue Influence," accessed October 17, 2017, www.panna.org/resources/undue-influence.

40. Skip Spitzer, "Industrial Agriculture and Corporate Power," *Global Pesticide Campaigner* 13, no. 2 (August 2003): 1.

41. Juliet Eilperin, Chris Mooney, and Steven Mufson, "New EPA Documents Reveal Even Deeper Proposed Cuts to Staff and Programs," *Washington Post,* March 31, 2017, www.washingtonpost.com/news/energy-environment/wp/2017/03/31/new-epa-documents-reveal-even-deeper-proposed-cuts-to-staff-and-programs/?utm_term=.a0730f3dadce; Oklahoma Office of the Attorney General, "Oklahoma Office of the Attorney General E. Scott Pruitt: About the Attorney General," accessed August 25, 2017, http://web.archive.org/web/20170108114336/https://www.ok.gov/oag/Media/About_the_AG/.

42. Elizabeth Bomberg, "Environmental Politics in the Trump Era: An Early Assessment," *Environmental Politics* 26, no. 5 (May 2017): 956–63, https://doi.org/10.1080/09644016.2017.1332543; Chlorpyrifos.org, "Companies That Manufacture Chlorpyrifos," accessed November 28, 2017, www.chlorpyrifos.org/chlorpyrifos-companies-that-manufacture-it.php; Coral Davenport, "Counseled by Industry, Not Staff, E.P.A. Chief Is Off to a Blazing Start," *New York Times,* July 1, 2017, www.nytimes.com/2017/07/01/us/politics/trump-epa-chief-pruitt-regulations-climate-change.html; Britt Paris et al., *Pursuing a Toxic Agenda: Environmental Injustice in the Early Trump Administration* (Environmental Data and Governance Initiative, 2017), https://envirodatagov.org/publication/pursuing-toxic-agenda/; Christopher Sellers et al., *The EPA under Siege: Trump's Assault in History and Testimony* (Environmental Data and Governance Initiative, June 2017), https://envirodatagov.org/publication/the-epa-under-siege/; Michael D. Shear, "Trump Discards Obama Legacy, One Rule at a Time," *New York Times,* May 1, 2017, www.nytimes.com/2017/05/01/us/politics/trump-overturning-regulations.html.

43. Center for Responsive Politics, "Agricultural Services/Products–Industry Profile: Summary, 2017," Opensecrets.org, accessed October 17, 2017, www.opensecrets.org/lobby/indusclient.php?id=A07&year=2017.

44. See Center for Responsive Politics, "Revolving Door," Opensecrets.org, accessed October 17, 2017, www.opensecrets.org/revolving/.

45. For example, see Pesticide Action Network, "Monsanto Collusion on Glyphosate and Cancer," *Pesticide Action Network* (blog), accessed October 17, 2017, www.panna.org/blog/monsanto-collusion-glyphosate-cancer; Carey Gillam, "Cancer Questions, Controversy and Chorus at EPA Glyphosate Meetings," *Huffington Post,* December 16, 2016, www.huffingtonpost.com/carey-gillam/cancer-questions-controve_b_13679052.html.

46. Harrison, *Pesticide Drift,* 51–84.

47. Judy Hatcher, "No More Bhopals," *Pesticide Action Network* (blog), December 3, 2014, accessed November 27, 2017, www.panna.org/blog/no-more-bhopals; Justin King, "Dow Sues Activists in India over Bhopal Protests," *Digital Journal,* February 9, 2014, www.digitaljournal.com/news/world/dow-sues-activists-in-india-over-bhopal-protest/article/369743.

48. Anna Lappe, "What Dow Chemical Doesn't Want You to Know about Your Water," *Grist,* June 9, 2011. http://grist.org/pollution/2011–06–08-what-dow-chemical-doesnt-want-you-to-know-about-your-water/.

DRIFT CATCHERS COMBATTING PESTICIDE POWER

1. United States Court of Appeals for the Ninth Circuit, No. 17–71636, ID: 11269636, Dkt Entry: 171, LULAC vs. Wheeler, "On Petition for Review of an Order of the Environmental Protection Agency, argued and submitted en banc March 26, 2019," filed April 19, 2019.

2. Brian Melley, "California Moves to Ban Chlorpyrifos, Widely Used Pesticide," Associated Press, May 8, 2019, accessed May 13, 2019, www.kqed.org /science/1941369/california-moves-to-ban-chlorpyrifos-widely-used-pesticide.

3. Meredith Minkler, "Using Participatory Action Research to Build Healthy Communities," *Public Health Reports* 115, nos. 2–3 (March–June 2000): 192. www .ncbi.nlm.nih.gov/pmc/articles/PMC1308710/pdf/pubhealthrepo0022–0089.pdf.

4. David Michaels and Celeste Monforton, "Manufacturing Uncertainty: Contested Science and the Protection of the Public's Health and Environment," *American Journal of Public Health* 95, no. S1 (July 2005): S40. https://doi.org/10.2105 /AJPH.2004.043059.

5. David B. Resnik, Brandon Konecny, and Grace E. Kissling, "Conflict of Interest and Funding Disclosure Policies of Environmental, Occupational, and Public Health Journals," *Journal of Occupational and Environmental Medicine* 59, no. 1 (January 2017), https://doi.org/10.1097/JOM.0000000000000910; Sheldon Krimsky and Tim Schwab, "Conflicts of Interest among Committee Members in the National Academies' Genetically Engineered Crop Study," *PLOS ONE* 12, no. 2 (February 28, 2017): e0172317, p. 7, https://doi.org/10.1371/journal.pone.0172317.

6. Wendy Wagner and Thomas McGarity, "Regulatory Reinforcement of Journal Conflict of Interest Disclosures: How Could Disclosure of Interests Work Better in Medicine, Epidemiology and Public Health?" *Journal of Epidemiology and Community Health* 63, no. 8 (August 1, 2009): 606. https://doi.org/10.1136 /jech.2008.085001.

7. Lex Horan, "Catching the Drift in Iowa," *Pesticide Action Network* (blog), April 30, 2015, accessed November 22, 2017, www.panna.org/blog/catching-drift-iowa.

8. Horan, "Catching the Drift in Iowa."

9. "United States Court of Appeals for the Ninth Circuit."

10. Horan, "Catching the Drift in Iowa."

DEVIL'S BARGAIN

Portions of this chapter previously appeared in Stephanie A. Malin and Kathryn T. De Master, "A Devil's Bargain: Rural Environmental Injustices and Hydraulic Fracturing on Pennsylvania's Farms," *Journal of Rural Studies* 47, part A (October 2016): 278–90, https://doi.org/10.1016/j.jrurstud.2015.12.015.

1. Jeffrey B. Jacquet and David L. Kay, "The Unconventional Boomtown: Updating the Impact Model to Fit New Spatial and Temporal Scales," *Journal of Rural and Community Development* 9, no. 1 (2014): 1–23.

2. US Energy Information Administration (EIA), "U.S. Remained Largest Producer of Petroleum and Natural Gas Hydrocarbons in 2014," principal contributor, Linda Dorman, *Today in Energy*, April 7, 2015, www.eia.gov/todayinenergy /detail.cfm?id=20692.

3. US EIA, "U.S. Remained."

4. US EIA, "U.S. Remained."

5. Jessica L. Semega, Kayla R. Fontenot, and Melissa A. Kollar, *Income and Poverty in the United States: 2016*, Current Population Reports, P60–259, US Department of Commerce, Economics and Statistics Administration, US Census Bureau (Washington, DC: US Government Printing Office, 2017), https://census.gov/content/dam/Census/library/publications/2017/demo/P60–259.pdf; Brian Bienkowski, "Poor in Pennsylvania? You're Fracked," *Environmental Health News,* May 6, 2015, http://taylorsvillebasin.com/wp-content/uploads/2015/12/2015–05–11-Fracking.docx.

6. Patrick J. Drohan et al., "Perspectives from the Field: Oil and Gas Impacts on Forest Ecosystems: Findings Gleaned from the 2012 Goddard Forum at Penn State University," *Journal of Environmental Practice* 14, no. 4 (December 2012): 394–99, https://doi.org/10.1017/S1466046612000300; see also Kyle A. Hoy et al., "Marcellus Shale Gas Development and Farming," *Agricultural and Resource Economics Review* 47, no. 3 (December 2018): 634–64,https://doi.org/10.1017/age.2017.28.

7. Ted Auch and Natasha Léger, "Health vs. Power—Risking America's Food for Energy," in Articles, Data and Analysis, Guest Commentaries, FracTracker Alliance, June 7, 2017, www.fractracker.org/2017/06/risking-americas-food-for-energy/.

8. For example, see the *60 Minutes* segment: CBS News, "Meet the 'Shaleionaires,'" *60 Minutes,* December 8, 2010, www.cbsnews.com/videos/extra-meet-the-shaleionaires/.

9. Jeremy Weber, Jason Brown, and John Pender, *Rural Wealth Creation and Emerging Energy Industries: Lease and Royalty Payments to Farm Households and Businesses,* RWP 13–07 (Federal Reserve Bank of Kansas City research working paper, Kansas City, MO: Federal Reserve Bank, June 1, 2013); see also Kyle A. Hoy et al., "Marcellus Shale Gas Development and Farming," *Agricultural and Resource Economics Review* 47, no. 3 (December 2018): 634–64, https://doi.org/10.1017/age.2017.28.

10. Bienkowski, "Poor in Pennsylvania?"

11. Compared to an average of 6,900 cubic feet/day by the second-place Eagle Ford shale region; US Energy Information Administration (EIA), *Drilling Productivity Report* (Washington, August 10, 2015), accessed September 9, 2015, www.eia.gov/petroleum/drilling/#tabsummary-2.

12. Robert Strauss, "Oil Makes a Comeback in Pennsylvania," *New York Times,* April 22, 2015, www.nytimes.com/2015/04/23/business/energy-environment/oil-makes-a-comeback-in-pennsylvania.html.

13. For example, see Richard S. Krannich and Albert E. Luloff, "Problems of Resource Dependency in US Rural Communities," *Progress in Rural Policy and Planning* 5, no. 18 (1991); William R. Freudenburg and Robert Gramling, "Linked to What? Economic Linkages in an Extractive Economy," *Society and Natural Resources* 11 no. 6 (1998): 569–86.

14. Craig R. Humphrey et al., "Theories in the Study of Natural Resource-Dependent Communities and Persistent Rural Poverty in the United States," in

Persistent Poverty in Rural America, ed. Rural Sociological Society (Boulder, CO: Westview Press, 1993), 136–72.

15. Kathryn J. Brasier et al., "Residents' Perceptions of Community and Environmental Impacts from Development of Natural Gas in the Marcellus Shale: A Comparison of Pennsylvania and New York Cases," *Journal of Rural Social Sciences* 26, no. 1 (2011): 32–61. www.researchgate.net/profile/Kathryn_Brasier/publication /267508934_Residents'_Perceptions_of_Community_and_Environmental_ Impacts_From_Development_of_Natural_Gas_in_the_Marcellus_Shale_A_Comparison_of_Pennsylvania_and_New_York_Cases/links/54510fd10cf2bf864cba88cc /Residents-Perceptions-of-Community-and-Environmental-Impacts-From-Development-of-Natural-Gas-in-the-Marcellus-Shale-A-Comparison-of-Pennsylvania-and-New-York-Cases.pdf.

16. US EIA, "U.S. Remained."

17. Samuel B. Boxerman, Joel F. Visser, and Michael Krantz, *Hydraulic Fracturing Regulation in the US: 2013 Update* (Practical Law: Multi-Jurisdictional Guide 2013), www.sidley.com/~/media/files/publications/2014/01/hydraulic%20fracturing%20 regulation%20in%20the%20us%202013%20u__/files/view%20article/fileattachment /plc%20hydraulic%20fracturing%20regulation%20in%20the%20us%2020__.pdf.

18. Larry Lev et al., "Values-Based Food Supply Chains," in *The Sage Encyclopedia of Food Issues,* vol. 3, ed. Ken Albala (Los Angeles: Sage, 2015), 1417–19.

19. Food and Water Watch, *Consolidation and Price Manipulation in the Dairy Industry: Fact Sheet* (Washington, DC, March 2011), www.foodandwaterwatch .org/sites/default/files/consolidation_price_manipulation_dairy_fs_march_2011 .pdf.

20. US Department of Agriculture, National Agricultural Statistics Service (NASS), "Dairy, Cattle, and Milk Production," 2012 Census of Agriculture Highlights, accessed March 15, 2015, www.agcensus.usda.gov/Publications/2012 /Online_Resources/Highlights/Dairy Cattle Milk_Prod/Dairy_Cattle_and_ Milk_Production_Highlights.pdf.

21. Food and Water Watch, *Consolidation and Price.*

22. US Department of Agriculture, Economic Research Service, "Farm and Wealth Statistics: Pennsylvania," accessed October 3, 2015, www.ers.usda.gov/data-products/farm-income-and-wealth-statistics/returns-to-operators-us-and-state. asp x#P80a07f8ba91b4b31918c3be5ae1eca3b_2_160iToRox38.

23. Matt Kelso, "Over 1.7 Million Active Oil and Gas Wells in the US," in Articles, Data and Analysis, Feature, FracTracker Alliance, March 4, 2014, accessed August 10, 2018, www.fractracker.org/2017/06/risking-americas-food-for-energy/.

24. Kelso, "Over 1.7 Million Active"; Barbara Warner and Jennifer Shapiro, "Fractured, Fragmented Federalism: A Study in Fracking Regulatory Policy," *Publius: The Journal of Federalism* 43, no. 3 (July 1, 2013): 474–96.

25. Robert W. Howarth, "Methane Emissions and Climatic Warming Risk from Hydraulic Fracturing and Shale Gas Development: Implications for Policy," *Energy and Emission Control Technologies 2015* 3 (October 8, 2015): 45–54, www.academia .edu/download/39165483/EECT-61539.pdf.

26. Justin L. Rubenstein and Alireza Babaie Mahani, "Myths and Facts on Waste Water Injection, Hydraulic Fracturing, Enhanced Oil Recovery, and Induced Seismicity," *Seismological Research Letters* 86, no. 4 (July–August 2015): 1060–67, https://doi.org/10.1785/0220150067.

27. John L. Adgate, Bernard D. Goldstein, and Lisa M. McKenzie, "Potential Public Health Hazards, Exposures and Health Effects from Unconventional Natural Gas Development," *Environmental Science and Technology* 48, no. 15 (February 2014): 8307–20; Lisa M. McKenzie et al., "Birth Outcomes and Maternal Residential Proximity to Natural Gas Development in Rural Colorado," *Environmental Health Perspectives* 122, no. 4 (April 1, 2014): 412–17, http://dx.doi.org/10.1289/ehp.1306722.

28. Simona L. Perry, "Development, Land Use, and Collective Trauma: The Marcellus Shale Gas Boom in Rural Pennsylvania," *Culture, Agriculture, Food and Environment* 34, no. 1 (June 2012): 81–92, https://doi.org/10.1111/j.2153-9561.2012.01066.x; Sara Wylie and Len Albright, "WellWatch: Reflections on Designing Digital Media for Multisited Para-Ethnography," *Journal of Political Ecology* 21 (2014): 320–48, www.academia.edu/download/38253785/WylieandAlbright.pdf.

29. Abrahm Lustgarten, "Unfair Share: How Oil and Gas Drillers Avoid Paying Royalties," *ProPublica,* August 13, 2013, www.propublica.org/article/unfair-share-how-oil-and-gas-drillers-avoid-paying-royalties.

30. Gerald S. Leventhal, "What Should Be Done with Equity Theory?" in *Social Exchange,* ed. K. J. Gergen, M. S. Greenberg, and R. H. Willis (Boston: Springer, 1980), 27–55, https://doi.org/10.1007/978-1-4613-3087-5_2.

FOOD AND WATER OVER FRACKING

1. Krishna Ramanujan, "Study Suggests Hydrofracking Is Killing Farm Animals, Pets," *Cornell Chronicle,* March 7, 2012, http://news.cornell.edu/stories/2012/03/reproductive-problems-death-animals-exposed-fracking.

2. Susan Phillips, "Burning Questions: Quarantined Cows Give Birth to Dead Calves," *StateImpact Pennsylvania,* September 27, 2011, https://stateimpact.npr.org/pennsylvania/2011/09/27/burning-questions-quarantined-cows-give-birth-to-dead-calves/.

FOOD WORKERS VERSUS FOOD GIANTS

1. Maria Gonzalez (real name withheld), from interview by Jose Oliva via telephone from Chicago, Illinois, December 5, 2017.

2. Tyson Foods Inc., *Tyson Fact Book: Facts about Tyson Foods at 2017 Fiscal Year End,* 4, accessed May 17, 2015, http://ir.tyson.com/investor-323 relations/investor-overview/tyson-factbook/; Claire Phoenix, "The World's Top 100 Food and Beverage

Companies of 2017," *Food Engineering,* September 6, 2017, accessed December 2017, www.foodengineeringmag.com/2017-top-100-food-and-beverage-companies.

3. Tyson Foods Inc., *Tyson Fact Book,* 2.

4. Tyson Foods Inc., "Who We Are—Our Partners—Farmers," accessed May, 10, 2019, www.tysonfoods.com/our-story/farmers.aspx.

5. Tyson Foods Inc., "Our Story: Locations," accessed December 10, 2017, www .tysonfoods.com/our-story/locations.aspx.

6. Ron Wood, "173 Hospitalized in Chlorine Gas Leak at Tyson Plant," *Arkansas Democrat Gazette,* June 27, 2011, www.arkansasonline.com/news/2011/jun/27 /chlorine-leak-tyson-plant-hospitalizes-several/?latest.

7. No-fault points systems are common in processing plants. The employer will provide a certain number of points to each employee for calling in sick or missing work. After the employee reaches a certain number of points they will be terminated or disciplined.

8. Food Chain Workers Alliance, *The Hands That Feed Us: Challenges and Opportunities for Workers along the Food Chain* (Los Angeles, 2012), 1.

9. Food Chain Workers Alliance, *Hands,* 1.

10. Unfortunately, no one has analyzed the total number of food system workers globally.

11. US economic census for 2012 for total sales for North American Industry Classification System (NAICS) codes 311, 722, and 445, US Department of Agriculture, National Agricultural Statistics Service, "U.S. National Level Data," in *2012 Census of Agriculture: United States Summary and State Data, Volume 1, Geographic Area Series, Part 51,* AC-12-A-51 (Washington, DC, May 2014): 2–13, www.agcensus .usda.gov/Publications/2012/Full_Report/Volume_1,_Chapter_1_US/st99_1_ 001_001.pdf; World Bank, "National Accounts Data, and OECD National Accounts Data Files," accessed November 15, 2017, http://data.worldbank.org /indicator/NY.GDP.MKTP.CD.

12. Food Chain Workers Alliance, *Hands,* 3.

13. Food Chain Workers Alliance, *Hands,* 3.

14. Jonathan Chew, "Report Alleges Walmart and Whole Foods Are Selling Shrimp Peeled by Slaves," *Fortune,* December 14, 2015, https://fortune.com/2015 /12/14/thailand-slaves-shrimp/.

15. Eric Holt-Giménez, "The World Food Crisis: What Is behind It and What We Can Do," *Hunger Notes,* October 23, 2008, www.worldhunger.org/holt-gimenez/.

16. Food and Water Watch, *Grocery Goliaths: How Food Monopolies Impact Consumers* (Washington, DC, December 2013), 4, 21, 22, www.foodopoly.org/wp-content/uploads/2016/02/RPT_1312_RetailCons-FWWweb.pdf.

17. Lisa Baertlein, "Tyson Wins Bid for Hillshire in Battle of Meat Titans," *Reuters,* June 8, 2014, www.reuters.com/article/330 2014/06/09/us-tyson-hillshire-brands-idUSKBN0EK02N20140609.

18. Tyson Foods Inc., *Tyson Fact Book,* 4.

19. Food Chain Workers Alliance, *Hands,* 19.

20. Food Chain Workers Alliance, *Hands,* 20.

21. Food Chain Workers Alliance, *Hands,* 26.

22. Yvonne Yen Liu and Dominique Apollon, *The Color of Food* (New York: Applied Research Center, February 2011), 7, http://reimaginerpe.org/files/food_justiceARC.pdf.

23. Sylvia A. Allegretto et al., *Fast Food, Poverty Wages: The Public Cost of Low-Wage Jobs in the Fast-Food Industry* (University of Illinois at Urbana-Champaign and University of California, Berkeley, Labor Center, October 15, 2013), 8, http://laborcenter.berkeley.edu/pdf/2013/fast_food_poverty_wages.pdf.

FOOD WORKERS TAKING ON GOLIATH

Portions of this chapter draw from Saru Jayaraman's *Forked: A New Standard for American Dining* (New York: Oxford University Press, 2016).

1. Teofilo Reyes, "One Fair Wage Supporting Restaurant Workers and Industry Growth," in *Investing in America's Workforce Improving Outcomes for Workers and Employers. Volume 2, Investing in Work,* ed. Stuart Andreason et al. (Kalamazoo, MI: W.E. Upjohn Institute for Employment Research, 2018), 27, www.investinwork.org/-/media/Files/volume-two/Volume%202%20-%20Investing%20in%20Work.pdf?la=en.

2. National Employment Law Project, "14 Cities and States Approved $15 Minimum Wage In 2015" (NELP news release, December 21, 2015), www.nelp.org/news-releases/14-cities-states-approved-15-minimum-wage-in-2015/.

3. Coalition of Immokalee Workers, "Fair Food Program: Frequently Asked Questions," www.ciw-online.org, 1, accessed December 1, 2018, www.ciw-online.org/Resources/12FFP_FAQs_Formatted.pdf.

4. Fatima Hussein, "How a Group of Food Service Workers Formed a Union Underground," *Indy Star,* March 30, 2017, www.indystar.com/story/news/2017/03/30/how-group-food-service-workers-formed-union-underground/99499038/.

5. Andrea Strong, "Restaurant Owners and Managers Cannot Keep Servers' Tips, per New Budget Bill," *Eater,* March 23, 2018, www.eater.com/2018/3/22/17151172/tipping-laws-trump-budget-bill-pooling-minimum-wages.

6. Henry Louis Gates Jr., "100 Amazing Facts about the Negro: Did African-American Slaves Rebel?" PBS, *The African Americans: Many Rivers to Cross* (blog), January 12, 2013, originally posted on The Root, accessed May 13, 2019, www.pbs.org/wnet/african-americans-many-rivers-to-cross/hi"story/did-african-american-slaves-rebel/.

7. Gates, "100 Amazing Facts."

8. Susan Ferris, Ricardo Sandoval, and Diana Hembree, *The Fight in the Fields: Cesar Chavez and the Farmworkers Movement* (New York: Harcourt Brace, 1997): 141–45.

9. Stephanie Hinnershitz, "We Ask Not for Mercy, but for Justice": The Cannery Workers and Farm Laborers' Union and Filipino Civil Rights in the United States, 1927–1937," *Journal of Social History* 47, no. 1 (2013): 132–52.

10. Coalition of Immokalee Workers, "Fair Food," 1.

11. Eric Schlosser, *Fast Food Nation: The Dark Side of the All-American Meal* (Boston: Houghton Mifflin Harcourt, 2001), 183–86.

12. UNITE HERE, "Food Service: 100,000 Food Service Members—And Growing!," accessed December 1, 2018, https://unitehere.org/industry/food-service/.

13. Noam Scheiber, "Push to Settle McDonald's Case, a Threat to Franchise Model," *New York Times,* March 19, 2018, www.nytimes.com/2018/03/19/business/economy/mcdonalds-labor.html.

14. Food Chain Workers Alliance, *The Hands That Feed Us: Challenges and Opportunities for Workers along the Food Chain* (Los Angeles, 2012), 1–2, http://foodchainworkers.org/wp-content/uploads/2012/06/Hands-That-Feed-Us-Report.pdf.

15. US Department of Labor, Bureau of Labor Statistics, Occupational Employment Statistics, *May 2017 National Occupational Employment and Wage Estimates United States* (Washington, DC, 2017), accessed May 13, 2019, www.bls.gov/oes/current/oes_nat.htm.

16. Restaurant Opportunities Centers United, *The Other NRA: Unmasking the Agenda of the National Restaurant Association* (New York, April 28, 2014), 3, 10, http://rocunited.org/wp-content/uploads/2014/04/TheOtherNRA_Report_FINAL2014.pdf.

17. Saru Jayaraman, *Forked: A New Standard for American Dining* (New York: Oxford University Press, 2016).

18. Jayaraman, *Forked.*

19. Jayaraman, *Forked.*

20. Restaurant Opportunities Centers United, "One Fair Wage Sweeping the Nation," September 18, 2018, accessed May 13, 2019, https://rocunited.org/2018/09/one-fair-wage-sweeping-nation/; Shannon Van Sant, "Voters Back Measure to Raise Minimum Wage for Tipped Workers," National Public Radio, June 20, 2018, www.npr.org/2018/06/20/621726991/d-c-voters-back-measure-to-raise-minimum-wage-for-tipped-workers.

21. US Department of Labor, *May 2017 National Occupational Employment.*

22. Jayaraman, *Forked,* 33.

23. Jayaraman, *Forked,* 33.

24. Jayaraman, *Forked,* 34.

25. Jayaraman, *Forked,* 33.

26. Jayaraman, *Forked,* 35.

27. Jayaraman, *Forked,* 9.

28. Restaurant Opportunities Centers United and Forward Together, *The Glass Floor: Sexual Harassment in the Restaurant Industry* (New York: Restaurant Opportunities Centers United, October 7, 2014): 2, https://rocunited.org/2014/10/new-report-the-glass-floor-sexual-harassment-in-the-restaurant-industry/.

29. Restaurant Opportunities Centers United, *Glass Floor,* 5.

30. Bloomberg BNA, "AFL-CIO Executive Council Issues Statements on Range of Issues during Summer Meeting," *Bloomberg Government,* August 1, 2014.

31. Sam Thielman, "One Conservative Group's Successful Infiltration of the Media," *Columbia Journalism Review*, June 21, 2018, www.cjr.org/analysis/77-referendum-astroturf-tipping.php; Claudia Koerner, "These Tipping Activists Deny Being Funded by the Restaurant Lobby," *Buzzfeed News*, June 27, 2018, www.buzzfeednews.com/article/claudiakoerner/rwa-restaurant-workers-america-grassroots-astroturf-berman.

32. Restaurant Opportunities Centers United, *Better Wages, Better Tips: Restaurants Flourish with One Fair Wage* (New York, February 12, 2018), 2, https://rocunited.org/2018/02/new-report-better-wages-better-tips-restaurants-flourish-one-fair-wage/.

33. Restaurant Opportunities Centers United, *Better Wages*, 6.

34. John Oliver, "Astroturfing," *Last Week Tonight with John Oliver*, HBO, August 12, 2018. www.youtube.com/watch?v=Fmh4RdIwswE.

FAST FOOD EMBODIED

1. Kate Northstone et al., "Are Dietary Patterns in Childhood Associated with IQ at 8 Years of Age? A Population-Based Cohort Study," *Journal of Epidemiology and Community Health* 66, no. 7 (2012): 624–28; S. Jay Olshansky et al., "A Potential Decline in Life Expectancy in the United States in the 21st Century," *New England Journal of Medicine* 352, no. 11 (2005): 1138–45, www.nejm.org/doi/full/10.1056/NEJMsr043743.

2. Anthony Winson, *The Industrial Diet: The Degradation of Food and the Struggle for Healthy Eating* (Vancouver: University of British Columbia Press, 2013), 42–75.

3. Eric Schlosser, *Fast Food Nation: The Dark Side of the All-American Meal* (Boston: Houghton Mifflin Harcourt, 2001), 13–30.

4. Charlene C. Price, "Trends in Eating Out," *Food Review* 20, no. 3 (1997): 18–19, https://ageconsearch.umn.edu/record/234489/files/sept97c.pdf.

5. Statistic Brain Research Institute, *Fast Food Eating Statistics 2016* (New York, 2016), accessed December 21, 2017, www.statisticbrain.com/fast-food-statistics/.

6. Andrew Jacobs and Matt Richtel, "How Big Business Got Brazil Hooked on Junk Food," *New York Times*, September 16, 2017, accessed December 1, 2017, www.nytimes.com/interactive/2017/09/16/health/brazil-obesity-nestle.html; Irene Braithwaite et al., "Fast-Food Consumption and Body Mass Index in Children and Adolescents: An International Cross-Sectional Study," *BMJ Open* 4, no. 12 (2014), accessed December 21, 2017, http://bmjopen.bmj.com/content/4/12/e005813.

7. Winson quoted in Jacobs and Richtel, "How Big Business Got Brazil Hooked on Junk Food."

8. Cynthia Ogden and Margaret Carroll, "Prevalence of Obesity among Children and Adolescents: United States, Trends 1963–1965 through 2007–2008" (National Center for Health Statistics Data Brief, November 2015), 5, accessed December 4, 2017, www.cdc.gov/nchs/data/hestat/obesity_child_07_08/obesity_child_07_08.pdf; Global Burden of Disease 2015 Obesity Collaborators, "Health

Effects of Overweight and Obesity in 195 Countries over 25 Years," *New England Journal of Medicine* 377, no. 1 (2017): 13–27, accessed December 6, 2017, https://dot.org/10.1056/NEJMoa1614362.

9. Zahra Bahadoran, Parvin Mirmiran, and Fereidoun Azizi, "Fast Food Pattern and Cardiometabolic Disorders: A Review of Current Studies," *Health Promotion Perspectives* 5, no. 4 (2015): 231–40, accessed December 6, 2017, https://doi.gov/10.15171/hpp.2015.028; David A. Alter and Karen Eny, "The Relationship between the Supply of Fast-Food Chains and Cardiovascular Outcomes," *Canadian Journal of Public Health* 96, no. 3 (May 2005): 173–77, accessed December 2, 2017. www.ncbi.nlm.nih.gov/pubmed/15913078.

10. World Obesity Federation, "World Obesity Day 2017: Treat Obesity Now and Avoid the Consequences Later," accessed December 21, 2017. www.obesityday.worldobesity.org/ourdata2017.

11. Michael Moss, "Bliss Point: The Extraordinary Science of Addictive Junk Food," *New York Times Magazine,* February 20, 2013, www.nytimes.com/2013/02/24/magazine/the-extraordinary-science-of-junk-food.html.

12. Tom Neltner, "The FDA Has Failed the Public by Letting Companies Determine 'Safe' Food Additives," *STAT,* September 7, 2016, www.statnews.com/2016/09/07/fda-food-safety-additives/.

13. Schlosser, *Fast Food Nation,* 124–28.

14. Lisa R. Young and Marion Nestle, "The Contribution of Expanding Portion Sizes to the US Obesity Epidemic," *American Journal of Public Health* 92, no. 2 (2002): 246–49, https://doi.org/10.2105/AJPH.92.2.246; Ashley N. Gearhardt et al., "Neural Correlates of Food Addiction," *Archives of General Psychiatry* 68, no. 8 (April 2011): 808, https://doi:10.1001/archgenpsychiatry.2011.32.

15. Biing-Hwan Lin and Joanne F. Guthrie, *Nutritional Quality of Food Prepared at Home and Away from Home, 1977–2008* (EIB-105, US Department of Agriculture, Economic Research Service, Washington, DC: US Department of Agriculture, December 2012), 5, www.ers.usda.gov/publications/pub-details/?pubid=43699; Eurídice Martínez Steele et al., "Ultra-processed Foods and Added Sugars in the US Diet: Evidence from a Nationally Representative Cross-Sectional Study," *BMJ Open* 6, no. 3 (2016), https://doi.org/10.1136/bmjopen-2015–009892.

16. Schlosser, *Fast Food Nation,* 130–31.

17. McDonald's Corporation, "Company History," McDonald's Culture and History, March 5, 2010, accessed December 9, 2017, https://Accessedarchive.org/web/20100305203439/http://www.mcdonalds.com/usa/work/companyhistory.html.

18. Michele Simon, *Appetite for Profit: How the Food Industry Undermines Our Health and How to Fight Back* (New York: Nation, 2006), 34.

19. Oerther Foods McDonald's, "Birthday Parties—Frequently Asked Questions," accessed August 28, 2016, http://mcfun.com/party-faqs/.

20. Conrad Phillip Kottak, *Cultural Anthropology* (Columbus, OH: McGraw-Hill, 2000), 468; McDonald's Wiki, "McDonald's PlayPlace," June 16, 2015, accessed December 6, 2017, http://mcdonalds.wikia.com/wiki/PlayPlace; Corporate Accountability, *Clowning with Kids' Health: The Case for Ronald McDonald's*

Retirement (Boston, 2017), 14, www.corporateaccountability.org/wp-content /uploads/2017/11/Clowning-With-Kids-Health.pdf.

21. Hayley Peterson, "Why the Average McDonald's Makes Twice as Much as Burger King," *Business Insider,* March 26, 2014, www.businessinsider.com/mcdonalds-doubles-burger-king-profit-2014–3; McDonald's Corporation, *Form 10-K, Annual Report Pursuant to Section 13 or 15(d) of the Securities Exchange Act of 1934,* 2016, 12, accessed December 15, 2017, http://corporate.mcdonalds.com/content/dam /AboutMcDonalds/Investors/2016%20Annual%20Report.pdf.

22. Susan Linn, *Consuming Kids: Protecting Our Children from the Onslaught of Marketing and Advertising* (New York: Anchor Books, 2005), 82.

23. Jim Metrock, "Channel One News Has Lost 11 Schools Each Week for the Last 364 Weeks," *Obligation,* July 13, 2012, accessed December 11, 2017, www.obligation .org/2010–07–13-channel-one-news-has-lost-11-schools-each-week-for-the-last-364-weeks.

24. AAP Committee on Communications, "Children, Adolescents, and Advertising," *American Academy of Pediatrics* 95, no. 2 (1995), http://pediatrics.aappublications .org/content/95/2/295.

25. Schlosser, *Fast Food Nation,* 51–58.

26. School and Library Show, "It's Book Time with Ronald McDonald," accessed August 19, 2015, http://findronald.com/index_files/Page335.htm; School Show, "Giving Back with Ronald McDonald," accessed August 19, 2015, http:// findronald.com/index_files/Page770.htm; "Where's Ronald McDonald?" accessed August 19, 2015, http://wheresronald.com/.

27. McDonald's Educates Scholarship Program, accessed August 15, 2015, www .mcdonaldseducates.com/ronald.html.

28. Ray Kroc, *Grinding It Out: The Making of McDonald's* (Chicago: Contemporary Books, 1977), 176.

29. S. Bryn Austin et al., "Clustering of Fast-Food Restaurants around Schools: A Novel Application of Spatial Statistics to the Study of Food Environments," *American Journal of Public Health* 95, no. 9 (September 2005): 1575–81, https://doi .org/10.2105/ajph.2004.056341.

30. Brennan Davis and Christopher Carpenter, "Proximity of Fast-Food Restaurants to Schools and Adolescent Obesity," *American Journal of Public Health* 99, no. 3 (2009): 505–10, https://doi.org/10.2105/ajph.2008.137638.

31. Yale Rudd Center for Food Policy and Obesity, *Fast Food Marketing 360° Briefs 2012–2013* (New Haven, 2013), 5, accessed September 8, 2018, www .fastfoodmarketing.org/media/fastfoodfacts_360marketingbriefs.pdf.

32. Berkeley Media Studies Group, "Health Equity and Junk Food Marketing: Talking about Targeting Kids of Color" (framing brief, Berkeley Media Studies Group, 2017), 2, accessed December 14, 2017, www.bmsg.org/resources/publications /health-equity-junk-food-marketing-talking-about-targeting-kids-color.

33. Center for Responsive Politics, "Food and Beverage Industry Profile: Summary, 2016," opensecrets.org, accessed December 14, 2017, www.opensecrets.org /lobby/indusclient.php?id=N01&year=2016.

34. Rob Waters, "Soda and Fast Food Lobbyists Push State Preemption Laws to Prevent Local Regulation," *Forbes,* June 21, 2017, www.forbes.com/sites/robwaters /2017/06/21/soda-and-fast-food-lobbyists-push-state-preemption-laws-to-prevent-local-regulation/#26362c44745d.

35. Michele Simon, "McDonald's and Coca-Cola—An Unhealthy Alliance," *Huffington Post,* September 13, 2012, www.huffingtonpost.com/michele-simon /mcdonalds-coca-cola_b_1874770.html.

36. Center for Responsive Politics, "Food and Beverage: Money to Congress, Summary 2016," opensecrets.org, November 27, 2017, accessed December 10, 2017, www.opensecrets.org/industries/summary.php?cycle=2016&ind=N01.

37. Center for Responsive Politics, "Food and Beverage: Top Contributors to Federal Candidates, Parties, and Outside Groups, Election Cycle 2016," opensecrets .org, November 27, 2017, accessed September 21, 2018, www.opensecrets.org/industries /contrib.php?ind=N01&Bkdn=Source&cycle=2016.

38. Center for Responsive Politics, "Food and Beverage: Money to Congress."

39. Simon, *Appetite for Profit,* 21–44.

40. Michele Simon, *Best Public Relations That Money Can Buy* (Washington, DC: Center for Food Safety, 2013), 3–8, www.centerforfoodsafety.org/files/cfs_ front_groups_79234.pdf.

41. Phillip H. Howard, *Concentration and Power in the Food System: Who Controls What We Eat?* (London: Bloomsbury, 2016), 17–35.

42. Saru Jayaraman, *Forked: A New Standard for American Dining* (New York: Oxford University Press, 2016).

43. Marion Nestle, "Corporate Funding of Food and Nutrition Research," *JAMA Internal Medicine* 176, no. 1 (2016): 13–14, https://jamanetwork.com/journals /jamainternalmedicine/fullarticle/2471609.

44. Dan Mitchell, "How 2 Women Are Planning to Take on the Powerful Meat Industry," *Fortune,* March 16, 2016, http://fortune.com/2016/03/16/plant-based-food-lobbying/.

45. Polina Marinova, "Millennials Are Driving an $18 Billion Food Revolution," *Fortune,* October 13, 2015, http://fortune.com/2015/10/13/food-revolution-millennials/.

MOVING A MCMOUNTAIN

1. Seeking Alpha, "McDonald's CEO Hosts 2013 Annual Shareholders' Meeting Conference (Transcript)," Seeking Alpha Transcripts, May 23, 2013, http://seekingalpha .com/article/1458281-mcdonalds-ceo-hosts-2013-annual-shareholders-meeting-confer-ence-transcript; Maria Godoy, "This 9-Year-Old Girl Told McDonald's CEO: Stop Tricking Kids," National Public Radio, May 23, 2013, www.npr.org/sections /thesalt/2013/05/23/186304643/this-9-year-old-girl-told-mcdonalds-ceo-stop-tricking-kids.

2. Seeking Alpha, "McDonald's CEO."

3. Godoy, "This 9-Year-Old."

4. Bruce Horovitz, "McDonald's CEO Bawled-out by 9-Year-Old," *USA Today,* May 23, 2013, www.usatoday.com/story/money/2013/05/23/mcdonalds-ceo-don-thompson-childhood-nutrition/2355129/; Associated Press, "As McDonald's Tries to Evolve Its Image, Criticism over Nutrition Persists at Annual Meeting," *Macleans.ca,* May 23, 2013, www.macleans.ca/economy/business/as-mcdonalds-tries-to-evolve-its-image-criticism-over-nutrition-persists-at-annual-meeting/; Pakistan Today News Desk, "This Girl, 9, Scolded McDonald's CEO," *Pakistan Today,* May 28, 2013, www.pakistantoday.com.pk/2013/05/28/entertainment/this-girl-9-scolded-mcdonalds-ceo/; ABC News, "Girl Confronts McDonald's CEO," *Good Morning America,* New York, May 25, 2013, https://archive.org/details/KGO_20130525_140000_ABC_News_Good_Morning_America/start/600/end/660.

5. Phillipa Ellwood et al., "Do Fast Foods Cause Asthma, Rhinoconjunctivitis and Eczema? Global Findings from the International Study of Asthma and Allergies in Childhood (ISAAC) Phase Three," *Thorax* 68, no. 4 (April 2013): 351–60, http://doi.org/10.1136/thoraxjnl-2012–202285.

6. Eric Schlosser, *Fast Food Nation: The Dark Side of the All-American Meal* (Boston: Houghton Mifflin Harcourt, 2001).

7. Maureen Morrison, "Is Ronald McDonald the New Joe Camel?" *Ad Age,* April 23, 2012, http://adage.com/article/news/ronald-mcdonald-joe-camel/234287/.

8. Crain's Chicago Business, "Ronald Sits Out of McDonald's 2012 Olympics Ads," *Chicago Business Today,* Chicago, April 18, 2012, www.youtube.com/watch?v=Yi1sQI9kipY.

9. Crain's Chicago Business, "Ronald Sits Out."

10. Seeking Alpha, "McDonald's CEO."

11. Casey Hinds, "How McTeacher's Nights and Coke Science Betray Us," *Beyond Chron,* October 14, 2015.

12. Morrison, "New Joe Camel?"; Mitchell Hamline School of Law, "Master Settlement Agreement," Public Health Law Center, accessed December 21, 2017, www.publichealthlawcenter.org/topics/tobacco-control/tobacco-control-litigation/master-settlement-agreement.

13. Michele Simon, *And Now a Word from Our Sponsors: Are America's Nutrition Professionals in the Pocket of Big Food?* (Oakland: Eat Drink Politics, January 2013), www.eatdrinkpolitics.com/wp-content/uploads/AND_Corporate_Sponsorship_Report.pdf.

14. "Doctors' Orders: Stop Marketing Junk Food to Kids; An Open Letter to McDonald's CEO Jim Skinner from More Than 550 Health Professionals and Institutions in All 50 States." www.odwyerpr.com/site_images/051811letter.pdf.

15. "Doctors' Orders."

16. Signatories, "Doctors' Orders: Stop Marketing Junk Food to Kids," accessed August 19, 2015, www.lettertomcdonalds.org/signatories.

17. Hannah B. Sahud et al., "Marketing Fast Food: Impact of Fast Food Restaurants in Children's Hospitals," *Pediatrics* 118, no. 6 (December 1, 2006), https://doi.org/10.1542/peds.2006–1228.

18. Michelle Fay Cortez, "McDonald's in Hospitals Targeted by Group Seeking Fast Food End," *Bloomberg,* April 11, 2012, www.bloomberg.com/news/articles /2012–04–11/mcdonald-s-in-hospitals-targeted-by-group-seeking-fast-food-end; Richard Gunderman, "Does McDonald's Belong in a Children's Hospital?" *Atlantic,* November 13, 2013, www.theatlantic.com/health/archive/2013/11/does-mcdonalds-belong-in-a-childrens-hospital/281398/; Michael Mayo, "Mayo Column: Do McDonald's and Hospitals Belong Together?" *South Florida SunSentinel,* April 16, 2012, www.sun-sentinel.com/news/fl-xpm-2012–04–16-fl-mcdonalds-mayocol-b041712–20120416-story.html.

19. Gordon, Elana. "Hospital Bids Bye-Bye to Big Macs, Others May Follow Suit," National Public Radio, December 27, 2012, www.npr.org/sections/thesalt /2012/12/17/167463286/hospital-bids-bye-bye-to-big-macs-others-may-follow-suit; Allison Aubrey, "So Long, Big Mac: Cleveland Clinic Ousts McDonald's from Cafeteria," National Public Radio, August 19, 2015, www.npr.org/sections/thesalt /2015/08/19/432885995/so-long-big-mac-cleveland-clinic-ousts-mcdonalds-from-cafeteria; Physicians Committee for Responsible Medicine, "Hospital Food Review," January 27, 2015, accessed August 28, 2016, www.pcrm.org/health/health-topics/hospital-food-review; Jenny Deam, "McDonald's at Ben Taub Will Not Reopen after Harvey," *Houston Chronicle,* August 17, 2018, www.houstonchronicle .com/news/houston-texas/houston/article/McDonald-s-at-Ben-Taub-will-not-reopen-after-13164791.php.

20. Julia Medew, "Health Experts Warn against Fast Food at Monash Children's Hospital," *Age,* December 28, 2014, www.theage.com.au/victoria/health-experts-warn-against-fast-food-at-monash-childrens-hospital-20141222–12c9et. html; Denis Campbell, "Ban Fast-Food Outlets from Hospitals, MPs Demand," *Guardian,* March 24, 2015, www.theguardian.com/society/2015/mar/25/ban-fast-food-outlets-nhs-hospitals-mps.

21. Physicians Committee, "Hospital Food Review."

22. Corporate Accountability, "The Olympics and McDonald's Sever Ties," *Corporate Accountability* (blog), June 16, 2017, accessed December 21, 2017, www .corporateaccountability.org/blog/the-olympics-and-mcdonalds-severs-ties/; Liana B. Baker and Karolos Grohmann, "McDonald's Ends Olympics Sponsorship Deal Early," *Reuters,* June 16, 2017, www.reuters.com/article/us-olympics-mcdonalds /mcdonalds-ends-olympics-sponsorship-deal-early-idUSKBN1971HB.

23. Mark Penn and E. Kinney Zalesne, *Microtrends: The Small Forces behind Tomorrow's Big Changes* (New York: Grand Central Publishing, 2007).

24. Penn and Zalesne, *Microtrends;* Associated Press, "McDonald's Unveils Panel for Food Advice," *Washington Post,* May 9, 2006, www.washingtonpost.com /wp-dyn/content/article/2006/05/09/AR2006050901167.html.

25. Associated Press, "McDonald's Unveils."

26. Kim Bhasin et al., "McDonald's Has Gained A New Ally by Sucking Up to This Group of Bloggers," *Business Insider,* May 7, 2012, www.businessinsider.com /how-mcdonalds-works-with-mom-bloggers-2012–5.

27. Michele Simon, *Clowning Around with Charity: How McDonald's Exploits Philanthropy and Targets Children* (Oakland: Eat Drink Politics, October 2013), 2, www.eatdrinkpolitics.com/wp-content/uploads/Clowning_Around_Charity_Report_Full.pdf.

28. Simon, *Clowning Around*, 14.

29. Bruce Horovitz, "McDonald's Slammed over Ronald McDonald House Giving," *USA Today,* October 29, 2013, www.usatoday.com/story/money/business/2013/10/29/mcdonalds-ronald-mcdonald-house/3189709/.

30. Quoted in Andrea Germanos, "McDonald's: Exploiting Charity to Deflect Criticism, Reap Benefits," *Common Dreams,* October 30, 2013, www.commondreams.org/news/2013/10/30/mcdonalds-exploiting-charity-deflect-criticism-reap-benefits.

31. Simon, *Clowning Around*, 2.

32. Corporate Accountability, "Three Million Teachers to McDonald's: We're Not Lovin' It," October 14, 2015, accessed December 21, 2017, www.corporateaccountability.org/media/3-million-teachers-mcdonalds-not-lovin/.

33. Campaign for a Commercial-Free Childhood, "3 Million Teachers to McDonald's: We're Not Lovin' It" (press release, October 14, 2015), accessed December 21, 2017, http://commercialfreechildhood.org/3-million-teachers-mcdonalds-were-not-lovin-it.

34. Allison Aubrey, "McTeacher's Nights: Teachers Unions Say No to School Fundraisers," National Public Radio, October 15, 2015, www.npr.org/sections/thesalt/2015/10/15/448960665/mcteachers-nights-teachers-unions-say-no-to-school-fundraisers; Greg Trotter, "Teachers Raising Money for Schools at McDonald's? Unions Want It to Stop," *Chicago Tribune,* October 14, 2015, www.chicagotribune.com/business/ct-mcdonalds-nea-mcteachers-nights-1015-biz-20151014-story.html; Sacha Pfeiffer, "Nonprofits Pressure McDonald's to End 'McTeacher's Night,'" *Boston Globe,* October 16, 2015, www.bostonglobe.com/business/2015/10/15/boston-nonprofits-pressure-mcdonald-ends-its-mcteacher-night-program/7HQToaty8suXULpDjIud6N/story.html.

35. McDonald's of St. Louis, "McTeacher's Night," October 3, 2017, accessed December 1, 2017, http://mcdonaldsstl.com/community/mcteachers-night/; Sriram Madhusoodanan and David Monahan, "L.A. Teachers to McDonald's: Stay Away from our Students," *Beyond Chron,* November 2, 2016, www.beyondchron.org/l-teachers-mcdonalds-stay-away-students/; Hannah Freedberg, "Victory! The Nation's Second-Largest School District Ends McTeacher's Nights," *Corporate Accountability* (blog), April 26, 2017, accessed December 21, 2017, www.corporateaccountability.org/blog/victory-the-nations-second-largest-school-district-end-mcteachers-nights/.

36. Howard Blume, "L.A. School Board Targets McTeacher's Nights, but Not All Fast-Food Fundraisers," *Los Angeles Times,* April 18, 2017, www.latimes.com/local/lanow/la-me-edu-los-angeles-schools-ban-mcteachers-20170418-story.html.

37. California Federation of Teachers, "Floor Debate," CFT Convention 2018, March 23–25, 2018, Orange County, accessed September 17, 2018, http://cft.org

/images/Convention/2018_Convention/Amendments_Resolutions-Convention-2018–02–20.pdf.

38. American Federation of Teachers, "Oppose Exploitation of Schools and Students by Corporate-Sponsored Fundraising Events" (American Federation of Teachers Union Resolution, February 7, 2019), accessed April 2, 2019, www.aft.org /resolution/oppose-exploitation-schools-and-students-corporate-sponsored-fundraising-events.

39. For more, see the report produced by Nicholas Freudenberg: Monica Gagnon, Nicholas Freudenberg, and Corporate Accountability, *Slowing Down Fast Food: A Policy Guide for Healthier Kids and Families* (Boston, 2012), accessed August 19, 2015, www.corporateaccountability.org/wp-content/uploads/2012/12 /slowing_down_fast_food_factsheet.pdf.

40. Sharon Bernstein, "San Francisco Bans Happy Meals," *Los Angeles Times,* November 2, 2010, http://articles.latimes.com/2010/nov/02/business/la-fi-happy-meals-20101103.

41. "Page 5," *San Francisco Examiner,* October 18, 2010, accessed August 19, 2015, http://edition.pagesuite-professional.co.uk/launch.aspx?eid=d45ac552–1945–46fd-b51f-cd2f5d7ef764.

42. Trevor Hunnicutt, "Happy Meal Ban Passed: San Francisco Says No to Toys," *Christian Science Monitor,* November 3, 2010, www.csmonitor.com/Business/Latest-News-Wires/2010/1103/Happy-Meal-ban-passed-San-Francisco-says-no-to-toys.

43. Maureen Morrison, "McDonald's Bows to Pressure with More Healthful Happy Meal," *Ad Age,* July 26, 2011, http://adage.com/article/news/mcdonald-s-bows-pressure-healthful-happy-meal/228939/.

44. Maureen Morrison, "Jack in the Box Eliminates Toys from Kids' Meals," *Ad Age,* June 21, 2016, http://adage.com/article/news/jack-box-eliminates-toys-kids-meals/228334/.

45. Sam Oches, "Arby's Revamps Kids' Meals," *QSR,* September 28, 2011, www .qsrmagazine.com/exclusives/arby-s-revamps-kids-meals.

46. Maureen Morrison, "Taco Bell Axes Kids Meals," *Ad Age,* July 22, 2013, http:// adage.com/article/news/taco-bell-axes-kids-meals/243244/; Bruce Horovitz, "Taco Bell Dropping Kids Meals, Toys," *USA Today,* July 22, 2013, www.usatoday.com/story /money/business/2013/07/22/taco-bell-kids-meals-toys-fast-food/2574959/.

47. Panera Bread Company, "Panera Bread Unveils Largest Clean Kids Menu of Any National Restaurant Chain, Offering 250+ Meal Combinations without Toys or Sugary Drinks" (press release, September 20, 2017), accessed December 21, 2017, https://globenewswire.com/news-release/2017/09/20/1125261/0/en/Panera-Bread-Unveils-Largest-Clean-Kids-Menu-of-Any-National-Restaurant-Chain-Offering-250-Meal-Combinations-Without-Toys-or-Sugary-Drinks.html; Allison Aubrey, "Fast Food Restaurants Announce Efforts to Serve Healthier Kids' Meals," National Public Radio, September 25, 2017, /www.npr.org/2017/09/25/553532517/fast-food-restaurants-announce-efforts-to-serve-healthier-kids-meals.

48. Jon C. Ogg, "Should McDonald's Be Worth More Than All Direct Competitors Combined?" 24/7 Wall St., April 29, 2019, accessed May 31, 2019,

https://247wallst.com/services/2019/04/29/in-2019-should-mcdonalds-be-worth-more-than-all-direct-competitors-combined/.

49. Patti Rundall, "Have You Signed This? If Not, Act Now to Safeguard the UN from Conflicts of Interest: July 10–11 2014," *Conflicts of Interest Coalition* (blog), November 12, 2015, http://coicoalition.blogspot.com/2015/11/have-you-signed-this-if-not-act-now-to.html; World Health Organization, "Sixty-Third World Health Assembly: Marketing of Food and Non-Alcoholic Beverages to Children" (World Health Organization recommendation, May 21, 2010), accessed August 19, 2015, http://apps.who.int/gb/ebwha/pdf_files/WHA63/A63_R14-en.pdf.

50. Food Marketing Workgroup, "Food Marketing in Other Countries," accessed August 28, 2016, www.foodmarketing.org/resources/food-marketing-101/food-marketing-in-other-countries/.

51. World Cancer Research Fund, Nourishing Database, accessed August 19, 2015, www.wcrf.org/int/policy/nourishing-framework; Consumers International, "Advertising to Children Now Illegal in Brazil," April 10, 2014, accessed August 19, 2015, www.consumersinternational.org/news-and-media/news/2014/04/advertising-to-children-now-technically-illegal-in-brazil/; Amy Guthrie, "Mexico Plays the Heavy on Food Ads," *Wall Street Journal,* August 24, 2014, www.wsj.com/articles/mexico-plays-the-heavy-on-junk-food-ads-1408645600.

52. Rick Cohen, "Gates Divestment Decision Leads to Less Than Happy Meal at Mickey D's (and ExxonMobil)," *Nonprofit Quarterly,* February 18, 2015, https://nonprofitquarterly.org/2015/02/18/gates-divestment-from-mcdonalds-lobbying-dark-money/.

53. Julie Jargon and Anna Prior, "McDonald's Expects Further Challenges: Fast Food Company Takes Steps to Repair Business Fundamentals," *Wall Street Journal,* July 22, 2014, www.wsj.com/articles/mcdonalds-profit-slips-amid-struggles-1406031165; Laura Lorenzetti, "Not Lovin' It," *Fortune,* August 25, 2014, http://fortune.com/2014/08/25/mcdonalds-struggling-to-stay-relevant-with-millennials/; Lisa Bertagnoli, "McDonald's Has a New Generational Problem: Kids," *Crain's Chicago Business,* September 6, 2014, www.chicagobusiness.com/article/20140906/ISSUE01/309069980/mcdonalds-has-a-new-generational-problem-kids.

54. Julie Jargon, "McDonald's Faces 'Millennial' Challenge," *Wall Street Journal,* August 25, 2014, www.wsj.com/articles/mcdonalds-faces-millennial-challenge-1408928743.

55. Maureen Morrison, "McDonald's Sets up Shop in Silicon Valley," *Ad Age,* June 4, 2014, http://adage.com/article/digital/mcdonald-s-sets-shop-silicon-valley/293500/; McDonald's Corporation, "Our Food, Your Questions," accessed August 19, 2015, www.mcdonalds.com/content/us/en/your_questions/our_food.html; Anjali Athavaley, "McDonald's CEO Don Thompson Leaving after Tumultuous Run," *Reuters,* January 29, 2015, www.reuters.com/article/us-mcdonalds-ceo-idUSKBN0L12PS20150129; Samantha Bokamp, "McDonald's No. 2 Executive Pete Bensen to Retire," *Chicago Tribune,* August 2, 2016, www.chicagotribune.com/business/ct-mcdonalds-executive-retirement-0803-biz-20160802-story.html; Lisa Baertlein, "McDonald's Replaces U.S. Chief for the Second Time in Two Years," *Reuters,* August 22, 2014, www.reuters.com

/article/us-mcdonalds-managementchanges-idUSKBN0GM1GT20140822; Ezequiel Minaya, "McDonald's U.S. Chief Mike Andres to Retire," *Wall Street Journal*, August 31, 2016, www.wsj.com/articles/mcdonalds-u-s-chief-mike-andres-to-retire-1472679393.

56. Center for Responsive Politics, "Annual Lobbying by McDonald's Corp," Opensecrets.org, accessed December 21, 2017, www.opensecrets.org/lobby/clientsum.php?id=D000000373; McDonald's Corporation, "McDonald's Reports Third Quarter 2014 Results," accessed December 21, 2017, http://news.mcdonalds.com/Corporate/news-stories/2014/McDonald-s-Reports-Third-Quarter-2014-Results.

57. Phil Wahba, "McDonald's Sales Bleed Continues Despite Turnaround Efforts," *Fortune*, April 22, 2015, http://fortune.com/2015/04/22/mcdonalds-sales-decline/.

HUNGER INCORPORATED

Portions of this chapter draw from author Andy Fisher's book *Big Hunger: The Unholy Alliance between Corporate America and Anti-Hunger Groups* (Cambridge: MIT Press, 2017) and have been reprinted courtesy of MIT Press.

1. Feeding America, *Feeding Families, Feeding Hope: 2015 Annual Report* (Chicago, 2015), inside cover, www.feedingamerica.org/sites/default/files/about-us/financials/2015-feeding-america-annual-report.pdf.

2. Quoted in Patrick Butler, "Food Banks Are a 'Slow Death to the Soul,'" *Guardian*, September 25, 2013, www.theguardian.com/society/2013/sep/25/food-banks-slow-death-soul.

3. Twenty-two percent of African American households are food insecure as compared to nine percent of white households, according to the US Department of Agriculture, Economic Research Service, "Food Security in the U.S.: Key Statistics and Graphics," accessed May 10, 2019, www.ers.usda.gov/topics/food-nutrition-assistance/food-security-in-the-us/key-statistics-graphics.aspx.

4. Feeding America, "Farm to Pantry PSA," accessed May 10, 2019, www.ispot.tv/ad/7SE4/feeding-america-farm-to-pantry.

5. Janet Poppendieck, *Sweet Charity? Emergency Food and the End of Entitlement* (New York: Penguin Books, 1999), 26–27.

6. Andrew Fisher, "Food Banks Feed People: Why Don't They Fight Hunger?" *New Food Economy*, October 26, 2017, https://newfoodeconomy.org/food-banks-hunger-board-members/.

7. BSR, *Analysis of U.S. Food Waste among Food Manufacturers, Retailers, and Wholesalers* (San Francisco, April 2013), 10–13, www.foodwastealliance.org/wp-content/uploads/2013/06/FWRA_BSR_Tier2_FINAL.pdf. This figure is calculated as follows: Retailers and processors donated 1.37 billion pounds of food. The estimated cost of tipping fees is $49/ton (based on calculations of total tipping fees /estimated nationwide cost), 13–14.

8. Congressional Budget Office, "HR 4719, Fighting Hunger Incentive Act of 2014," accessed May 10, 2019, www.cbo.gov/publication/45425; Congressional Budget Office, *An Update to the Budget and Economic Outlook: Fiscal Years 2012 to 2022.* Washington, DC, August 22, 2012. www.cbo.gov/publication/43539.

9. Feeding America, *Feeding America: Financial Statements, Years Ended June 30, 2017 and 2016* (Chicago, 2017), accessed May 10, 2019, www.feedingamerica.org /sites/default/files/2018–10/2017-audit_0.PDF.

10. Catherine Candisky and Jim Siegel, "Food Banks Group Bows to Donor's Pressure on Payday-Lending Bill," *Columbus Dispatch,* May 2, 2008, www.dispatch .com/content/stories/local/2008/05/02/foodbanks.html.

11. Smithfield Foods, "Smithfield Foods Donates More then 42,000 Pounds of Protein to Support Veteran Food Drive and Mid-South Food Bank" (press release, November 15, 2018), accessed May 10, 2019, www.smithfieldfoods.com/newsroom /press-releases-and-news/smithfield-foods-donates-more-than-42000-pounds-of-protein-to-support-veteran-food-drive-and-mid-south-food-bank.

12. Erica Hellerstein and Ken Fine, "A Million Tons of Feces and an Unbearable Stench: Life Near Industrial Pig Farms," *Guardian,* September 20, 2017, www .theguardian.com/us-news/2017/sep/20/north-carolina-hog-industry-pig-farms.

13. Alfred Lubrano, "Tsunami of Free Food for the Hungry Is Coming: Will It Be Too Much to Handle?" *Philadelphia Inquirer,* October 1, 2018, www2.philly.com /philly/news/food-poverty-farmers-tariffs-trump-administration-philabundance-share-pennsylvania-20181001.html.

14. Alan Rappeport, "Kraft Warns on US Food Stamp Cut Plans," *Financial Times,* September 9, 2012, www.ft.com/cms/s/0/7ed1db42-f932–11e1–945b-00144feabdco.html.

15. Michele Simon, *Food Stamps: Follow the Money; Are Corporations Profiting from Hungry Americans?* (Oakland: Eat Drink Politics, June 2012), 17, www .eatdrinkpolitics.com/wp-content/uploads/FoodStampsFollowtheMoneySimon .pdf; Krissy Clark and Henry Grabar, "The Secret Life of a Food Stamp Might Become a Little Less Secret," *Slate,* August 5, 2014, www.slate.com/blogs/moneybox /2014/08/05/how_much_walmart_gets_in_food_stamp_dollars_the_answer_ may_be_forthcoming.html.

16. US Senate, "Lobbying Disclosure Act Database," accessed August 21, 2016, http://soprweb.senate.gov/index.cfm?event=selectfields. I placed Pepsi under the beverages category, though it does market a number of snack foods, including Fri-toLay products. I placed Kraft under the manufacturer category, although it also produces the CapriSun sweetened beverage line.

17. Christina Wong, "SNAP Restaurant Meals Program" (unpublished manu-script), no longer accessible.

18. Simon, *Food Stamps,* 3.

19. Robert Pear, "Soft Drink Industry Fights Proposed Food Stamp Ban," *New York Times,* April 29, 2011, www.nytimes.com/2011/04/30/us/politics/30food.html; Food Research and Action Center (FRAC), "Coalition Statement on Preserving

Food Choice in SNAP/Food Stamps" (Washington, DC, May 24, 2010), 1–2, accessed June 14, 2011, www.frac.org/pdf/foodchoicemay1ofinal.pdf.

20. FRAC, "Coalition Statement," 1–2.

21. Center on Budget and Policy Priorities, "A Quick Guide to SNAP Eligibility and Benefits," SNAP Basics, accessed August 21, 2016, www.cbpp.org/research /food-assistance/a-quick-guide-to-snap-eligibility-and-benefits.

22. Elise Gould, "Raising Wages Is Key to Improving Incomes of Low-Income Americans," Economic Policy Institute Economic Snapshot, June 17, 2014, accessed May 10, 2019, www.epi.org/publication/raising-wages-key-improving-incomes-income/.

23. Economic Policy Institute, "The Economy Can Afford to Raise the Minimum Wage to $12.00 by 2020" (press release, April 30, 2015), accessed May 10, 2019, www.epi.org/press/the-economy-can-afford-to-raise-the-minimum-wage-to-12–00-by-2020/.

24. Joshua Leftin et al., *Dynamics of Supplemental Nutrition Assistance Program Participation from 2008 to 2012: Current Perspectives on SNAP Participation* (Washington, DC: US Department of Agriculture, Food and Nutrition Service, Office of Research and Analysis, December 2014), x, www.fns.usda.gov/sites/default/files /ops/Dynamics2008–2012.pdf.

25. Joel Berg, "A New Poor People's Movement Must Have Leadership from Poor People," *Talk Poverty,* May 20, 2014, https://talkpoverty.org/2014/05/20/jberg/.

PROGRESS OVER POVERTY THROUGH POLITICAL POWER

1. Saru Jayaraman and Food Chain Workers Alliance, *Shelved: How Wages and Working Conditions for California's Food Retail Workers Have Declined as the Industry Has Thrived* (Berkeley: Food Labor Research Center, June 2014), http://laborcenter.berkeley.edu/pdf/2014/Food-Retail-Report.pdf.

2. Bayard Rustin, "From Protest to Politics: The Future of the Civil Rights Movement," *Commentary Magazine,* February, 1965, www.commentarymagazine .com/articles/from-protest-to-politics-the-future-of-the-civil-rights-movement/.

THE CORPORATE STOCK IN TRADE

1. María Elena Martínez-Torres and Peter M. Rosset, "La Vía Campesina: The Birth and Evolution of a Transnational Social Movement," *Journal of Peasant Studies* 37, no. 1 (2010): 163, https://doi.org/10.1080/03066150903498804.

2. Madeleine Fairbairn, "Framing Resistance: International Food Regimes and the Roots of Food Sovereignty," in *Food Sovereignty: Reconnecting Food, Nature et Community,* ed. Hannah Wittman, Annette A. Desmarais, and Nettie Wiebe (Oakland: Food First Books, 2010), 17.

3. Henry Bernstein, *Class Dynamics of Agrarian Change,* Agrarian Change and Peasant Studies Series (Halifax, NS: Fernwood, 2010), 81.

4. Harriet Friedmann, "The Political Economy of Food: A Global Crisis," *New Left Review* 197 (1993): 29–57.

5. Eric Holt Giménez and Annie Shattuck, "Food Crises, Food Regimes and Food Movements: Rumblings of Reform or Tides of Transformation?" *Journal of Peasant Studies* 38, no. 1 (2011): 111, https://doi.org/10.1080/03066150.2010.538578.

6. Friedmann, "Political Economy of Food," 52.

7. David Goodman and Michael Watts, eds., *Globalising Food: Agrarian Questions and Global Restructuring* (London: Routledge, 1997), 13.

8. Lawrence Busch, "Can Fairy Tales Come True? The Surprising Story of Neoliberalism and World Agriculture," *Sociologia Ruralis* 50, no. 4 (2010): 331; Julie Guthman, "The Polanyian Way? Voluntary Food Labels as Neoliberal Governance," *Antipode* 39, no. 3 (2007): 456–78, https://doi.org/10.1111/j.1467-8330.2007.00535.x.

9. Philip McMichael, "A Food Regime Analysis of the 'World Food Crisis,'" *Agriculture and Human Values* 26, no. 4 (2009), 286–87.

10. José Bové and Francois Dufour, *The World Is Not for Sale* (London and New York: Verso, 2001), 55.

11. McMichael, "Food Regime Analysis," 289.

12. Timothy Wise, *Eating Tomorrow: Agribusiness, Family Farmers, and the Battle for the Future of Food* (New York: New Press, 2019), 220.

13. Mike Davis, *Planet of Slums* (London: Verso, 2006).

14. There's a story told by MIT economics professor and New York Times columnist Paul Krugman in his book *Peddling Prosperity: Economic Sense and Nonsense in the Age of Diminished Expectations* (New York: Norton, 1994), xi: An Indian-born economist was explaining his personal theory of reincarnation to his graduate economics class. "If you are a good economist, a virtuous economist," he said, "you are reborn as a physicist. But if you are an evil, wicked economist, you are reborn as a sociologist."

15. Paul A. Samuelson, "The Way of an Economist," in *International Economic Relations: Proceedings of the Third Congress of the International Economic Association,* ed. Paul A. Samuelson, (London: Macmillan, 1969), 1–11. It's tremendously interesting to see the cultural capital that the economics industry gains by the association of its annual gong—sponsored not by the Nobel Foundation but by the Bank of Sweden—with the Nobel Prizes for literature, the sciences, and literature. Yves Gingras ("Beautiful Mind, Ugly Deception: The Bank of Sweden Prize in Economics Science," *Post-Autistic Economics Review* 17, no. 4 [December 4, 2002], article 4, www.paecon.net/PAEReview/issue17/Gingras17.htm) suggests that this kind of magical authority wouldn't be possible if, say, Samuelson were the winner of the million-dollar Bank of Sweden Adam Smith Prize in Economics. Then again, the fact that Henry Kissinger has won the Nobel Prize rather deflates the entire affair.

16. Paul Anthony Samuelson and Robert C. Merton, *The Collected Scientific Papers of Paul A. Samuelson,* vol. 3 (Cambridge: MIT Press, 1991), 683.

17. World Trade Organization, "Understanding the WTO: Basics—The Case for Open Trade," accessed May 10, 2019, www.wto.org/english/thewto_e/whatis_e /tif_e/fact3_e.htm.

18. To use the title of Douglas Irwin's fine 1996 book, *Against the Tide: An Intellectual History of Free Trade* (Princeton: Princeton University Press, 1996).

19. Walden Bello, "NGO's Take on WTO in the Battle of Seattle," *Business World,* November 23, 1999, https://focusweb.org/ngos-take-on-wto-in-the-battle-of-seattle/.

20. Peter Rosset, *Food Is Different: Why We Must Get the WTO out of Agriculture,* Global Issues (Halifax, NS: Fernwood, 2006), 18.

21. Raj Patel and Jason W. Moore, *A History of the World in Seven Cheap Things: A Guide to Capitalism, Nature, and the Future of the Planet* (Oakland: University of California Press, 2017).

22. See especially Ha-Joon Chang, *Kicking Away the Ladder: Development Strategy in Historical Perspective* (London: Anthem, 2002), Ha-Joon Chang, "Kicking Away the Ladder: The 'Real' History of Free Trade," *Foreign Policy in Focus,* December 30, 2003, accessed May 10, 2019, http://fpif.org/kicking_away_the_ladder_the_real_history_of_free_trade/, and Paul Bairoch, *Economics and World History—Myths and Paradoxes* (Brighton: Wheatsheaf, 1993).

23. As cited by Andre Gunder Frank, *Capitalism and Underdevelopment in Latin America: Historical Studies of Chile and Brazil,* revised and enlarged edition (New York: Monthly Review Press, 1969), 164. We're grateful to Chang, "Real History," for reminding us of it. We've had some trouble finding the original source for this quote—Frank's source is unreferenced.

24. Rosset, *Food Is Different,* 21.

25. Ben Lilliston, "NAFTA Renegotiation: What's at Stake for Food, Farmers and the Land?" Institute for Agriculture and Trade Policy (IATP), August 15, 2017, accessed May 10, 2019, www.iatp.org/nafta-renegotiation.

26. Narayani Lasala-Blanco, "Las negociaciones del maíz en el Tratado de Libre Comercio de América del Norte," Licenciada en Relaciones Internacionales, Centro de Estudios Internacionales (thesis, El Colegio de México, 2003).

27. Timothy Wise, "Agricultural Dumping under NAFTA: Estimating the Costs of U.S. Agricultural Policies to Mexican Producers," Mexican Rural Development Research Report, Working Papers Series 09–08, Tufts Global Development and Environment Institute, Tufts University, 2009, 6, accessed May 10, 2019, https://ageconsearch.umn.edu/record/179078/files/09-08AgricDumping.pdf.

28. Institute for Agriculture and Trade Policy, "Biofuels and Tortillas: A US-Mexico Tale of Chances and Challenges," March 16, 2007, 3, accessed May 10, 2019, http://np-net.pbworks.com/f/Spieldoch+%282007%29+Biofuels+and+Tortillas%2C+IATP.pdf.

29. Wise, *Eating Tomorrow,* 219.

30. Christopher Burns, "The Number of Midsize Farms Declined from 1992 to 2012, but Their Household Finances Remain Strong," *Amber Waves—USDA Economic and Research Service,* December 5, 2016, US Department of Agriculture, Economic

Research Service, accessed May 10, 2019, www.ers.usda.gov/amber-waves/2016/december/the-number-of-midsize-farms-declined-from-1992-to-2012-but-their-household-finances-remain-strong/.

31. Lilliston, "NAFTA Renegotiation," citing Gregory Meyer, "US Farmers Rattled by Trump's Mexico Plans," *Financial Times,* February 7, 2017, www.ft.com/content/7016f032-ecf9-11e6-930f-061b01e23655.

32. Philip H. Howard, *Concentration and Power in the Food System: Who Controls What We Eat?* (New York: Bloomsbury, 2016).

33. William Heffernan, expert testimony in "NAFTA: Fueling Market Concentration in Agriculture," Institute for Agriculture and Trade Policy, March 2010, 2, accessed May 10, 2019, www.iatp.org/sites/default/files/451_2_107275.pdf.

34. David Gaukrodger and Kathryn Gordon, *Investor-State Dispute Settlement: A Scoping Paper for the Investment Policy Community,* OECD Working Papers on International Investment, No. 2012/03 (Paris: OECD, December 31, 2012), accessed May 10, 2019, www.oecd-ilibrary.org/finance-and-investment/investor-state-dispute-settlement_5k46b1r85j6f-en.

35. In the case of the 2004 ADM/Tate and Lyle decision, the ADM win of $37 million was $33.5 million + $3.5 million interest; see Public Citizen, "Table of Foreign Investor-State Cases and Claims under NAFTA and Other U.S. 'Trade' Deals," August 2018, accessed May 10, 2019, www.citizen.org/sites/default/files/investor-state-chart_16.pdf.

36. On top of the $77.3 million award, the tribunal ordered Mexico to pay for the tribunal's costs and half of Cargill's own legal fees, for a total of $90.7 million; see Public Citizen, "Table of Foreign Investor-State Cases," 34–35.

37. Tina Rosenberg, "How One of the Most Obese Countries on Earth Took on the Soda Giants," *Guardian,* November 3, 2015.

38. Lawrence Summers, "Voters Deserve Responsible Nationalism Not Reflex Globalism," *Financial Times,* July 9, 2016.

39. Christopher Bacon, "Confronting the Coffee Crisis: Can Fair Trade, Organic, and Specialty Coffees Reduce Small-Scale Farmer Vulnerability in Northern Nicaragua?" *World Development* 33, no. 3 (March 2005): 497–511, https://doi.org/10.1016/j.worlddev.2004.10.002; see also Daniel Jaffee, *Brewing Justice: Fair Trade Coffee, Sustainability, and Survival* (Oakland: University of California Press, 2014).

40. Ian Scoones et al., "Emancipatory Rural Politics: Confronting Authoritarian Populism," Forum on Authoritarian Populism and the Rural World, *Journal of Peasant Studies* 45, no. 1 (June 19, 2017), 3, https://doi.org/10.1080/03066150.2017.1339693.

FOOD SOVEREIGNTY IN JAPAN AND BEYOND

1. Jill McCluskey et al., "Bovine Spongiform Encephalopathy in Japan: Consumers' Food Safety Perceptions and Willingness to Pay for Tested Beef," *Australian Journal of Agricultural and Resource Economics* 49, no. 2 (June 2005): 197–209, https://doi.org/10.1111/j.1467-8489.2005.00282.x.

2. Yuka Sumi, Yasumasa Oode, and Hiroshi Tanaka, "Chinese Dumpling Scare Hits Japan—A Case of Methamidophos Food Poisoning," *Journal of Toxicological Sciences* 33, no. 4 (2008): 485–86, https://doi.org/10.2131/jts.33.485.

3. Dominic Smith and Paul Riethmuller, "Consumer Concerns about Food Safety in Australia and Japan," *International Journal of Social Economics* 26, no. 6 (1999): 724–42, https://doi.org/10.1108/03068299910227237.

4. Jacob Chamberlain, "Farmers Protest Japan's Push to Join 'Trans-Pacific Partnership,'" *Common Dreams,* March 13, 2013, accessed May 10, 2019, www .commondreams.org/news/2013/03/13/farmers-protest-japans-push-join-trans-pacific-partnership.

5. KYODO, "TPP Negotiators Work to Revise Trade Deal after U.S. Withdrawal," *Japan Times,* September 21, 2017.

6. Moreover, it seems likely that far from abandoning free trade, the Trump administration is simply going to pursue multiple sets of bilateral free trade agreements. These bilateral "FTs" tend to give the US even more leverage over less powerful partners.

7. Jennifer Clapp, "Food Self-Sufficiency: Making Sense of It, and When It Makes Sense," *Food Policy* 66 (January 1, 2017): 89, https://doi.org/10.1016/j .foodpol.2016.12.001.

8. La Vía Campesina, "Food Sovereignty: A Right for All," *Nyéléni Bulletin,* February 6, 2007, https://nyeleni.org/spip.php?article125.

9. Curro Moreno, "La internacional de nuestros días se klama La Vía Campesina," *Kaosenlared,* August 12, 2017, accessed May 10, 2019, http:// kaosenlared.net/la-internacional-dias-se-llama-la-via-campesina/.

10. Marc Edelman, "Food Sovereignty: Forgotten Genealogies and Future Regulatory Challenges," *Journal of Peasant Studies* 41, no. 6 (November 2, 2014): 960–65, https://doi.org/10.1080/03066150.2013.876998.

11. Hannah Wittman, Annette A. Desmarais, and Nettie Wiebe, "The Origins and Potential of Food Sovereignty," in *Food Sovereignty: A New Rights Framework for Food and Nature?,* ed. Hannah Wittman, Annette A. Desmarais, and Nettie Wiebe (Oakland: Food First Books, 2010), 2–3.

12. Mark Landler, "Trump Offers a Selective View of Sovereignty in U.N. Speech," *New York Times,* September 19, 2017.

13. La Vía Campesina, "VIIth International Conference, La Vía Campesina: Euskal Herria Declaration," *Vía Campesina English,* July 26, 2017, accessed May 10, 2019, https://viacampesina.org/en/viith-international-conference-la-via-campesina-euskal-herria-declaration/.

14. This is in contrast to many other regions of the world, where during agrarian transitions, farmer numbers fall while farm sizes expand. While land concentration is happening to some extent on the island, the stronger trend is to move out of agriculture altogether, and promote importing as a food security strategy.

15. Ruth Ozeki, *A Tale for the Time Being: A Novel* (New York: Penguin Books, 2013), 259.

16. Ozeki, *Tale,* 107.

1. See for example Sidney G. Tarrow, *Power in Movement: Social Movements and Contentious Politics,* 3rd ed. (New York: Cambridge University Press, 2011), and Doug McAdam, Sidney Tarrow, and Charles Tilly, "To Map Contentious Politics," *Mobilization: An International Quarterly* 1, no. 1 (March 1996): 17–34.

BIBLIOGRAPHY

AAP Committee on Communications. "Children, Adolescents, and Advertising." *American Academy of Pediatrics* 95, no. 2 (1995): 295–97.

ABC News. "Girl Confronts McDonald's CEO." *Good Morning America*. May 25, 2013. https://archive.org/details/KGO_20130525_140000_ABC_News_Good_Morning_America/start/600/end/660.

Adams, Walter, and James W. Brock. *The Bigness Complex: Industry, Labor, and Government in the American Economy.* 2nd ed. Stanford, CA: Stanford Economics and Finance, 2004.

Adgate, John L., Bernard D. Goldstein, and Lisa M. McKenzie. "Potential Public Health Hazards, Exposures and Health Effects from Unconventional Natural Gas Development." *Environmental Science and Technology* 48, no. 15 (February 2014): 8307–20.

Alkon, Alison Hope, and Julie Guthman. *The New Food Activism: Opposition, Cooperation, and Collective Action.* Oakland: University of California Press, 2017.

Allegretto, Sylvia A., Marc Doussard, Dave Graham-Squire, Ken Jacobs, Dan Thompson, and Jeremy Thomspon. *Fast Food, Poverty Wages: The Public Cost of Low-Wage Jobs in the Fast-Food Industry.* University of Illinois at Urbana-Champaign and University of California, Berkeley, Labor Center. October 15, 2013. http://laborcenter.berkeley.edu/pdf/2013/fast_food_poverty_wages.pdf.

Als-Nielsen, Bodil, Wendong Chen, Christian Gluud, and Lise L. Kjaergard. "Association of Funding and Conclusions in Randomized Drug Trials: A Reflection of Treatment Effect or Adverse Events?" *Journal of the American Medical Association* 290, no. 7 (August 2003): 921–28. https://doi.org/10.1001/jama.290.7.921.

Alter, David A., and Karen Eny. "The Relationship between the Supply of Fast-Food Chains and Cardiovascular Outcomes." *Canadian Journal of Public Health* 96, no. 3 (May 2005): 173–77. Accessed December 2, 2017. www.ncbi.nlm.nih.gov/pubmed/15913078.

American Federation of Teachers. "Oppose Exploitation of Schools and Students by Corporate-Sponsored Fundraising Events." American Federation of

Teachers Union Resolution. February 7, 2019. Accessed April 2, 2019. www.aft
.org/resolution/oppose-exploitation-schools-and-students-corporate-sponsored-
fundraising-events.

"Antitrust Probe of Monsanto May Turn on Anti-Stacking Provisions." *Corporate
Crime Reporter,* May 10, 2010. www.corporatecrimereporter.com/monsanto051010
.htm.

Associated Press. "As McDonald's Tries to Evolve Its Image, Criticism over Nutrition Persists at Annual Meeting," *Macleans.ca,* May 23, 2013. www.macleans.ca
/economy/business/as-mcdonalds-tries-to-evolve-its-image-criticism-over-
nutrition-persists-at-annual-meeting/.

———. "McDonald's Unveils Panel for Food Advice." *Washington Post,* May 9,
2006. www.washingtonpost.com/wp-dyn/content/article/2006/05/09
/AR2006050901167.html.

Athavaley, Anjali. "McDonald's CEO Don Thompson Leaving after Tumultuous
Run." *Reuters,* January 29, 2015. www.reuters.com/article/us-mcdonalds-ceo-
idUSKBN0L12PS20150129.

Attorneys General of Montana, Iowa, Maine, Maryland, Mississippi, New Hampshire, New Mexico, Ohio, Oklahoma, Oregon, South Dakota, Tennessee, Vermont, and West Virginia. Comments regarding competition in the agriculture
industry, submitted to the US Departments of Justice and Agriculture on March
11, 2010. www.justice.gov/sites/default/files/atr/legacy/2010/09/14/AGW-15683-
a.pdf.

Atwood, Donald, and Claire Paisley-Jones. *Pesticides Industry Sales and Usage:
2008–2012 Market Estimates.* Washington, DC: US Environmental Protection
Agency, Office of Chemical Safety and Pollution Prevention, Office of Pesticide
Programs, Biological and Economic Analysis Division, 2017. www.epa.gov/sites
/production/files/2017–01/documents/pesticides-industry-sales-usage-2016_0
.pdf.

Aubrey, Allison. "Fast Food Restaurants Announce Efforts to Serve Healthier
Kids' Meals." National Public Radio, September 25, 2017. www.npr.org/2017
/09/25/553532517/fast-food-restaurants-announce-efforts-to-serve-healthier-kids-
meals.

———. "So Long, Big Mac: Cleveland Clinic Ousts McDonald's from Cafeteria."
National Public Radio, August 19, 2015. www.npr.org/sections/the-
salt/2015/08/19/432885995/so-long-big-mac-cleveland-clinic-ousts-mcdonalds-from-
cafeteria.

———. "McTeacher's Nights: Teachers Unions Say No to School Fundraisers,
National Public Radio, October 15, 2015. www.npr.org/sections/thesalt
/2015/10/15/448960665/mcteachers-nights-teachers-unions-say-no-to-school-
fundraisers.

Auch, Ted, and Natasha Léger. "Health vs. Power—Risking America's Food for
Energy." In Articles, Data and Analysis, Guest Commentaries, FracTracker Alliance. June 7, 2017. www.fractracker.org/2017/06/risking-americas-food-for-
energy/.

Austin, S. Bryn, Steven J. Melly, Brisa N. Sanchez, Aarti Patel, Stephen Buka, and Steven L. Gortmaker. "Clustering of Fast-Food Restaurants around Schools: A Novel Application of Spatial Statistics to the Study of Food Environments." *American Journal of Public Health* 95, no. 9 (September 2005): 1575–81. https://doi.org/10.2105/ajph.2004.056341.

Avery, Dennis T. *Saving the Planet with Pesticides and Plastic.* Indianapolis: Hudson Institute, 2000.

Aviv, Rachel. "A Valuable Reputation." *New Yorker,* February 10, 2014. www.newyorker.com/magazine/2014/02/10/a-valuable-reputation.

Bacon, Christopher. "Confronting the Coffee Crisis: Can Fair Trade, Organic, and Specialty Coffees Reduce Small-Scale Farmer Vulnerability in Northern Nicaragua?" *World Development* 33, no. 3 (March 2005): 497–511. https://doi.org/10.1016/j.worlddev.2004.10.002.

Baertlein, Lisa. "McDonald's Replaces U.S. Chief for the Second Time in Two Years." *Reuters,* August 22, 2014. www.reuters.com/article/us-mcdonalds-managementchanges-idUSKBN0GM1GT20140822.

———. "Tyson Wins Bid for Hillshire in Battle of Meat Titans." *Reuters,* June 8, 2014. www.reuters.com/article/330 2014/06/09/us-tyson-hillshire-brands-idUSKBN0EK02N20140609.

Bahadoran, Zahra, Parvin Mirmiran, and Fereidoun Azizi. "Fast Food Pattern and Cardiometabolic Disorders: A Review of Current Studies." *Health Promotion Perspectives* 5, no. 4 (2015): 231–40. Accessed December 6, 2017. https://doi.org/10.15171/hpp.2015.028.

Bairoch, Paul. *Economics and World History: Myths and Paradoxes.* Brighton: Wheatsheaf, 1993.

Baker, Liana B., and Karolos Grohmann. "McDonald's Ends Olympics Sponsorship Deal Early," *Reuters,* June 16, 2017. www.reuters.com/article/us-olympics-mcdonalds/mcdonalds-ends-olympics-sponsorship-deal-early-idUSKBN1971HB.

Barker, Debbie, Bill Freese, and George Kimbrell. *Seed Giants vs. U.S. Farmers.* Washington, DC: Center for Food Safety, 2013. www.centerforfoodsafety.org/reports/1770/seed-giants-vs-us-farmers#.

Bartels, Larry M. *Unequal Democracy: The Political Economy of the New Gilded Age.* Princeton: Princeton University Press, 2009.

Bayer AG. "Feeding a Growing World Population." Bayer Crop Science UK, 2007. Accessed November 28, 2017. https://cropscience.bayer.co.uk/tools-and-services/stewardship-food-and-environment/producing-more-using-less/feeding-a-growing-world-population/.

Bell, Michael. *Farming for Us All: Practical Agriculture and the Cultivation of Sustainability.* University Park: Pennsylvania State University Press, 2004.

Bello, Walden. "NGO's Take on WTO in the Battle of Seattle." *Business World,* November 23, 1999. https://focusweb.org/ngos-take-on-wto-in-the-battle-of-seattle/.

Berg, Joel. "A New Poor People's Movement Must Have Leadership from Poor People." *Talk Poverty,* May 20, 2014. https://talkpoverty.org/2014/05/20/jberg/.

Berkeley Media Studies Group. "Health Equity and Junk Food Marketing: Talking about Targeting Kids of Color." Framing brief, Berkeley Media Studies Group, 2017. Accessed December 14, 2017. www.bmsg.org/wp-content/uploads/2017/11/bmsg_target_marketing_framing_brief.pdf.

Berne Declaration. *Agropology: A Handful of Corporations Control World Food Production.* Zurich: EcoNexus, September 2013. www.econexus.info/sites/econexus/files/Agropoly_Econexus_BerneDeclaration_wide-format.pdf.

Bernstein, Henry. *Class Dynamics of Agrarian Change.* Agrarian Change and Peasant Studies Series. Halifax, NS: Fernwood, 2010.

Bernstein, Sharon. "San Francisco Bans Happy Meals." *Los Angeles Times,* November 2, 2010. http://articles.latimes.com/2010/nov/02/business/la-fi-happy-meals-20101103.

Bertagnoli, Lisa. "McDonald's Has a New Generational Problem: Kids." *Crain's Chicago Business,* September 6, 2014. www.chicagobusiness.com/article/20140906/ISSUE01/309069980/mcdonalds-has-a-new-generational-problem-kids.

Bhasin, Kim. "McDonald's Has Gained a New Ally by Sucking Up to This Group of Bloggers." *Business Insider,* May 7, 2012. www.businessinsider.com/how-mcdonalds-works-with-mom-bloggers-2012-5.

Bienkowski, Brian. "Poor in Pennsylvania? You're Fracked." *Environmental Health News,* May 6, 2015. http://taylorsvillebasin.com/wp-content/uploads/2015/12/2015-05-11-Fracking.docx.

Bloomberg BNA. "AFL-CIO Executive Council Issues Statements on Range of Issues during Summer Meeting." *Bloomberg Government,* August 1, 2014.

Blume, Howard. "L.A. School Board Targets McTeacher's Nights, but Not All Fast-Food Fundraisers." *Los Angeles Times,* April 18, 2017. www.latimes.com/local/lanow/la-me-edu-los-angeles-schools-ban-mcteachers-20170418-story.html.

Bokamp, Samantha. "McDonald's No. 2 Executive Pete Bensen to Retire." *Chicago Tribune,* August 2, 2016. www.chicagotribune.com/business/ct-mcdonalds-executive-retirement-0803-biz-20160802-story.html.

Bomberg, Elizabeth. "Environmental Politics in the Trump Era: An Early Assessment." *Environmental Politics* 26, no. 5 (May 2017): 956–63. https://doi.org/10.1080/09644016.2017.1332543.

Bosso, Christopher. *Pesticides and Politics: The Life Cycle of a Public Issue.* Pittsburgh: University of Pittsburgh Press, 1987.

Bové, José, and François Dufour. *The World Is Not for Sale.* London and New York: Verso, 2001.

Bowman v. Monsanto Company, No. 11–796 (U.S. May 13, 2013). Boxerman, Samuel B., Joel F. Visser, and Michael Krantz. *Hydraulic Fracturing Regulation in the US: 2013 Update.* Practical Law: Multi-Jurisdictional Guide 2013. www.sidley.com/~/media/files/publications/2014/01/hydraulic-fracturing-regulation-in-the-us-2013-u__/files/view-article/fileattachment/plc-hydraulic-fracturing-regulation-in-the-us-20__.pdf.

Braithwaite, Irene, Alistair W. Stewart, Robert J. Hancox, Richard Beasley, Rinki Murphy, and Edwin A. Mitchell. "Fast-Food Consumption and Body Mass Index in Children and Adolescents: An International Cross-Sectional Study." *BMJ Open* 4, no. 12 (2014). https://doi.org/10.1136/bmjopen-2014–005813.

Brasier, Kathryn J., Matthew R. Filteau, Diane K. McLaughlin, Jeffrey Jacquet, Richard C. Stedman, Timothy W. Kelsey, and Stephan J. Goetz. "Residents' Perceptions of Community and Environmental Impacts from Development of Natural Gas in the Marcellus Shale: A Comparison of Pennsylvania and New York Cases." *Journal of Rural Social Sciences* 26, no. 1 (2011): 32–61. www .researchgate.net/profile/Kathryn_Brasier/publication/267508934_Residents'_ Perceptions_of_Community_and_Environmental_Impacts_From_Develop-ment_of_Natural_Gas_in_the_Marcellus_Shale_A_Comparison_of_Penn-sylvania_and_New_York_Cases/links/54510fd10cf2bf864cba88cc/Residents-Perceptions-of-Community-and-Environmental-Impacts-From-Development-of-Natural-Gas-in-the-Marcellus-Shale-A-Comparison-of-Pennsylvania-and-New-York-Cases.pdf.

Brown, Phil. *Toxic Exposures: Contested Illnesses and the Environmental Health Movement.* New York: Columbia University Press, 2007.

BSR (Business for Social Responsibility). *Analysis of U.S. Food Waste among Food Manufacturers, Retailers, and Wholesalers.* San Francisco, April 2013. www .foodwastealliance.org/wp-content/uploads/2013/06/FWRA_BSR_Tier2_ FINAL.pdf.

Burns, Christopher. "The Number of Midsize Farms Declined from 1992 to 2012, but Their Household Finances Remain Strong." *Amber Waves—USDA Economic and Research Service,* December 5, 2016. US Department of Agriculture, Economic Research Service. Accessed May 10, 2019. www.ers.usda.gov/amber-waves/2016/december/the-number-of-midsize-farms-declined-from-1992-to-2012-but-their-household-finances-remain-strong/.

Busch, Lawrence. "Can Fairy Tales Come True? The Surprising Story of Neoliberalism and World Agriculture." *Sociologia Ruralis* 50, no. 4 (2010): 331–51.

Butler, Patrick. "Food Banks Are a 'Slow Death to the Soul.'" *Guardian,* September 25, 2013. www.theguardian.com/society/2013/sep/25/food-banks-slow-death-soul.

California Department of Pesticide Regulation (DPR). *Pesticide Air Monitoring Results Conducted by the Air Resources Board, 1986–2000.* Sacramento: California Department of Pesticide Regulation, 2002.

California Federation of Teachers. "Floor Debate." CFT Convention 2018, March 23–25, 2018, Orange County. Accessed September 17, 2018. http://cft.org/images /Convention/2018_Convention/Amendments_Resolutions-Convention-2018-02-20.pdf.

Campaign for a Commercial-Free Childhood. "Three Million Teachers to McDon-ald's: We're Not Lovin' It." Press release. October 14, 2015. Accessed December 21, 2017. https://commercialfreechildhood.org/3-million-teachers-mcdonalds-were-not-lovin-it.

Campbell, Denis. "Ban Fast-Food Outlets from Hospitals, MPs Demand." *Guardian,* March 24, 2015. www.theguardian.com/society/2015/mar/25/ban-fast-food-outlets-nhs-hospitals-mps.

Candisky, Catherine, and Jim Siegel. "Food Banks Group Bows to Donor's Pressure on Payday-Lending Bill." *Columbus Dispatch,* May 2, 2008. www.dispatch.com/content/stories/local/2008/05/02/foodbanks.html.

Carolan, Michael S. "Do You See What I See? Epistemic Barriers to Sustainable Agriculture." *Rural Sociology* 71, no. 2 (2006): 232–60.

———. "Saving Seeds, Saving Culture: A Case Study of a Heritage Seed Bank." *Society and Natural Resources* 20, no. 8 (July 19, 2007): 739–50. https://doi.org/10.1080/08941920601091345.

CBS News. "Meet the 'Shaleionaires.'" *60 Minutes.* December 8, 2010. www.cbsnews.com/videos/extra-meet-the-shaleionaires/.

Center for Media and Democracy. "Dennis Avery." 2017. Accessed October 17, 2017. www.sourcewatch.org/index.php/Dennis_Avery.

Center for Responsive Politics. "Agricultural Services/Products–Industry Profile: Summary, 2017." Opensecrets.org. Accessed October 17, 2017. www.opensecrets.org/lobby/indusclient.php?id=A07&year=2017.

———. "Annual Lobbying by McDonald's Corp." Opensecrets.org. Accessed December 21, 2017, www.opensecrets.org/lobby/clientsum.php?id=D000000373

———. "Food and Beverage: Money to Congress, Summary 2016." Opensecrets.org. Accessed December 10, 2017. www.opensecrets.org/industries/summary.php?cycle=2016&ind=N01.

———. "Food and Beverage: Top Contributors to Federal Candidates, Parties, and Outside Groups, Election Cycle 2016." Opensecrets.org. November 27, 2017. Accessed September 21, 2018. www.opensecrets.org/industries/contrib.php?ind=N01&Bkdn=Source&cycle=2016.

———. "Food and Beverage Industry Profile: Summary, 2016." Opensecrets.org. Accessed December 14, 2017. www.opensecrets.org/lobby/indusclient.php?id=N01&year=2016.

———. "Revolving Door." Opensecrets.org. Accessed October 17, 2017. www.opensecrets.org/revolving/.

Center on Budget and Policy Priorities. "A Quick Guide to SNAP Eligibility and Benefits." SNAP Basics. Accessed August 21, 2016. www.cbpp.org/research/food-assistance/a-quick-guide-to-snap-eligibility-and-benefits.

Chamberlain, Jacob. "Farmers Protest Japan's Push to Join 'Trans-Pacific Partnership.'" *Common Dreams,* March 13, 2013. Accessed May 10, 2019. www.commondreams.org/news/2013/03/13/farmers-protest-japans-push-join-trans-pacific-partnership.

Chang, Ha-Joon. *Kicking Away the Ladder: Development Strategy in Historical Perspective.* London: Anthem, 2002.

———. "Kicking Away the Ladder: The 'Real' History of Free Trade." *Foreign Policy in Focus,* December 30, 2003. Accessed May 10, 2019. http://fpif.org/kicking_away_the_ladder_the_real_history_of_free_trade/.

Chew, Jonathan. "Report Alleges Walmart and Whole Foods Are Selling Shrimp Peeled by Slaves." *Fortune,* December 14, 2015. https://fortune.com/2015/12/14/thailand-slaves-shrimp/.

Citizens United v. Federal Election Commission, 558 U.S. 310 (2010).

Clapp, Jennifer. "Food Self-Sufficiency: Making Sense of It, and When It Makes Sense." *Food Policy* 66 (January 1, 2017): 88–96. https://doi.org/10.1016/j.foodpol.2016.12.001.

Clark, Krissy, and Henry Grabar. "The Secret Life of a Food Stamp Might Become a Little Less Secret." *Slate,* August 5, 2014. www.slate.com/blogs/moneybox/2014/08/05/how_much_walmart_gets_in_food_stamp_dollars_the_answer_may_be_forthcoming.html.

Coalition of Immokalee Workers. "Fair Food Program: Frequently Asked Questions." Accessed December 1, 2018. www.ciw-online.org/Resources/12FFP_FAQs_Formatted.pdf.

Cohen, Rick. "Gates Divestment Decision Leads to Less Than Happy Meal at Mickey D's (and ExxonMobil)." *Nonprofit Quarterly,* February 18, 2015. https://nonprofitquarterly.org/2015/02/18/gates-divestment-from-mcdonalds-lobbying-dark-money/.

Collins, Jane L. *Threads: Gender, Labor, and Power in the Global Apparel Industry.* Chicago: University of Chicago Press, 2003.

Congressional Budget Office. "HR 4719, Fighting Hunger Incentive Act of 2014," accessed May 10, 2019, www.cbo.gov/publication/45425.

———. *An Update to the Budget and Economic Outlook: Fiscal Years 2012 to 2022.* Washington, DC, August 22, 2012. www.cbo.gov/publication/43539.

Consumers International. "Advertising to Children Now Illegal in Brazil." April 10, 2014. Accessed August 28, 2016. www.consumersinternational.org/news-and-media/news/2014/04/advertising-to-children-now-technically-illegal-in-brazil/.

Corporate Accountability. "3 Million Teachers to McDonald's: We're Not Lovin' It." October 14, 2015. Accessed December 21, 2017. www.corporateaccountability.org/media/3-million-teachers-mcdonalds-not-lovin/.

———. *Clowning with Kids' Health: The Case for Ronald McDonald's Retirement.* Boston, 2017. www.corporateaccountability.org/wp-content/uploads/2017/11/Clowning-With-Kids-Health.pdf.

———. "The Olympics and McDonald's Sever Ties." *Corporate Accountability* (blog). June 16, 2017. Accessed December 21, 2017. www.corporateaccountability.org/blog/the-olympics-and-mcdonalds-severs-ties/.

Cortez, Michelle Fay. "McDonald's in Hospitals Targeted by Group Seeking Fast Food End." *Bloomberg,* April 11, 2012. www.bloomberg.com/news/articles/2012-04-11/mcdonald-s-in-hospitals-targeted-by-group-seeking-fast-food-end.

Crain's Chicago Business. "Ronald Sits Out of McDonald's 2012 Olympics Ads." *Chicago Business Today,* April 18, 2012. www.youtube.com/watch?v=Yi1sQI9kipY.

CropLife America. "Our Values." Accessed October 17, 2017. www.croplifeamerica.org/our-values/.

Dansereau, Carol. "MITC in Our Air: Air Monitoring Results, Poisoning Cases, and the Need for Action to Protect Workers and Families." Farm Worker Pesticide Project, 2009. www.fwpp.org.

Davenport, Coral. "Counseled by Industry, Not Staff, E.P.A. Chief Is Off to a Blazing Start." *New York Times,* July 1, 2017. www.nytimes.com/2017/07/01/us/politics/trump-epa-chief-pruitt-regulations-climate-change.html.

Davis, Brennan, and Christopher Carpenter. "Proximity of Fast-Food Restaurants to Schools and Adolescent Obesity." *American Journal of Public Health* 99, no. 3 (March 2009): 505–10. https://doi.org/10.2105/ajph.2008.137638.

Davis, Mike. *Planet of Slums.* London: Verso, 2006.

Deam, Jenny. "McDonald's at Ben Taub Will Not Reopen after Harvey." *Houston Chronicle,* August 17, 2018. www.houstonchronicle.com/news/houston-texas/houston/article/McDonald-s-at-Ben-Taub-will-not-reopen-after-13164791.php.

Dillon, Matthew. "Monsanto Buys Seminis." *New Farm,* February 22, 2005. http://newfarm.rodaleinstitute.org/features/2005/0205/seminisbuy/.

———. "Organic Vegetable Farmer–WARNING–You May Be Engaging in Contract Agreements with Monsanto." *Seed Broadcast Blog,* March 16, 2010. http://blog.seedalliance.org/2010/03/16/organic-vegetable-farmers-warning-you-may-be-engaging-in-contract-agreements-with-monsanto/.

"Doctors' Orders: Stop Marketing Junk Food to Kids; An Open Letter to McDonald's CEO Jim Skinner from More Than 550 Health Professionals and Institutions in All 50 States." Accessed August 28, 2016. www.odwyerpr.com/site_images/051811letter.pdf.

Drohan, Patrick J., James C. Finley, Paul Roth, Thomas M. Schuler, Susan L. Stout, Margaret C. Brittingham, and Nels C. Johnson. "Perspectives from the Field: Oil and Gas Impacts on Forest Ecosystems: Findings Gleaned from the 2012 Goddard Forum at Penn State University." *Journal of Environmental Practice* 14, no. 4 (December 2012): 394–99. https://doi.org/10.1017/S1466046612000300.

Du Boff, Richard B., and Edward S. Herman. "Mergers, Concentration, and the Erosion of Democracy." *Monthly Review,* May 1, 2001. http://monthlyreview.org/2001/05/01/mergers-concentration-and-the-erosion-of-democracy/.

Dupraz, Emily. *Monsanto and the Per Se Illegal Rule for Bundled Discounts.* SSRN Scholarly Paper. Rochester, NY: Social Science Research Network, April 1, 2012. http://papers.ssrn.com/abstract=2032615.

Economic Policy Institute. "The Economy Can Afford to Raise the Minimum Wage to $12.00 by 2020." Press release. April 30, 2015. Accessed May 10, 2019. www.epi.org/press/the-economy-can-afford-to-raise-the-minimum-wage-to-12-00-by-2020/.

Edelman, Marc. "Food Sovereignty: Forgotten Genealogies and Future Regulatory Challenges." *Journal of Peasant Studies* 41, no. 6 (November 2, 2014): 959–78. https://doi.org/10.1080/03066150.2013.876998.

Eilperin, Juliet, Chris Mooney, and Steven Mufson. "New EPA Documents Reveal Even Deeper Proposed Cuts to Staff and Programs." *Washington Post,* March 31, 2017. www.washingtonpost.com/news/energy-environment/wp/2017/03/31/new-epa-documents-reveal-even-deeper-proposed-cuts-to-staff-and-programs/?utm_term=.a0730f3dadce.

Ellwood, Philippa, M. Innes Asher, Luis García-Marcos, Hywel Williams, Ulrich Keil, Colin Robertson, and Gabriele Nagel. "Do Fast Foods Cause Asthma, Rhinoconjunctivitis and Eczema? Global Findings from the International Study of Asthma and Allergies in Childhood (ISAAC) Phase Three." *Thorax* 68, no. 4 (April 2013): 351–60. http://doi.org/10.1136/thoraxjnl-2012–202285.

ETC Group. *Breaking Bad: Big Ag Mega-Mergers in Play.* Montreal, December 15, 2015. www.etcgroup.org/content/breaking-bad-big-ag-mega-mergers-play.

———. *Gene Giants Seek "Philanthrogopoly."* Montreal, March 7, 2013. www.etcgroup.org/content/gene-giants-seek-philanthrogopoly.

———. *Putting the Cartel before the Horse . . . and Farm, Seeds, Soil and Peasants Etc.: Who Will Control the Agricultural Inputs?* Montreal, September 4, 2013. www.etcgroup.org/putting_the_cartel_before_the_horse_2013.

Faber, Daniel. *Capitalizing on Environmental Injustice: The Polluter-Industrial Complex in the Age of Globalization.* Lanham, MD: Rowman and Littlefield, 2008.

Fairbairn, Madeleine. "Framing Resistance: International Food Regimes and the Roots of Food Sovereignty." In *Food Sovereignty: Reconnecting Food, Nature and Community,* edited by Hannah Wittman, Annette A. Desmarais, and Nettie Wiebe, 15–32. Oakland: Food First Books, 2010.

Feeding America. "Farm to Pantry PSA." Accessed August 21, 2016. www.feedingamerica.org/assets/video/video-farm-to-pantry-psa.html.

———. *Feeding America: Statements, Years Ended June 30, 2017 and 2016.* Chicago, 2017. Accessed May 10, 2019. www.feedingamerica.org/sites/default/files/2018–10/2017-audit_0.PDF.

———. *Feeding Families, Feeding Hope: 2015 Annual Report.* Chicago, 2015. www.feedingamerica.org/sites/default/files/about-us/financials/2015-feeding-america-annual-report.pdf.

Ferris, Susan, Ricardo Sandoval, and Diana Hembree. *The Fight in the Fields: Cesar Chavez and the Farmworkers Movement.* New York: Harcourt Brace, 1997.

First National Bank of Boston v. Bellotti, 435 U.S. 765 (1978).

Fisher, Andrew. *Big Hunger: The Unholy Alliance between Corporate America and Anti-Hunger Groups.* Cambridge: MIT Press, 2017.

Fisher, Andrew. "Food Banks Feed People: Why Don't They Fight Hunger?" *New Food Economy,* October 25, 2017. https://newfoodeconomy.org/food-banks-hunger-board-members/.

Food and Agricultural Policy Research Institute, University of Missouri (FAPRI-MU). *U.S. Baseline Briefing Book: Projections for Agricultural and Biofuel Markets.* Columbia, MO, March 2016. www.fapri.missouri.edu/wp-content/uploads/2016/03/FAPRI-MU-Report-02–16.pdf.

Food and Water Watch. *Consolidation and Price Manipulation in the Dairy Industry: Fact Sheet.* Washington, DC, March 2011. www.foodandwaterwatch.org/sites/default/files/consolidation_price_manipulation_dairy_fs_march_2011.pdf.

————. *Grocery Goliaths: How Food Monopolies Impact Consumers.* Washington, DC, December 2013. www.foodopoly.org/wp-content/uploads/2016/02 /RPT_1312_RetailCons-FWWweb.pdf.

————. *Public Research, Private Gain.* Washington, DC: Food and Water Watch, 2012.

Food Chain Workers Alliance. *The Hands That Feed Us: Challenges and Opportunities for Workers along the Food Chain.* Los Angeles, 2012. http://foodchainworkers .org/wp-content/uploads/2012/06/Hands-That-Feed-Us-Report.pdf.

Food Marketing Workgroup. "Food Marketing in Other Countries." Accessed August 28, 2016. www.foodmarketing.org/resources/food-marketing-101 /food-marketing-in-other-countries/.

Food Research and Action Center. "Coalition Statement on Preserving Food Choice in SNAP/Food Stamps." Washington, DC, May 24, 2010. Accessed June 14, 2011. www.frac.org/pdf/foodchoicemay10final.pdf.

Fowler, Cary, and Patrick R. Mooney. *Shattering: Food, Politics, and the Loss of Genetic Diversity.* Tucson: University of Arizona Press, 1990.

Frank, Andre Gunder. *Capitalism and Underdevelopment in Latin America: Historical Studies of Chile and Brazil.* Revised and enlarged edition. New York: Monthly Review Press, 1969.

Fraser, Rebekah. "Seed Research: Seed Cleaning Takes a Bath." *Growing Magazine,* 2009. www.growingmagazine.com/article-3671.aspx.

Freedberg, Hannah. "Victory! The Nation's Second-Largest School District Ends McTeacher's Nights." Corporate Accountability, April 26, 2017. Accessed December 21, 2017. www.corporateaccountability.org/blog/victory-the-nations- second-largest-school-district-end-mcteachers-nights/.

Freudenburg, William R., and Robert Gramling. "Linked to What? Economic Linkages in an Extractive Economy." *Society and Natural Resources* 11, no. 6 (1998): 569–86.

Friedmann, Harriet. "The Political Economy of Food: A Global Crisis." *New Left Review* 197 (1993): 29–57.

Gagnon, Monica, Nicholas Freudenberg, and Corporate Accountability. *Slowing Down Fast Food: A Policy Guide for Healthier Kids and Families.* Boston: Corporate Accountability, 2012. Accessed August 28, 2016. www.stopcorporateabuse .org/resource/slowing-down-fast-food-policy-guide-healthier-kids-and-families.

Galt, Ryan E. "Overlap of US FDA Residue Tests and Pesticides Used on Imported Vegetables: Empirical Findings and Policy Recommendations." *Food Policy* 34 (2009): 468–76.

————. "Scaling Up Political Ecology: The Case of Illegal Pesticides on Fresh Vegetables Imported into the United States, 1996–2006." *Annals of the Association of American Geographers* 100, no. 2 (2010): 327–55.

Gates, Henry Louis Jr. "100 Amazing Facts about the Negro: Did African-American Slaves Rebel?" PBS, *The African Americans: Many Rivers to Cross* (blog). January 12, 2013, originally posted on The Root. Accessed May 13, 2019. www.pbs.org

/wnet/african-americans-many-rivers-to-cross/history/did-african-american-slaves-rebel/.

Gaukrodger, David, and Kathryn Gordon. *Investor-State Dispute Settlement: A Scoping Paper for the Investment Policy Community*. OECD Working Papers on International Investment, No. 2012/03. Paris: OECD, December 31, 2012. Accessed May 10, 2019. www.oecd-ilibrary.org/finance-and-investment /investor-state-dispute-settlement_5k46b1r85j6f-en.

Gearhardt, Ashley N., Sonja Yokum, Patrick T. Orr, Eric Stice, William R. Corbin, and Kelly D. Brownell. "Neural Correlates of Food Addiction." *Archives of G eneral Psychiatry* 68, no. 8 (August 2011): 808–16. https://doi.org/10.1001 /archgenpsychiatry.2011.32.

Gennaro, Valerio, and Lorenzo Tomatis. "Business Bias: How Epidemiologic Studies May Underestimate or Fail to Detect Increased Risks of Cancer and Other Diseases." *International Journal of Occupational and Environmental Health* 11, no. 4 (July 2013): 356–59. https://doi.org/10.1179/oeh.2005.11.4.356.

Germanos, Andrea. "McDonald's: Exploiting Charity to Deflect Criticism, Reap Benefits." *Common Dreams,* October 30, 2013. www.commondreams.org /news/2013/10/30/mcdonalds-exploiting-charity-deflect-criticism-reap-benefits.

Gilens, Martin. *Affluence and Influence: Economic Inequality and Political Power in America*. Princeton: Princeton University Press, 2012.

Gillam, Carey. "Cancer Questions, Controversy and Chorus at EPA Glyphosate Meetings." *Huffington Post,* December 16, 2016. www.huffingtonpost.com/carey-gillam/cancer-questions-controve_b_13679052.html.

———. "New 'Monsanto Papers' Add to Questions of Regulatory Collusion, Scientific Mischief." *Huffington Post,* August 1, 2017. www.huffingtonpost.com /entry/newly-released-monsanto-papers-add-to-questions-of_us_597fc800e4 b0d187a5968fbf.

Giménez, Eric Holt, and Annie Shattuck. "Food Crises, Food Regimes and Food Movements: Rumblings of Reform or Tides of Transformation?" *Journal of Peasant Studies* 38, no. 1 (2011): 109–44. https://doi.org/10.1080/03066150.2010 .538578.

Gingras, Yves. "Beautiful Mind, Ugly Deception: The Bank of Sweden Prize in Economics Science." *Post-Autistic Economics Review* 17, no. 4 (December 4, 2002), article 4. www.paecon.net/PAEReview/issue17/Gingras17.htm.

Glenna, Leland. "The Purpose-Driven University: The Role of University Research in the Era of Science Commercialization." Agriculture, Food and Human Values Society 2017 Presidential Address. Clinton, SC: AFHVS, 2017.

Glenna, Leland, John Tooker, J. Rick Welsh, and David Ervin. "Intellectual Property, Scientific Independence, and the Efficacy and Environmental Impacts of Genetically Engineered Crops: Intellectual Property, Scientific Independence." *Rural Sociology* 80, no. 2 (June 2015): 147–72. https://doi.org/10.1111/ruso.12062.

Global Burden of Disease 2015 Obesity Collaborators. "Health Effects of Overweight and Obesity in 195 Countries over 25 Years." *New England Journal of*

Medicine 377, no. 1 (July 2017): 13–27. Accessed December 6, 2017. https://dot .org/10.1056/NEJMoa1614362.

Godoy, Maria. "This 9-Year-Old Girl Told McDonald's CEO: Stop Tricking Kids." National Public Radio, May 23, 2013. www.npr.org/sections/thesalt/2013/05 /23/186304643/this-9-year-old-girl-told-mcdonalds-ceo-stop-tricking-kids.

Goodman, David, and Michael Watts, eds. *Globalising Food: Agrarian Questions and Global Restructuring.* London: Routledge, 1997.

Gordon, Elana. "Hospital Bids Bye-Bye to Big Macs, Others May Follow Suit," National Public Radio, December 27, 2012. www.npr.org/sections/thesalt /2012/12/17/167463286/hospital-bids-bye-bye-to-big-macs-others-may-follow-suit.

Gould, Elise. "Raising Wages Is Key to Improving Incomes of Low-Income Americans." Economic Policy Institute Economic Snapshot, June 17, 2014. Accessed May 10, 2019. www.epi.org/publication/raising-wages-key-improving-incomes-income/.

Goulson, Dave. "Review: An Overview of the Environmental Risks Posed by Neonicotinoid Insecticides." *Journal of Applied Ecology* 50, no. 4 (August 2013): 977–87. doi:10.1111/1365–2664.12111.

GRAIN. "New Mega-Treaty in the Pipeline: What Does RCEP Mean for Farmers' Seeds in Asia?" *Against the Grain,* March 7, 2016. www.grain.org/article /entries/5405-new-mega-treaty-in-the-pipeline-what-does-rcep-mean-for-farmers-seeds-in-asia.

Gray, Michael E. "Relevance of Traditional Integrated Pest Management (IPM) Strategies for Commercial Corn Producers in a Transgenic Agroecosystem: A Bygone Era?" *Journal of Agricultural and Food Chemistry* 59, no. 11 (June 8, 2011): 5852–58. https://doi.org/10.1021/jf102673s.

Gunderman, Richard. "Does McDonald's Belong in a Children's Hospital?" *Atlantic,* November 13, 2013. www.theatlantic.com/health/archive/2013/11/does-mcdonalds-belong-in-a-childrens-hospital/281398/.

Guthman, Julie. "The Polanyian Way? Voluntary Food Labels as Neoliberal Governance." *Antipode* 39, no. 3 (June 2007): 456–78. https://doi.org/10.1111 /j.1467–8330.2007.00535.x.

———. *Agrarian Dreams: The Paradox of Organic Farming in California.* Berkeley: University of California Press, 2004.

Guthrie, Amy. "Mexico Plays the Heavy on Food Ads." *Wall Street Journal,* August 24, 2014. www.wsj.com/articles/mexico-plays-the-heavy-on-junk-food-ads-1408645600.

Hamilton, Lisa. "Linux for Lettuce," *VQR,* May 14, 2014.

Harrison, Jill Lindsey. *Pesticide Drift and the Pursuit of Environmental Justice.* Cambridge: MIT Press, 2011.

Harrison, Jill Lindsey, and Sarah E. Lloyd. "Illegality at Work: Deportability and the Productive New Era of Immigration Enforcement." *Antipode* 44, no. 2 (2012): 365–85.

Hatcher, Judy. "No More Bhopals." *Pesticide Action Network* (blog). December 3, 2014. Accessed November 27, 2017. www.panna.org/blog/no-more-bhopals.

Hauter, Wenonah. *Foodopoly: The Battle over the Future of Food and Farming in America*. New York: New Press, 2012.

Hayes, Tyrone B. "There Is No Denying This: Defusing the Confusion about Atrazine." *BioScience* 54, no. 12 (December 2004): 1138–49. https://doi.org/10.1641/0006-3568(2004)054[1138:TINDTD]2.0.CO;2.

Heffernan, William. "Concentration of Ownership and Control in Agriculture." In *Hungry for Profit: The Agribusiness Threat to Farmers, Food, and the Environment*, edited by Fred Magdoff, John Bellamy Foster, and Frederick H. Buttel, 61–75. New York: Monthly Review Press, 2000.

———. Expert Testimony in "NAFTA: Fueling Market Concentration in Agriculture." Institute for Agriculture and Trade Policy, March 2010. Accessed May 10, 2019. www.iatp.org/sites/default/files/451_2_107275.pdf.

Heffernan, William, with Mary Hendrickson and Robert Gronski. *Consolidation in the Food and Agriculture System*. Report to National Farmers Union. Columbia: University of Missouri, February 5, 1999. www.foodcircles.missouri.edu/whstudy.pdf.

Hellerstein, Erica, and Ken Fine. "A Million Tons of Feces and an Unbearable Stench: Life Near Industrial Pig Farms." *Guardian*, September 20, 2017. www.theguardian.com/us-news/2017/sep/20/north-carolina-hog-industry-pig-farms.

Hendrickson, Mary, and William Heffernan, *Concentration of Agricultural Markets*. Columbia: Department of Rural Sociology, University of Missouri, 2005.

Hightower, Jim. *Hard Tomatoes, Hard Times*. Cambridge: Schenkman, 1973.

Hinds, Casey. "How McTeacher's Nights and Coke Science Betray Us." *Beyond Chron*, October 14, 2015.

Hinnershitz, Stephanie. "'We Ask Not for Mercy, but for Justice': The Cannery Workers and Farm Laborers' Union and Filipino Civil Rights in the United States, 1927–1937." *Journal of Social History* 47, no. 1 (2013): 132–52.

Holt-Giménez, Eric. "The World Food Crisis: What Is behind It and What We Can Do." *Hunger Notes*, October 23, 2008. www.worldhunger.org/holt-gimenez/.

Horan, Lex. "Catching the Drift in Iowa." *Pesticide Action Network* (blog). April 30, 2015. Accessed November 22, 2017. www.panna.org/blog/catching-drift-iowa.

Horovitz, Bruce. "McDonald's CEO Bawled-Out by 9-Year-Old," *USA Today*, May 23, 2013. www.usatoday.com/story/money/2013/05/23/mcdonalds-ceo-don-thompson-childhood-nutrition/2355129/.

———. "McDonald's Slammed over Ronald McDonald House Giving." *USA Today*, October 29, 2013. www.usatoday.com/story/money/business/2013/10/29/mcdonalds-ronald-mcdonald-house/3189709/.

———. "Taco Bell Dropping Kids Meals, Toys," *USA Today*, July 22, 2013. www.usatoday.com/story/money/business/2013/07/22/taco-bell-kids-meals-toys-fast-food/2574959/.

Howard, Clare. "Pest Control: Syngenta's Secret Campaign to Discredit Atrazine's Critics." *100 Reporters*, June 17, 2013. https://100r.org/2013/06/pest-control-syngentas-secret-campaign-to-discredit-atrazines-critics/.

Howard, Philip H. *Concentration and Power in the Food System: Who Controls What We Eat?* New York: Bloomsbury, 2016.

———. "Intellectual Property and Consolidation in the Food System." *Crop Science* 55, no. 6 (2015): 2489–95.

———. "Organic Industry Structure: Acquisitions and Alliances, Top 100 Food Producers in North America." Poster. Michigan State University, January 2016. https://msu.edu/~howardp/OrganicJan16.pdf.

———. "Too Big to Ale? Globalization and Consolidation in the Beer Industry." In *The Geography of Beer: Regions, Environment, and Society,* edited by Mark W. Patterson and Nancy Hoast Pullen, 155–65. New York: Springer, 2014.

———. "Transnational Corporations." In *Achieving Sustainability: Visions, Principles and Practices,* edited by Debra Rowe, 737–42. Detroit: Macmillan, 2014.

———. "Visualizing Consolidation in the Global Seed Industry: 1996–2008." *Sustainability* 1, no. 4 (December 8, 2009): 1266–87. doi:10.3390/su1041266.

Howarth, Robert W. "Methane Emissions and Climatic Warming Risk from Hydraulic Fracturing and Shale Gas Development: Implications for Policy." *Energy and Emission Control Technologies 2015* 3 (October 8, 2015): 45–54. www.academia.edu/download/39165483/EECT-61539.pdf.

Hoy, Kyle A., Irene M. Xiarchos, Timothy W. Kelsey, Kathryn J. Brasier, and Leland L. Glenna. "Marcellus Shale Gas Development and Farming." *Agricultural and Resource Economics Review* 47, no. 3 (December 2018): 633–64. https://doi.org/10.1017/age.2017.28.

Hubbard, Kristina. *Out of Hand: Farmers Face the Consequences of a Consolidated Seed Industry.* Report for the Farmer to Farmer Campaign on Genetic Engineering. Washington, DC: National Family Farm Coalition, December 2009. www.farmertofarmercampaign.com/Out%20of%20Hand.FullReport.pdf.

Hubbard, Kristina, and Jared Zystro. *State of Organic Seed, 2016.* Port Townsend, WA: Organic Seed Alliance, 2016.

Humphrey, Craig R., Gigi Berardi, Matthew S. Carroll, Sally Fairfax, Louise Fortmann, C. Geisler, Thomas Johnson, Jonathan Kusel, R. G. Lee, and Seth Macinko. "Theories in the Study of Natural Resource-Dependent Communities and Persistent Rural Poverty in the United States." In *Persistent Poverty in Rural America,* edited by Rural Sociology Society, 136–72. Boulder, CO: Westview Press, 1993.

Hunnicutt, Trevor. "Happy Meal Ban Passed: San Francisco Says No to Toys." *Christian Science Monitor,* November 3, 2010. www.csmonitor.com/Business/Latest-News-Wires/2010/1103/Happy-Meal-ban-passed-San-Francisco-says-no-to-toys.

Hunter, Wenonah. *Foodopoly: The Battle over the Future of Food and Farming in America.* New York: New Press, 2012.

Hussein, Fatima. "How a Group of Food Service Workers Formed a Union Underground." *Indy Star,* March 30, 2017. www.indystar.com/story/news/2017/03/30/how-group-food-service-workers-formed-union-underground/99499038/.

Institute for Agriculture and Trade Policy (IATP). "Biofuels and Tortillas: A US-Mexico Tale of Chances and Challenges." March 16, 2007. Accessed May 10, 2019. http://np-net.pbworks.com/f/Spieldoch+%282007%29+Biofuels+and+Tortillas%2C+IATP.pdf.

International Panel of Experts on Sustainable Food Systems and Pat Mooney. *Too Big to Feed: Exploring the Impacts of Mega-Mergers, Consolidation, Concentration of Power in the Agri-Food Sector.* Brussels: IPEC-Food, October 2017. Accessed October 17, 2017. www.ipes-food.org/_img/upload/files/Concentration_FullReport.pdf.

Irwin, Douglas A. *Against the Tide: An Intellectual History of Free Trade.* Princeton: Princeton University Press, 1996.

Jacobs, Andrew, and Matt Richtel. "How Big Business Got Brazil Hooked on Junk Food." *New York Times,* September 16, 2017. Accessed December 1, 2017. www.nytimes.com/interactive/2017/09/16/health/brazil-obesity-nestle.html.

Jacquet, Jeffrey B., and David L. Kay. "The Unconventional Boomtown: Updating the Impact Model to Fit New Spatial and Temporal Scales." *Journal of Rural and Community Development* 9, no. 1 (2014): 1–23.

Jaffee, Daniel. *Brewing Justice: Fair Trade Coffee, Sustainability, and Survival.* Oakland: University of California Press, 2014.

Jargon, Julie, and Anna Prior. "McDonald's Expects Further Challenges." *Wall Street Journal,* July 22, 2014. www.wsj.com/articles/mcdonalds-profit-slips-amid-struggles-1406031165.

———. "McDonald's Faces 'Millennial' Challenge." *Wall Street Journal,* August 24, 2014. www.wsj.com/articles/mcdonalds-faces-millennial-challenge-1408928743.

Jayaraman, Saru. *Forked: A New Standard for American Dining.* New York: Oxford University Press, 2016.

Jayaraman, Saru, and Food Chain Workers Alliance. *Shelved: How Wages and Working Conditions for California's Food Retail Workers Have Declined as the Industry Has Thrived.* Berkeley: Food Labor Research Center, June 2014. http://laborcenter.berkeley.edu/pdf/2014/Food-Retail-Report.pdf.

Kegley, Susan, Anne Katten, and Marion Moses. 2003. *Secondhand Pesticides: Airborne Pesticide Drift in California.* San Francisco: Pesticide Action Network.

Kelso, Matt. "Over 1.7 Million Active Oil and Gas Wells in the US." In Articles, Data and Analysis, Feature. FracTracker Alliance. March 4, 2014. Accessed August 10, 2018. www.fractracker.org/2017/06/risking-americas-food-for-energy/.

King, Justin. "Dow Sues Activists in India over Bhopal Protests." *Digital Journal,* February 9, 2014. www.digitaljournal.com/news/world/dow-sues-activists-in-india-over-bhopal-protest/article/369743.

Kleinman, Daniel Lee. *Impure Cultures: University Biology and the World of Commerce.* Madison: University of Wisconsin Press, 2003.

Kloppenburg, Jack Ralph Jr. *First the Seed: The Political Economy of Plant Biotechnology, 1492–2000.* 2nd ed. Madison: University of Wisconsin Press, 2004. http://hdl.handle.net/2027/heb.06255.

———. "Planetary Patriots or Sophisticated Scoundrels?" *Biotechnology and Development Monitor* 16 (September 1993): 24.

———. "Re-Purposing the Master's Tools: The Open Source Seed Initiative and the Struggle for Seed Sovereignty." *Journal of Peasant Studies* 41, no. 6 (November 2, 2014): 1225–46. doi:10.1080/03066150.2013.875897.

Koerner, Claudia. "These Tipping Activists Deny Being Funded by the Restaurant Lobby." *Buzzfeed News*, June 27, 2018. www.buzzfeednews.com/article/claudiakoerner/rwa-restaurant-workers-america-grassroots-astroturf-berman.

Korten, David. *When Corporations Rule the World*. Sterling, VA: Kumerian Press, 1995.

Kottak, Conrad Phillip. *Cultural Anthropology*. Columbus, OH: McGraw-Hill, 2000.

Krannich, Richard S., and Albert E. Luloff. "Problems of Resource Dependency in US Rural Communities." *Progress in Rural Policy and Planning* 5, no. 18 (1991): 569–86.

Krimsky, Sheldon. *Science in the Private Interest: Has the Lure of Profits Corrupted Biomedical Research?* Lanham, MD: Rowman and Littlefield, 2003.

Krimsky, Sheldon, and Tim Schwab. "Conflicts of Interest among Committee Members in the National Academies' Genetically Engineered Crop Study." *PLOS ONE* 12, no. 2 (February 28, 2017): e0172317. https://doi.org/10.1371/journal.pone.0172317.

Kroc, Ray. *Grinding It Out: The Making of McDonald's*. Chicago: Contemporary Books, 1977.

Kroma, Margaret, and Cornelia Butler Flora. "Greening Pesticides: A Historical Analysis of the Social Construction of Farm Chemical Advertisements." *Agriculture and Human Values* 20, no. 1 (2003): 21–35.

Krugman, Paul R. *Peddling Prosperity: Economic Sense and Nonsense in the Age of Diminished Expectations*. New York: Norton, 1994.

KYODO. "TPP Negotiators Work to Revise Trade Deal after U.S. Withdrawal." *Japan Times*, September 21, 2017.

Landler, Mark. "Trump Offers a Selective View of Sovereignty in U.N. Speech." *New York Times*, September 19, 2017.

Lappe, Anna. "What Dow Chemical Doesn't Want You to Know about Your Water." *Grist*, June 9, 2011. http://grist.org/pollution/2011-06-08-what-dow-chemical-doesnt-want-you-to-know-about-your-water/.

Lasala-Blanco, Narayani. "Las negociaciones del maíz en el Tratado de Libre Comercio de América del Norte." Thesis, El Colegio de México, 2003.

La Vía Campesina. "VIIth International Conference, La Vía Campesina: Euskal Herria Declaration." *Vía Campesina English*, July 26, 2017. Accessed May 10, 2019. https://viacampesina.org/en/viith-international-conference-la-via-campesina-euskal-herria-declaration/.

——— "Food Sovereignty: A Right for All." *Nyéléni Bulletin*, February 6, 2007. https://nyeleni.org/spip.php?article125.

Leftin, Joshua, Nancy Wemmerus, James Mabli, Thomas Godfrey, and Stephen Tordella. *Dynamics of Supplemental Nutrition Assistance Program Participation from 2008 to 2012: Current Perspectives on SNAP Participation.* Washington, DC: US Department of Agriculture, Food and Nutrition Service, Office of Research and Analysis, December 2014. www.fns.usda.gov/sites/default/files/ops/Dynamics 2008–2012.pdf.

Leonard, Christopher. *The Meat Racket: The Secret Takeover of America's Food Business.* New York: Simon and Schuster, 2014.

Lev, Larry, George W. Stevenson, Kate Clancy, Robert P. King, and Marcia Ostrom. Values-Based Food Supply Chains." In *The Sage Encyclopedia of Food Issues,* vol. 3, edited by Ken Albala, 1417–19. Los Angeles: Sage, 2015.

Leventhal, Gerald S. "What Should Be Done with Equity Theory?" In *Social Exchange,* edited by K. J. Gergen, M. S. Greenberg, and R. H. Willis, 27–55. Boston: Springer, 1980. https://doi.org/10.1007/978-1-4613-3087-5_2.

Lewontin, Richard C. "The Maturing of Capitalist Agriculture: Farmer as Proletarian." In *Hungry for Profit: The Agribusiness Threat to Farmers, Food, and the Environment,* edited by Fred Magdoff, John Bellamy Foster, and Frederick H. Buttel, 93–106. New York: Monthly Review Press, 2000.

Lilliston, Ben. "NAFTA Renegotiation: What's at Stake for Food, Farmers and the Land?" Institute for Agriculture and Trade Policy (IATP). August 15, 2017. Accessed May 10, 2019. www.iatp.org/nafta-renegotiation.

Lim, Daryl. "Self-Replicating Technologies and the Challenge for the Patent and Antitrust Laws." *Cardozo Arts and Entertainment Law Journal* 32, no. 1 (2013): 131–223.

Lin, Biing-Hwan, and Joanne F. Guthrie. *Nutritional Quality of Food Prepared at Home and Away from Home, 1977–2008.* EIB-105, US Department of Agriculture, Economic Research Service. Washington, DC: US Department of Agriculture, December 2012. www.ers.usda.gov/publications/pub-details/?pubid= 43699.

Linn, Susan. *Consuming Kids: Protecting Our Children from the Onslaught of Marketing and Advertising.* New York: Anchor Books, 2005.

Lorenzetti, Laura. "Not Lovin' It." *Fortune,* August 25, 2014. http://fortune .com/2014/08/25/mcdonalds-struggling-to-stay-relevant-with-millennials/.

Lubrano, Alfred. "Tsunami of Free Food for the Hungry Is Coming: Will It Be Too Much to Handle?" *Philadelphia Inquirer,* October 1, 2018. www2.philly.com /philly/news/food-poverty-farmers-tariffs-trump-administration-philabundance- share-pennsylvania-20181001.html.

Luna, Jessie K. "Getting out of the Dirt: Racialized Modernity and Environmental Inequality in the Cotton Sector of Burkina Faso." *Environmental Sociology* 4, no. 2 (November 2017): 221–34. https://doi.org/10.1080/23251042.2017.1396657.

Lustgarten, Abrahm. "Unfair Share: How Oil and Gas Drillers Avoid Paying Royalties." *ProPublica,* August 13, 2013. www.propublica.org/article/unfair-share- how-oil-and-gas-drillers-avoid-paying-royalties.

Madhusoodanan, Sriram, and David Monahan. "L.A. Teachers to McDonald's: Stay Away from Our Students," *Beyond Chron,* November 2, 2016. www .beyondchron.org/l-teachers-mcdonalds-stay-away-students/.

Malin, Stephanie A., and Kathryn T. De Master. "A Devil's Bargain: Rural Environmental Injustices and Hydraulic Fracturing on Pennsylvania's Farms." *Journal of Rural Studies* 47, part A (October 2016): 278–90. https://doi.org/10.1016/j.jrurstud.2015.12.015.

Marinova, Polina. "Millennials Are Driving an $18 Billion Food Revolution." *Fortune,* October 13, 2015. http://fortune.com/2015/10/13/food-revolution-millennials/.

Martínez-Torres, María Elena, and Peter M. Rosset. "La Vía Campesina: The Birth and Evolution of a Transnational Social Movement." *Journal of Peasant Studies* 37, no. 1 (2010): 149–75. https://doi.org/10.1080/03066150903498804.

Mascarenhas, Michael, and Lawrence Busch. "Seeds of Change: Intellectual Property Rights, Genetically Modified Soybeans and Seed Saving in the United States." *Sociologia Ruralis* 46, no. 2 (April 2006): 122–38. doi:10.1111/j.1467-9523.2006.00406.x.

Matson, James, Minli Tang, and Sarah Wynn. *Intellectual Property and Market Power in the Seed Industry: The Shifting Foundation of Our Food System.* SSRN Scholarly Paper. Rochester, NY: Social Science Research Network, September 1, 2012. http://papers.ssrn.com/abstract=2153098.

Mayo, Michael. "Mayo Column: Do McDonald's and Hospitals Belong Together?" *South Florida SunSentinel,* April 16, 2012. www.sun-sentinel.com/news/fl-xpm-2012-04-16-fl-mcdonalds-mayocol-b041712-20120416-story.html.

McAdam, Doug, Sidney Tarrow, and Charles Tilly. "To Map Contentious Politics." *Mobilization: An International Quarterly* 1, no. 1 (March 1996): 17–34.

McCluskey, Jill J., Kristine M. Grimsrud, Hiromi Ouchi, and Thomas I. Wahl. "Bovine Spongiform Encephalopathy in Japan: Consumers' Food Safety Perceptions and Willingness to Pay for Tested Beef." *Australian Journal of Agricultural and Resource Economics* 49, no. 2 (2005): 197–209. https://doi.org/10.1111/j.1467-8489.2005.00282.x.

McDonald's Corporation. "Company History." McDonald's Culture and History. March 5, 2010. Accessed December 9, 2017. https://Accessedarchive.org/web/20100305203439/http://www.mcdonalds.com/usa/work/companyhistory.html.

———. *Form 10-K, Annual Report Pursuant to Section 13 or 15(d) of the Securities Exchange Act of 1934, 2016.* Accessed December 15, 2017. http://corporate.mcdonalds.com/content/dam/AboutMcDonalds/Investors/2016%20Annual%20Report.pdf.

———. Investor call. December 10, 2014.

———. "McDonald's Reports Third Quarter 2014 Results." Accessed December 21, 2017. http://news.mcdonalds.com/Corporate/news-stories/2014/McDonald-s-Reports-Third-Quarter-2014-Results.

———. "Our Food, Your Questions." Accessed December 21, 2017. www.mcdonalds.com/us/en-us/about-our-food/our-food-your-questions.html.McDonald's Educates. "In Your Community: Ronald McDonald." Mcdonaldseducates.com. Accessed December 21, 2017. http://web.archive.org/web/20150314183028/http://www.mcdonaldseducates.com:80/ronald.html.

McDonald's of St. Louis. "McTeacher's Night." October 3, 2017. Accessed December 1, 2017. http://mcdonaldsstl.com/community/mcteachers-night/.

McDonald's Wiki. "McDonald's PlayPlace." June 16, 2015. Accessed December 6, 2017. http://mcdonalds.wikia.com/wiki/PlayPlace.

McKenzie, Lisa M., Ruixin Guo, Roxana Z. Witter, David A. Savitz, Lee S. Newman, and John L. Adgate. "Birth Outcomes and Maternal Residential Proximity to Natural Gas Development in Rural Colorado." *Environmental Health Perspectives* 122, no. 4 (April 1, 2014): 412–17. https://doi.org/10.1289/ehp.1306722.

McMahon, Karen. "Mycogen Purchases Cargill Seed." *Farm Industry News,* February 1, 2001. http://farmindustrynews.com/mycogen-purchases-cargill-seed.

McMichael, Philip. "A Food Regime Analysis of the 'World Food Crisis.'" *Agriculture and Human Values* 26, no. 4 (2009): 281–95.

Medew, Julia. "Health Experts Warn against Fast Food at Monash Children's Hospital." *Age,* December 28, 2014. www.theage.com.au/victoria/health-experts-warn-against-fast-food-at-monash-childrens-hospital-20141222-12c9et.html.

Meek, Andy. "Down and Out in Covington." *Memphis Daily News,* June 22, 2006. www.memphisdailynews.com/editorial/Article.aspx?id=30496.

Melley, Brian. "California Moves to Ban Chlorpyrifos, Widely Used Pesticide." Associated Press, May 8, 2019. Accessed May 13, 2019. www.kqed.org/science/1941369/california-moves-to-ban-chlorpyrifos-widely-used-pesticide.

Metrock, Jim. "Channel One News Has Lost 11 Schools Each Week for the Last 364 Weeks." Obligation.org, July 13, 2012. Accessed December 11, 2017. www.obligation.org/2010-07-13-channel-one-news-has-lost-11-schools-each-week-for-the-last-364-weeks.

Michaels, David, and Celeste Monforton. "Manufacturing Uncertainty: Contested Science and the Protection of the Public's Health and Environment." *American Journal of Public Health* 95, no. S1 (July 2005): S39–48. https://doi.org/10.2105/AJPH.2004.043059.

Mills, K., and S. E. Kegley. *Air Monitoring for Chlorpyrifos in Lindsay, California: June–July 2004 and July–August 2005.* Technical report. Pesticide Action Network. 2006. Accessed May 15, 2019. www.pesticideresearch.com/site/docs/Lindsay-CP_7_18_06.pdf.

Minaya, Ezequiel. "McDonald's U.S. Chief Mike Andres to Retire." *Wall Street Journal,* August 31, 2016. www.wsj.com/articles/mcdonalds-u-s-chief-mike-andres-to-retire-1472679393.

Minkler, Meredith. "Using Participatory Action Research to Build Healthy Communities." *Public Health Reports* 115, nos. 2–3 (March–June 2000): 191–97. www.ncbi.nlm.nih.gov/pmc/articles/PMC1308710/pdf/pubhealthrep00022-0089.pdf.

Mitchell, Dan. "How 2 Women Are Planning to Take on the Powerful Meat Industry." *Fortune,* March 16, 2016. http://fortune.com/2016/03/16/plant-based-food-lobbying/.

Mitchell Hamline School of Law. "Master Settlement Agreement." Public Health Law Center. Accessed December 21, 2017. www.publichealthlawcenter.org/topics/tobacco-control/tobacco-control-litigation/master-settlement-agreement.

Monbiot, George. "Taming Corporate Power: The Key Political Issue of Our Age." *Guardian,* December 8, 2014. www.theguardian.com/commentisfree/2014 /dec/08/taming-corporate-power-key-political-issue-alternative.

Moreno, Curro. "La internacional de nuestros días se llama La Vía Campesina." *Kaosenlared,* August 12, 2017. Accessed May 10, 2019. http://kaosenlared.net /la-internacional-dias-se-llama-la-via-campesina/.

Moretti, Irene Musselli. "Tracking the Trend towards Market Concentration: The Case of the Agricultural Input Industry." Geneva: United Nations Conference on Trade and Development, April 20, 2006. http://unctad.org/en/docs /ditccom200516_en.pdf.

Morrison, Maureen. "Is Ronald McDonald the New Joe Camel?" *Ad Age,* April 23, 2012. http://adage.com/article/news/ronald-mcdonald-joe-camel/234287/.

———. "Jack in the Box Eliminates Toys from Kids' Meals," *Ad Age,* June 21, 2011. http://adage.com/article/news/jack-box-eliminates-toys-kids-meals/228334/.

———. "McDonald's Bows to Pressure with More Healthful Happy Meal." *Ad Age,* July 26, 2011. http://adage.com/article/news/mcdonald-s-bows-pressure-healthful-happy-meal/228939/.

———. "McDonald's Sets up Shop in Silicon Valley." *Ad Age,* June 4, 2014. http:// adage.com/article/digital/mcdonald-s-sets-shop-silicon-valley/293500/.

———. "Taco Bell Axes Kids Meals." *Ad Age,* July 22, 2013. http://adage.com /article/news/taco-bell-axes-kids-meals/243244/.

Moss, Michael. "Bliss Point: The Extraordinary Science of Addictive Junk Food." *New York Times Magazine,* February 20, 2013. www.nytimes.com/2013/02/24 /magazine/the-extraordinary-science-of-junk-food.html.

National Employment Law Project. "14 Cities and States Approved $15 Minimum Wage in 2015." NELP news release. December 21, 2015. www.nelp.org /news-releases/14-cities-states-approved-15-minimum-wage-in-2015/.

Neltner, Tom. "The FDA Has Failed the Public by Letting Companies Determine 'Safe' Food Additives." *STAT,* September 7, 2016. www.statnews.com /2016/09/07/fda-food-safety-additives/.

Nestle, Marion. "Corporate Funding of Food and Nutrition Research." *JAMA Internal Medicine* 176, no. 1 (2016): 13–14. https://doi.org/10.1001 /jamainternmed.2015.6667.

Neubauer, Chuck. "Monsanto Chief Accuses Rival DuPont of Deceit." *Washington Times,* August 18, 2009. www.washingtontimes.com/news/2009/aug/18 /monsanto-chief-accuses-rival-dupont-of-deceit/.

New America. "America's Monopoly Problem: What Should the Next President Do about It?" Capitol Visitors Center, Washington, DC, June 29, 2016.

Nitzan, Jonathan, and Shimshon Bichler. *Capital as Power: A Study of Order and Creorder.* London: Routledge, 2009.

Northstone Kate, Carol Joinson, Pauline Emmett, Andy Ness, and Tomáš Paus. "Are Dietary Patterns in Childhood Associated with IQ at 8 Years of Age? A Population-Based Cohort Study." *Journal of Epidemiology and Community Health* 66, no. 7 (2012): 624–28.

O'Brien, Mary. *Making Better Environmental Decisions: An Alternative to Risk Assessment.* Cambridge: MIT Press, 2000.

Oches, Sam. "Arby's Revamps Kids' Meals." *QSR,* September 28, 2011. www.qsrmagazine.com/exclusives/arby-s-revamps-kids-meals.

Oerther Foods McDonald's. "Birthday Parties—Frequently Asked Questions." Accessed August 28, 2016. http://mcfun.com/party-faqs/.

Ogden, Cynthia, and Margaret Carroll. "Prevalence of Obesity among Children and Adolescents: United States, Trends 1963–1965 through 2007–2008." National Center for Health Statistics Data Brief. November 2015. Accessed December 4. 2017 www.cdc.gov/nchs/data/hestat/obesity_child_07_08/obesity_child_07_08.pdf.

Ogg, Jon C. "Should McDonald's Be Worth More Than All Direct Competitors Combined?" 24/7 Wall St., April 29, 2019. Accessed May 31, 2019. https://247wallst.com/services/2019/04/29/in-2019-should-mcdonalds-be-worth-more-than-all-direct-competitors-combined/.

Oklahoma Office of the Attorney General. "Oklahoma Office of the Attorney General E. Scott Pruitt: About the Attorney General." 2017. Accessed August 25, 2017. http://web.archive.org/web/20170108114336/https://www.ok.gov/oag/Media/About_the_AG/.

Oliver, John. "Astroturfing." *Last Week Tonight with John Oliver.* HBO. August 12, 2018. www.youtube.com/watch?v=Fmh4RdIwswE.

Olshansky, S. Jay, Douglas J. Passaro, Ronald C. Hershow, Jennifer Layden, Bruce A. Carnes, Jacob Brody, Leonard Hayflick, Robert N. Butler, David B. Allison, and David S. Ludwig. "A Potential Decline in Life Expectancy in the United States in the 21st Century." *New England Journal of Medicine* 352, no. 11 (2005): 1138–45. www.nejm.org/doi/full/10.1056/NEJMsr043743.

O'Malley, Michael. "Pesticides." In *Current Occupational and Environmental Medicine,* 5th ed., edited by Joseph LaDou and Robert Harrison, 573–616. New York: Lange Medical Books, 2014.

Ozeki, Ruth. *A Tale for the Time Being: A Novel.* New York: Penguin Books, 2013.

Padulosi, Stefano, Judith Thompson, and Per Rudebjer. *Fighting Poverty, Hunger and Malnutrition with Neglected and Underutilized Species (NUS): Needs, Challenges and the Way Forward.* Rome: Bioversity International, 2013. www.bioversityinternational.org/e-library/publications/detail/fighting-poverty-hunger-and-malnutrition-with-neglected-and-underutilized-species-nus-needs-challenges-and-the-way-forward/.

"Page 5." *San Francisco Examiner,* October 18, 2010. Accessed August 28, 2016. http://edition.pagesuite-professional.co.uk/launch.aspx?eid=d45ac552-1945-46fd-b51f-cd2f5d7ef764.

Pakistan Today News Desk. "This Girl, 9, Scolded McDonald's CEO," *Pakistan Today,* May 28, 2013. www.pakistantoday.com.pk/2013/05/28/this-girl-9-scolded-mcdonalds-ceo/.

Panera Bread Company. "Panera Bread Unveils Largest Clean Kids Menu of Any National Restaurant Chain, Offering 250+ Meal Combinations without Toys or Sugary Drinks." Press release. September 20, 2017. Accessed December 21, 2017.

https://globenewswire.com/news-release/2017/09/20/1125261/0/en/Panera-Bread-Unveils-Largest-Clean-Kids-Menu-of-Any-National-Restaurant-Chain-Offering-250-Meal-Combinations-Without-Toys-or-Sugary-Drinks.html.

Panousis, Jim. "Ag's Largest Advertisers." *AgriMarketing* 46, no. 6 (2008): 33.

Pardey, Philip, Bonwoo Koo, Jennifer Drew, Jeffrey Horwich, and Carol Nottenburg. "The Evolving Landscape of Plant Varietal Rights in the United States, 1930–2008." Nature Biotechnology 31, no. 1 (2013): 25.

Paris, Britt, Lindsey Dillon, Jennifer Pierre, Irene V. Pasquetto, Emily Marquez, Sara Wylie, Michelle Murphy, Phil Brown, Rebecca Lave, Chris Sellers, Becky Mansfield, Leif Fredrickson, and Nicholas Shapiro. *Pursuing a Toxic Agenda: Environmental Injustice in the Early Trump Administration.* Environmental Data and Governance Initiative. September 2017. https://envirodatagov.org/publication/pursuing-toxic-agenda/.

Park, Alex. "10 Supreme Court Rulings—Before Hobby Lobby—That Turned Corporations into People." *Mother Jones,* July 10, 2014. www.motherjones.com/politics/2014/07/how-supreme-court-turned-corporations-people-200-year-saga/.

Patel, Raj, and Jason W. Moore. *A History of the World in Seven Cheap Things: A Guide to Capitalism, Nature, and the Future of the Planet.* Oakland: University of California Press, 2017.

Patel, Rajeev, Robert J. Torres, and Peter Rosset. "Genetic Engineering in Agriculture and Corporate Engineering in Public Debate: Risk, Public Relations, and Public Debate over Genetically Modified Crops." *International Journal of Occupational and Environmental Health* 11, no. 4 (2005): 428–36.

Paul, Helena, and Ricarda Steinbrecher. *Hungry Corporations: Transnational Biotech Companies Colonise the Food Chain.* London: Zed Books, 2003.

Pear, Robert. "Soft Drink Industry Fights Proposed Food Stamp Ban." *New York Times,* April 29, 2011. www.nytimes.com/2011/04/30/us/politics/30food.html.

Penn, Mark, and E. Kinney Zalesne. *Microtrends: The Small Forces behind Tomorrow's Big Changes.* New York: Grand Central Publishing, 2007.

Perry, Simona. "Development, Land Use, and Collective Trauma: The Marcellus Shale Gas Boom in Rural Pennsylvania." *Culture, Agriculture, Food, Environment* 34, no. 1 (June 2012): 81–92. https://doi.org/10.1111/j.2153–9561.2012.01066.x.

Pesticide Action Network. "Monsanto Collusion on Glyphosate and Cancer." *Pesticide Action Network* (blog). Accessed October 17, 2017. www.panna.org/blog/monsanto-collusion-glyphosate-cancer.

———. "Undue Influence." Accessed October 17, 2017. www.panna.org/resources/undue-influence.

Peterson, Hayley. "Why the Average McDonald's Makes Twice as Much as Burger King." *Business Insider,* March 26, 2014. www.businessinsider.com/mcdonalds-doubles-burger-king-profit-2014-3.

Pfeiffer, Sacha. "Nonprofits Pressure McDonald's to End 'McTeacher's Night.'" *Boston Globe,* October 16, 2015. www.bostonglobe.com/business/2015/10/15/boston-nonprofits-pressure-mcdonald-ends-its-mcteacher-night-program/7HQToaty8suXULpDjIud6N/story.html.

Phillips, Susan. "Burning Questions: Quarantined Cows Give Birth to Dead Calves." *StateImpact Pennsylvania,* September 27, 2011. https://stateimpact.npr .org/pennsylvania/2011/09/27/burning-questions-quarantined-cows-give-birth-to-dead-calves/.

Philpott, Tom. "DOJ Mysteriously Quits Monsanto Antitrust Investigation." *Mother Jones,* December 1, 2012. www.motherjones.com/tom-philpott/2012/11 /dojs-monsantoseed-industry-investigation-ends-thud.

Phoenix, Claire. "The World's Top 100 Food and Beverage Companies of 2017." *Food Engineering,* September 6, 2017. Accessed December 2017. www.food engineeringmag.com/2017-top-100-food-and-beverage-companies.

Physicians Committee for Responsible Medicine. "Hospital Food Review." January 27, 2015. Accessed August 28, 2016. www.pcrm.org/health/health-topics /hospital-food-review.

Pimentel, David, and Lois Levitan. "Pesticides: Amounts Applied and Amounts Reaching Pests." *Bioscience* 36 (1986): 86–91.

Pitt, David. "DuPont Wins Fight for South African Seed Company." *Associated Press,* July 31, 2013. www.stltoday.com/business/local/dupont-wins-fight-for-south-african-seed-company/article_7dfca80c-a480-5a56-9b42-16a21d52bfaf.html.

Pollack, Andrew. 2009. "Crop Scientists Say Biotechnology Seed Companies Are Thwarting Research." *New York Times,* February 19, 2009.

Poppendieck, Janet. *Sweet Charity? Emergency Food and the End of Entitlement,* 1999. New York: Penguin, 1999.

Pray, Carl, and Keith Fuglie. "Agricultural Research by the Private Sector." *Annual Review of Resource Economics* 7 (October 2015): 399–424.

Price, Charlene C. "Trends in Eating Out." *Food Review* 20, no. 3 (1997): 18–19. https://ageconsearch.umn.edu/record/234489/files/sept97c.pdf.

Public Citizen. "Table of Foreign Investor-State Cases and Claims under NAFTA and Other U.S. 'Trade' Deals." August 2018. Accessed May 10, 2019. www.citizen .org/sites/default/files/investor-state-chart_16.pdf.

Raffensperger, Carolyn, and Joel Tickner, eds. *Protecting Public Health and the Environment: Implementing the Precautionary Principle.* Washington, DC: Island Press, 1999.

Ramanujan, Krishna. "Study Suggests Hydrofracking Is Killing Farm Animals, Pets." *Cornell Chronicle,* March 7, 2012. http://news.cornell.edu/stories/2012/03 /reproductive-problems-death-animals-exposed-fracking.

Rampton, Sheldon, and John Stauber. *Trust Us, We're Experts! How Industry Manipulates Science and Gambles with Your Future.* New York: Jeremy P. Tarcher, 2002.

Rappeport, Alan. "Kraft Warns on US Food Stamp Cut Plans." *Financial Times,* September 9, 2012. www.ft.com/cms/s/0/7ed1db42-f932-11e1-945b-00144feabdc0 .html.

Reganold, John P., and Jonathan M. Wachter. "Organic Agriculture in the Twenty-First Century." *Nature Plants* 2 (February 2016): 1–8.

Resnik, David B., Brandon Konecny, and Grace E. Kissling. "Conflict of Interest and Funding Disclosure Policies of Environmental, Occupational, and Public

Health Journals." *Journal of Occupational and Environmental Medicine* 59, no. 1 (January 2017): 28–33. https://doi.org/10.1097/JOM.0000000000000910.

Restaurant Opportunities Centers United. *Better Wages, Better Tips: Restaurants Flourish with One Fair Wage.* New York, February 13, 2018. https://rocunited. org/2018/02/new-report-better-wages-better-tips-restaurants-flourish-one-fair-wage/.

———. "One Fair Wage Sweeping the Nation." September 18, 2018. Accessed May 13, 2019, https://rocunited.org/2018/09/one-fair-wage-sweeping-nation.

———. *The Other NRA: Unmasking the Agenda of the National Restaurant Association.* New York, April 28, 2014. http://rocunited.org/wp-content/uploads /2014/04/TheOtherNRA_Report_FINAL2014.pdf.

Restaurant Opportunities Centers United and Forward Together. *The Glass Floor: Sexual Harassment in the Restaurant Industry.* New York: Restaurant Opportunities Centers United, October 7, 2014. https://rocunited.org/2014/10/new-report-the-glass-floor-sexual-harassment-in-the-restaurant-industry/.

Reyes, Teofilo. "One Fair Wage Supporting Restaurant Workers and Industry Growth." In *Investing in America's Workforce Improving Outcomes for Workers and Employers. Volume 2, Investing in Work,* edited by Stuart Andreason, Todd Greene, Heath Prince, and Carl E. Van Horn, 27–42. Kalamazoo, MI: W.E. Upjohn Institute for Employment Research, 2018). www.investinwork.org/-/media/Files/volume-two/Volume%202%20-%20Investing%20in%20Work .pdf?la=en.

Rosenberg, Tina. "How One of the Most Obese Countries on Earth Took on the Soda Giants." *Guardian,* November 3, 2015.

Ross, Zev. *Toxic Fraud: Deceptive Advertising by Pest Control Companies in California.* Californians for Pesticide Reform and California Public Interest Research Group, 1998. http://pesticidereform.org/article.php?id=13.

Rosset, Peter. *Food Is Different: Why We Must Get the WTO out of Agriculture.* Global Issues. Halifax, NS: Fernwood, 2006.

Rubenstein, Justin L., and Alireza Babaie Mahani. "Myths and Facts on Waste Water Injection, Hydraulic Fracturing, Enhanced Oil Recovery, and Induced Seismicity." *Seismological Research Letters* 86, no. 4 (July–August 2015): 1060–67. https://doi.org/10.1785/0220150067.

Rundall, Patti. "Have You Signed This? If Not, Act Now to Safeguard the UN from Conflicts of Interest: July 10–11 2014." *Conflicts of Interest Coalition* (blog). November 12, 2015. http://coicoalition.blogspot.com/2015/11/have-you-signed-this-if-not-act-now-to.html.

Russell, Edmund. *War and Nature: Fighting Humans and Insects with Chemicals from World War I to Silent Spring.* Cambridge: Cambridge University Press, 2001.

Rustin, Bayard. "From Protest to Politics: The Future of the Civil Rights Movement." *Commentary Magazine,* February 1965. www.commentarymagazine.com /articles/from-protest-to-politics-the-future-of-the-civil-rights-movement/.

Sahud, Hannah B., Helen J. Binns, William L. Meadow, and Robert R. Tanz. "Marketing Fast Food: Impact of Fast Food Restaurants in Children's Hospitals." *Pediatrics* 118, no. 6 (December 2006): 2290–97.

Sampat, Bhaven N. 2006. "Patenting and US Academic Research in the 20th Century: The World before and after Bayh-Dole." *Research Policy* 35, no. 6 (June 2006): 772–89.

Samuelson, Paul A. "The Way of an Economist." In *International Economic Relations: Proceedings of the Third Congress of the International Economic Association,* edited by Paul A. Samuelson, 1–11. London: Macmillan, 1969.

Samuelson, Paul A., and Robert C. Merton. *The Collected Scientific Papers of Paul A. Samuelson.* Vol. 3. Cambridge: MIT Press, 1991.

Santa Clara County v. Southern Pacific Railroad Company, 118 U.S. 394 (1886).

Saul, Nick, and Andrea Curtis. *The Stop: How the Fight for Good Food Transformed a Community and Inspired a Movement.* New York: Melville House, 2013.

Sbicca, Joshua. *Food Justice Now! Deepening the Roots of Social Struggle.* Minneapolis: University of Minnesota Press, 2018.

Schafer, Sara. "Behind the Seed Scene." AgWeb—The Home Page of Agriculture, July 27, 2012. Accessed August 16, 2016. www.agweb.com/article/behind_the_seed_scene/.

Schapiro, Mark. "Seeds of Disaster." *Mother Jones* 7, no. 10 (December 1982), 11–15, 36–37.

Scheiber, Noah. "Push to Settle McDonald's Case, a Threat to Franchise Model." *New York Times,* March 19, 2018. www.nytimes.com/2018/03/19/business/economy/mcdonalds-labor.html.

Schlosser, Eric. *Fast Food Nation: The Dark Side of the All-American Meal.* Boston: Houghton Mifflin Harcourt, 2001.

Schlozman, Kay Lehman, Sidney Verba, and Henry E. Brady. *The Unheavenly Chorus: Unequal Political Voice and the Broken Promise of American Democracy.* Princeton: Princeton University Press, 2012.

School and Community Show. "Go Active with Ronald McDonald." Accessed August 28, 2016. www.findronald.com/index_files/Page326.htm.

School and Library Show. "It's Book Time with Ronald McDonald." Accessed August 28, 2016. http://findronald.com/index_files/Page335.htm.

School Show. "Giving Back with Ronald McDonald." Accessed August 28, 2016. http://findronald.com/index_files/Page770.htm.

Schurman, Rachel, and William A. Munro. *Fighting for the Future of Food: Activists versus Agribusiness in the Struggle over Biotechnology.* Minneapolis: University of Minnesota Press, 2010.

Scoones, Ian, Marc Edelman, Saturnino M. Borras, Ruth Hall, Wendy Wolford, and Ben White. "Emancipatory Rural Politics: Confronting Authoritarian Populism." Forum on Authoritarian Populism and the Rural World. *Journal of Peasant Studies* 45, no. 1 (June 19, 2017): 1–20. https://doi.org/10.1080/03066150.2017.1339693.

Seeking Alpha. "McDonald's CEO Hosts 2013 Annual Shareholders' Meeting Conference (Transcript)." Seeking Alpha Transcripts, Seekingalpha.com. May 23, 2013. http://seekingalpha.com/article/1458281-mcdonalds-ceo-hosts-2013-annual-shareholders-meeting-conference-transcript.

Sellers, Christopher, Lindsey Dillon, Jennifer Liss Ohayon, Nick Shapiro, Marianne Sullivan, Chris Amoss, Stephen Bocking, Phil Brown, Vanessa De la Rosa, Jill Harrison, Sara Johns, Katherine Kulik, Rebecca Lave, Michelle Murphy, Liza Piper, Lauren Richter, and Sara Wylie. *The EPA under Siege: Trump's Assault in History and Testimony.* Environmental Data and Governance Initiative. June 2017. https://envirodatagov.org/publication/the-epa-under-siege/.

Semega, Jessica L., Kayla R. Fontenot, and Melissa A. Kollar. *Income and Poverty in the United States: 2016.* Current Population Reports, P60–259. US Department of Commerce, Economics and Statistics Administration, US Census Bureau. Washington, DC: US Government Printing Office, 2017. https://census.gov /content/dam/Census/library/publications/2017/demo/P60–259.pdf.

Shear, Michael D. "Trump Discards Obama Legacy, One Rule at a Time." *New York Times,* May 1, 2017. www.nytimes.com/2017/05/01/us/politics/trump-overturning-regulations.html.

Signatories. "Doctors' Orders: Stop Marketing Junk Food to Kids." Accessed August 28, 2016. www.lettertomcdonalds.org/signatories.

Simon, Michele. *And Now a Word from Our Sponsors: Are America's Nutrition Professionals in the Pocket of Big Food?* Oakland: Eat Drink Politics, January 2013. www.eatdrinkpolitics.com/wp-content/uploads/AND_Corporate_Sponsorship_Report.pdf.

———. *Appetite for Profit: How the Food Industry Undermines Our Health and How to Fight Back.* New York: Nation, 2006.

———. *Best Public Relations That Money Can Buy—A Guide to Food Industry Front Groups.* Washington, DC: Center for Food Safety, 2013. www.centerforfoodsafety .org/files/cfs_front_groups_79234.pdf.

———. *Clowning Around with Charity: How McDonald's Exploits Philanthropy and Targets Children.* Oakland: Eat Drink Politics, October 2013. www .eatdrinkpolitics.com/wp-content/uploads/Clowning_Around_Charity_Report_ Full.pdf.

———. *Food Stamps: Follow the Money; Are Corporations Profiting from Hungry Americans?* Oakland: Eat Drink Politics, June 2012. www.eatdrinkpolitics.com /wp-content/uploads/FoodStampsFollowtheMoneySimon.pdf.

———. "McDonald's and Coca-Cola—An Unhealthy Alliance." *Huffpost,* September 13, 2012. www.huffpost.com/entry/mcdonalds-coca-cola_b_1874770.

Smith, Dominic, and Paul Riethmuller. "Consumer Concerns about Food Safety in Australia and Japan." *International Journal of Social Economics* 26, no. 6 (1999): 724–42. https://doi.org/10.1108/03068299910227237.

Smith, Pam. "The Business of Seed." AgWeb—The Home Page of Agriculture, July 29, 2011. Accessed June 29, 2012. www.agweb.com/article/the_business_of_seed/.

Smithfield Foods. "Smithfield Foods Donates More then 42,000 Pounds of Protein to Support Veteran Food Drive and Mid-South Food Bank." Press release. November 15, 2018. Accessed May 10, 2019. www.smithfieldfoods.com/newsroom /press-releases-and-news/smithfield-foods-donates-more-than-42000-pounds-of-protein-to-support-veteran-food-drive-and-mid-south-food-bank.

Spitzer, Skip. "Industrial Agriculture and Corporate Power." *Global Pesticide Campaigner* 13, no. 2 (August 2003): 1.

Statistic Brain Research Institute. *Fast Food Eating Statistics 2016*. New York, 2016. Accessed December 21, 2017. www.statisticbrain.com/fast-food-statistics/.

Steele, Eurídice Martínez, Larissa Galastri Baraldi, Maria Laura da Costa Louzada, Jean-Claude Moubarac, Dariush Mozaffarian, and Carlos Augusto Monteiro. "Ultra-Processed Foods and Added Sugars in the US Diet: Evidence from a Nationally Representative Cross-Sectional Study." *BMJ Open* 6, no. 3 (2016). https://doi.org/10.1136/bmjopen-2015–009892.

Stevens, Sarah, and Peter Jenkins. *Heavy Costs: Weighing the Value of Neonicotinoid Insects in Agriculture*. Washington, DC: Center for Food Safety, March 2014. www.centerforfoodsafety.org/files/neonic-efficacy_digital_29226 .pdf.

Stitt, Paul A. *Fighting the Food Giants*. Manitowoc, WI: Natural Press, 1980.

Stoll, Steven. *The Fruits of Natural Advantage: Making the Industrial Countryside in California*. Berkeley: University of California Press, 1998.

Strauss, Robert. "Oil Makes a Comeback in Pennsylvania." *New York Times,* April 22, 2015. www.nytimes.com/2015/04/23/business/energy-environment/oil-makes-a-comeback-in-pennsylvania.html.

Strong, Andrea. "Restaurant Owners and Managers Cannot Keep Servers' Tips, per New Budget Bill." *Eater,* March 23, 2018. www.eater.com/2018/3/22/17151172 /tipping-laws-trump-budget-bill-pooling-minimum-wages.

Sumi, Yuka, Yasumasa Oode, and Hiroshi Tanaka. "Chinese Dumpling Scare Hits Japan—A Case of Methamidophos Food Poisoning." *Journal of Toxicological Sciences* 33, no. 4 (2008): 485–86. https://doi.org/10.2131/jts.33.485.

Summers, Lawrence. "Voters Deserve Responsible Nationalism Not Reflex Globalism." *Financial Times,* July 9, 2016.

Tarrow, Sidney G. *Power in Movement: Social Movements and Contentious Politics.* 3rd ed. New York: Cambridge University Press, 2011.

Thielman, Sam. "One Conservative Group's Successful Infiltration of the Media." *Columbia Journalism Review,* June 21, 2018. www.cjr.org/analysis/77-referendum-astroturf-tipping.php.

Thornton, Joe. *Pandora's Poison: Chlorine, Health, and a New Environmental Strategy*. Cambridge: MIT Press, 2000.

Tracy, William F., Julie C. Dawson, Virginia M. Moore, and Jillene Fisch. *Intellectual Property Rights and Public Plant Breeding: Recommendations, and Proceedings of a Conference on Best Practices for Intellectual Property Protection of Publicly Developed Plant Germplasm*. Raleigh, NC, August 12–13, 2016.

Tracy, William, and Michael Sligh, eds. *Proceedings of the 2014 Summit on Seeds & Breeds for 21st Century Agriculture*. Pittsboro, NC: Rural Advancement Foundation International, 2014.

Trotter, Greg. "Teachers Raising Money for Schools at Mcdonald's? Unions Want It to Stop." *Chicago Tribune,* October 14, 2015. www.chicagotribune.com/business /ct-mcdonalds-nea-mcteachers-nights-1015-biz-20151014-story.html.

Tupper, Karl, Susan Kegley, Sara Bjorkvist, and Andrew Wang. *Air Monitoring in Hastings, Florida, October 1–December 6, 2007*. Technical report. Pesticide Action Network, 2008. www.pesticideresearch.com/site/docs/DriftCatcher/FL-TechReport9–22–08-finalSM.pdf.

Tupper, Karl, Susan Kegley, Andrew Wang, Alex Lowe, Reanna Greene, and Karen Ford. *Air Monitoring for Pesticides in Hastings, Florida, December 6–14, 2006*. Technical Report. Pesticide Action Network, 2007. www.pesticideresearch.com /site/docs/DriftCatcher/HastingsFL02_19_08wc.pdf.

Tyson Foods Inc. *Annual Report 2017*. http://s1.q4cdn.com/900108309/files/doc_ financials/2017/Q4/Tyson-2017-10K.pdf.

———. "Our Story: Locations." Accessed December 15, 2017. www.tysonfoods .com/our-story/locations.aspx.

———. *Tyson Fact Book: Facts about Tyson Foods at 2017 Fiscal Year End*. Accessed May 17, 2015. http://ir.tyson.com/investor-323 relations/investor-overview /tyson-factbook/.

———. "Who We Are—Our Partners—Farmers." Accessed May, 10, 2019. www .tysonfoods.com/our-story/farmers.aspx.

United States Court of Appeals for the Ninth Circuit, No. 17–71636. ID: 11269636. Dkt Entry: 171. LULAC vs. Wheeler. "On Petition for Review of an Order of the Environmental Protection Agency, argued and submitted en banc March 26, 2019." Filed April 19, 2019.

UNITE HERE. "Food Service: 100,000 Food Service Members—And Growing!" Accessed December 1, 2018. https://unitehere.org/industry/food-service/.

US Department of Agriculture, Agricultural Marketing Service. *Pesticide Data Program Annual Summary, Calendar Year 2015*. Washington, DC, 2015.

US Department of Agriculture, Economic Research Service. "Commodity Costs and Returns," May 2, 2016. www.ers.usda.gov/data-products/commodity-costs-and-returns.aspx.

———. "Farm and Wealth Statistics: Pennsylvania." Accessed October 3, 2015. www .ers.usda.gov/data-products/farm-income-and-wealth-statistics/returns-to-operators-us-and-state. aspx#P80a07f8ba91b4b31918c3be5ae1eca3b_2_160iToR0x38.

———. "Food Security in the U.S.: Key Statistics and Graphics." Accessed May 10, 2019. www.ers.usda.gov/topics/food-nutrition-assistance/food-security-in-the-us/key-statistics-graphics.aspx.

US Department of Agriculture, National Agricultural Statistics Service (NASS). "Dairy, Cattle, and Milk Production." 2012 Census of Agriculture Highlights. Accessed March 15, 2015. www.agcensus.usda.gov/Publications/2012/Online_

Resources/Highlights/Dairy_Cattle_Milk_Prod/Dairy_Cattle_and_Milk_ Production_Highlights.pdf.

———. "U.S. National Level Data." In *2012 Census of Agriculture: United States Summary and State Data. Volume 1, Geographic Area Series, Part 51.* AC-12-A-51. Washington, DC, May 2014. www.agcensus.usda.gov/Publications/2012/Full_ Report/Volume_1,_Chapter_1_US/st99_1_001_001.pdf.

US Department of Justice. *Competition and Agriculture: Voices from the Workshops on Agriculture and Antitrust Enforcement in Our 21st Century Economy and Thoughts on the Way Forward.* Washington, DC, 2012.

US Department of Labor, Bureau of Labor Statistics, Occupational Employment Statistics. *May 2017 National Occupational Employment and Wage Estimates United States.* Washington, DC, 2017. Accessed May 13, 2019, www.bls.gov/oes /current/oes_nat.htm.

US Energy Information Administration (EIA). *Drilling Productivity Report.* Washington, DC, August 10, 2015. Accessed September 9, 2015. www.eia.gov/petroleum /drilling/#tabssummary-2.

———. "U.S. Remained Largest Producer of Petroleum and Natural Gas Hydrocarbons in 2014." Principal contributor, Linda Dorman. *Today in Energy,* April 7, 2015. www.eia.gov/todayinenergy/detail.cfm?id=20692.

US Senate. "Lobbying Disclosure Act Database." Accessed August 21, 2016. http:// soprweb.senate.gov/index.cfm?event=selectfields.

Van Sant, Shannon. "Voters Back Measure to Raise Minimum Wage for Tipped Workers." National Public Radio, June 20, 2018. www.npr.org/2018/06/20 /621726991/d-c-voters-back-measure-to-raise-minimum-wage-for-tipped-workers.

Wagner, Wendy, and Thomas McGarity. "Regulatory Reinforcement of Journal Conflict of Interest Disclosures: How Could Disclosure of Interests Work Better in Medicine, Epidemiology and Public Health?" *Journal of Epidemiology and Community Health* 63, no. 8 (August 1, 2009): 606–7. https://doi.org/10.1136 /jech.2008.085001.

Wahba, Phil. "McDonald's Sales Bleed Continues Despite Turnaround Efforts." *Fortune,* April 22, 2015. http://fortune.com/2015/04/22/mcdonalds-sales-decline/.

Warner, Barbara, and Jennifer Shapiro. "Fractured, Fragmented Federalism: A Study in Fracking Regulatory Policy." *Publius: The Journal of Federalism* 43, no. 3 (July 1, 2013): 474–96.

Washburn, Jennifer. *University Inc: The Corporate Corruption of Higher Education.* New York: Basic Books, 2005.

Waters, Rob. "Soda and Fast Food Lobbyists Push State Preemption Laws to Prevent Local Regulation." *Forbes,* June 21, 2017. www.forbes.com/sites/robwaters /2017/06/21/soda-and-fast-food-lobbyists-push-state-preemption-laws-to-prevent-local-regulation/#26362c44745d.

Weber, Jeremy, Jason Brown, and John Pender. *Rural Wealth Creation and Emerging Energy Industries: Lease and Royalty Payments to Farm Households and*

Businesses. RWP 13–07, Federal Reserve Bank of Kansas City research working paper. Kansas City, MO: Federal Reserve Bank, June 1, 2013. https://dx.doi.org/10.2139/ssrn.2307667.

"Where's Ronald McDonald?" Wheresronald.com. Accessed August 28, 2016. http://wheresronald.com.

Whiteside, Kerry H. *Precautionary Politics: Principle and Practice in Confronting Environmental Risk.* Cambridge: MIT Press, 2006.

Winne, Mark. *Closing the Food Gap: Resetting the Table in the Land of Plenty.* Boston: Beacon, 2008.

Winson, Anthony. *The Industrial Diet: The Degradation of Food and the Struggle for Healthy Eating.* Vancouver: University of British Columbia Press, 2013.

Winters, Patrick. "Syngenta to Buy Biotech Seedmaker Devgen for $523 Million." *Bloomberg,* September 21, 2012. www.bloomberg.com/news/articles/2012–09–21/syngenta-agrees-to-buy-biotech-rival-devgen-for-523-million-1-.

Wise, Timothy. *Agricultural Dumping under NAFTA: Estimating the Costs of U.S. Agricultural Policies to Mexican Producers.* Mexican Rural Development Research Report. Working Papers Series 09–08. Tufts Global Development and Environment Institute, Tufts University, 2009. Accessed May 10, 2019. https://ageconsearch.umn.edu/record/179078/files/09–08AgricDumping.pdf.

———. *Eating Tomorrow: Agribusiness, Family Farmers, and the Battle for the Future of Food.* New York: New Press, 2019.

Wong, Christina. "SNAP Restaurant Meals Program." Unpublished manuscript.

Wood, Ron. "173 Hospitalized in Chlorine Gas Leak at Tyson Plant." *Arkansas Democrat Gazette,* June 27, 2011. www.arkansasonline.com/news/2011/jun/27/chlorine-leak-tyson-plant-hospitalizes-several/?latest.

Woodcock, Ben A., Nicholas J. B. Isaac, James M. Bullock, David B. Roy, David G. Garthwaite, Andrew Crowe, and Richard F. Pywell. "Impacts of Neonicotinoid Use on Long-Term Population Changes in Wild Bees in England." *Nature Communications* 7 (August 16, 2016): 1–8. https://doi.org/10.1038/ncomms12459.

World Cancer Research Fund. Nourishing database. Accessed August 28, 2016, www.wcrf.org/int/policy/nourishing-database.

World Health Organization. "Sixty-Third World Health Assembly: Marketing of Food and Non-Alcoholic Beverages to Children." World Health Organization recommendation, May 21, 2010. Accessed August 28, 2016. http://apps.who.int/gb/ebwha/pdf_files/WHA63/A63_R14-en.pdf.

World Obesity Federation. "World Obesity Day 2017: Treat Obesity Now and Avoid the Consequences Later." Accessed December 21, 2017. www.obesityday.worldobesity.org/ourdata2017.

World Trade Organization. "Understanding the WTO: Basics—The Case for Open Trade." World Trade Organization, 2015. Accessed May 10, 2019. www.wto.org/english/thewto_e/whatis_e/tif_e/fact3_e.htm.

Wylie, Sara, and Len Albright. "WellWatch: Reflections on Designing Digital Media for Multisited Para-Ethnography." *Journal of Political Ecology* 21 (2014): 320–48. www.academia.edu/download/38253785/WylieandAlbright.pdf.

Yale Rudd Center for Food Policy and Obesity. *Fast Food Marketing: 360° Briefs, 2012–2013* (New Haven, 2013). Accessed September 8, 2018. www.fastfoodmarketing .org/media/fastfoodfacts_360marketingbriefs.pdf.

Yen Liu, Yvonne, and Dominique Apollon. *The Color of Food.* New York: Applied Research Center, February 2011. http://reimaginerpe.org/files/food_ justiceARC.pdf.

Young, Lisa R., and Marion Nestle. "The Contribution of Expanding Portion Sizes to the US Obesity Epidemic." *American Journal of Public Health* 92, no. 2 (February 2002): 246–49. https://doi.org/10.2105/AJPH.92.2.246.

CONTRIBUTORS

JAMES (JIM) ARABY is currently the Director of Strategic Campaigns for United Food and Commercial Workers Union (UFCW) local 5. Before joining UFCW 5, Mr. Araby was the Executive Director of UFCW Western States Council, where he helped lead coalitions in California to pass first-in-the-nation laws on paid sick days, banning plastic bags, worker retention in the grocery industry, and regulating medical cannabis. Mr. Araby is married and has two children, and lives in Briones, California.

KATHRYN DE MASTER is a rural sociologist in the Department of Environmental Science, Policy, and Management at the University of California, Berkeley, where her research focuses on the changing structures of agriculture in the US and internationally. Raised on a small farm in northwest Montana, she is an avid advocate for community-driven rural conservation and regenerative farming systems.

ANDY FISHER cofounded and led the Community Food Security Coalition, which played a seminal role in coalescing the food movement. His book, *Big Hunger: The Unholy Alliance between Corporate America and Anti-Hunger Groups,* was published in 2017. Andy now serves as the Executive Director of the Ecological Farming Association in Santa Cruz, California.

SETH A. GLADSTONE is the Deputy Communications Director at Food and Water Watch. Previously he served as Communications Director for the Sports and Arts in Schools Foundation, as Press Officer for former New York City council speaker Gifford Miller, and as a deputy state director for John Kerry's 2004 presidential campaign. Seth lives in New York's Hudson Valley.

WENDI GOSLINER is a Senior Researcher and Policy Advisor at the Nutrition Policy Institute, UC Division of Agriculture and Natural Resources, and a Lecturer at UC Berkeley's School of Public Health. She is a nutrition expert who works at the nexus of research, public policy, and community-based interventions to eliminate health disparities and improve population nutrition, food security, and health.

JILL LINDSEY HARRISON is Associate Professor of Sociology at the University of Colorado, Boulder. Her research focuses on environmental justice, workplace inequalities, and immigration politics. Her publications include *Pesticide Drift and the Pursuit of Environmental Justice* (2011, MIT Press), *From the Inside Out: The Fight for Environmental Justice within Government Agencies* (2019, MIT Press), and articles in various academic journals.

WENONAH HAUTER is the Founder and Executive Director of Food and Water Watch and Food and Water Action. She is the author of *Frackopoly: The Battle for the Future of Energy and the Environment* and *Foodopoly: The Battle over the Future of Food and Farming in America*. Hauter holds a degree in applied anthropology from the University of Maryland and a degree in sociology from James Madison University.

JUDY HERTZ worked as a community organizer in Chicago for twenty years, including ten years as Executive Director of Chicago's largest neighborhood-based tenants' rights organization, Rogers Park Tenants Committee. During her time there, she helped to pass the Chicago Tenants' Bill of Rights, and helped launch the Lead Elimination Action Drive, which improved Chicago's response to lead paint poisoning. Judy was also a founding board member of the National Organizers Alliance.

PHILIP H. HOWARD is an Associate Professor in the Department of Community Sustainability at Michigan State University. He is the author of *Concentration and Power in the Food System* (2016, Bloomsbury), former president of the Agriculture, Food and Human Values Society, and currently a member of the International Panel of Experts on Sustainable Food Systems.

KRISTINA "KIKI" HUBBARD is Director of Advocacy and Communications for Organic Seed Alliance (OSA). Her work spans nearly twenty years in the areas of antitrust, biotechnology, consolidation, intellectual property, and organic regulation. At OSA, Hubbard works to advance seed systems that are democratic and just, support environmental and human health, and foster biodiversity in our seed and food.

MARCIA ISHII-EITEMAN is a Senior Scientist and Director of the Grassroots Science Program at Pesticide Action Network. She has written extensively on the ecological, social, and political dimensions of food and agriculture and was a lead author of the UN-sponsored International Assessment of Agricultural Knowledge, Science and Technology for Development.

SARU JAYARAMAN is the Director of the Food Labor Research Center at the University of California, Berkeley, an Assistant Adjunct Professor of Public Policy at UC Berkeley, and the President of Restaurant Opportunities Centers United (ROC United), a revolutionary initiative to achieve workplace equity for low-wage food service workers nationwide. Following 9/11, Ms. Jayaraman cofounded ROC together with displaced World Trade Center workers; ROC United now has more than eighteen thousand worker members, two hundred employer partners, and several thousand consumer members in a dozen states nationwide.

AYUMI KINEZUKA is an organic tea farmer with degrees in psychology and sociology from the University of California, Berkeley. After completing her degrees, she returned to Japan, where her family is one of the pioneers of the global organic farming movement. After her family's farm was hit with fallout from the Fukushima meltdown, Kinezuka led the long struggle to return to the high standards of Japanese organic tea. She is guided by a passion to connect people, agriculture, and nature.

ANNA LAPPÉ is a national best-selling author and passionate advocate for food justice and sustainability. A James Beard Foundation Leadership honoree, Anna is the coauthor or author of three books, the most recent of which is *Diet for a Hot Planet: The Climate Crisis at the End of Your Fork and What You Can Do about It*. Anna currently codirects Real Food Media, which is housed at Corporate Accountability.

JOANN LO is the Codirector of the Food Chain Workers. Joann graduated with a degree in environmental biology from Yale University. She cofounded the Garment Worker Center, featured in the Emmy-winning documentary *Made in L.A.* Joann was a codirector of Enlace, an alliance of worker centers and unions. Joann was awarded the 2017 James Beard Foundation Leadership Award.

KELLE LOUAILLIER is President Emeritus of Corporate Accountability, a member-powered organization that for more than forty years has stopped transnational corporations from devastating democracy, trampling human rights, and destroying our planet. Since its inception as the Infant Formula Action Coalition (INFACT), the organization has effectively challenged a range of food industry abuses. Louaillier was on the leadership team that stewarded the organization through boycotts of Kraft and Nabisco. Also under her leadership, Corporate Accountability launched interrelated campaigns on food, water, and climate change that are shifting the landscape on corporate control and food democracy.

KRISTINE MADSEN is an Associate Professor at UC Berkeley's School of Public Health and the Faculty Director for the Berkeley Food Institute. She is a pediatrician and research scientist with expertise in the design and evaluation of interventions related to pediatric obesity, cardiovascular risk, and health disparities.

STEPHANIE A. MALIN is an environmental sociologist in Colorado State University's Department of Sociology. She specializes in sociological and ecological impacts of natural resource extraction, environmental justice and health, and governance.

EMILY MARQUEZ has a research background in comparative endocrinology, reproductive development, and endocrine disruption and is currently a Staff Scientist at Pesticide Action Network (PAN). Emily works in PAN's Grassroots Science Program, managing PAN air-monitoring work using the Drift Catcher with community partners.

MAYWA MONTENEGRO DE WIT is a President's Postdoctoral Fellow at the University of California, Davis. With a background in molecular biology and science journalism, she combines political ecology, geography, and science and technology studies to examine the knowledge politics underpinning struggles for seeds.

MARION NESTLE is Professor and Chair of the Department of Nutrition and Food Studies at New York University. Author of *Nutrition in Clinical Practice*

(1985), she has served as a nutrition policy advisor to the Department of Health and Human Services and as a member of nutrition and science advisory committees to the U.S. Department of Agriculture and the Food and Drug Administration. She is the author of *Safe Food: Bacteria, Biotechnology, and Bioterrorism* (California, 2003), *Pet Food Politics: The Chihuahua in the Coal Mine* (California, 2010), and *Why Calories Count: From Science to Politics* (California, 2012), among other books.

JOSE OLIVA is the Codirector of the Food Chain Workers Alliance and has served in several leadership positions for Restaurant Opportunities Center. He was the Executive Director of Casa Guatemala, where he began to organize Chicago day laborers. He founded the Chicago Interfaith Workers' Center and was the coordinator for the Workers' Alliance for a Just Economy. Jose is a 2017 James Beard Award recipient.

RAJ PATEL is an award-winning writer, activist, and scholar, and a member of the International Panel of Experts on Sustainable Food Systems. In 2009 he joined the advisory board of Corporate Accountability International's Value the Meal campaign, and in 2016 he was recognized with a James Beard Foundation Leadership Award. Raj regularly writes for the *Guardian* and has contributed to the *Financial Times, Los Angeles Times, New York Times,* and *San Francisco Chronicle.* His first of several notable books was *Stuffed and Starved: The Hidden Battle for the World Food System.*

KRISTIN SCHAFER has held many roles at the Pesticide Action Network (PAN) and is currently the Executive Director of PAN. Before joining PAN in 1996, Kristin worked for the World Resources Institute's Sustainable Agriculture Program, as a Communications Specialist for the EPA, and as an Agro-forestry Extension Officer with the Peace Corps in Kenya.

Food Research Lab (Japan): and contamination testing, 193–94; as non-corporate community based science, 194–95; and policy advocacy, 195–96; and the "Positive List" regulatory system, 194

food sovereignty: as alternative to international free trade, 197; American exceptionalism disguised as, 198–99; defined, 197; vs. globalization and racist-nationalist populism, 196–97; interdependence focus of, 200; in Japanese contexts, 198; and trade dumping impact on peasants, 197

food sovereignty movements: against the TPP (in Japan), 194–96; confronting nationalism and patriarchy, 198–99; and food movements, 196–97; and Food Research Lab (Japan), 194; and food sufficiency (defined), 193, 197; La Vía Campesina, 175, 189, 191, 197, 199; and nationalism vs. international anti-corporatist solidarity, 198–200; and Nouminren (in Japan), 177, 192–93, 197–201; as reaction to trade policy, 197; and *time being* values, 200–201

Food Stamps: Follow the Money, 153

food stamps. *See* SNAP program

food system consolidation: and corporate decision-making, 3; extent of control over food production, 102; and factory farms (animal abuses), 131; industrialization and globalization of, 1–2; and international trade, 178–80; and labor exploitation, 102, 161–63; limits of consumption-based alternatives, 5–6; and small and mid-size farmers, 61–62, 69, 78, 80–81, 186–87; and Tyson Foods Inc., 102; in the US with NAFTA, 186–87; and vertical integration of supply chains, 2–3, 80, 132, 160–61, 182, 205. *See also* international capitalist food system; *specific trade agreements*

food system marketing and branding: through charities, 127, 136–38; and corporate citizenship messaging, 2, 4; and food bank philanthropy, 150; impact on children's health, 134; and McDonald's in hospitals, 134–35

food system workers: of color, 104; and exploitation, 101–2, 181–82; and food insecurity, 76, 101, 161–62, 163; and gender discrimination, 7, 104–5; in grocery stores, 161; health and safety issues (injuries and working while sick), 100, 101, 103–4; historical struggles of, 107–8; and sick day benefits, 9, 110, 113, 116, 160, 167; and unionization, 107, 108–9; use of food stamps, 101, 151; and wage inequities, 102–3

Forbes, 142

Fortuna Energy (later Talisman Energy), 92, 93

FRAC (Food Research & Action Center), 151, 153

Frack Action, 87

fracking. *See* hydraulic fracturing

Freedom, 90, 156–57

free trade, 176, 180–84, 184*fig.*, 187–90, 192–93; and comparative advantage, 180–82; externalities, 190; and the Green Revolution, 178; modern institutions of, 176; nation-based opposition to, 187–90; and Nouminren (Japan), 177, 192–93; and the state, 178–80. *See also* GATT; ISDS; NAFTA; TPP; World Trade Organization

free trade, 176, 180–84, 184*fig.*, 187–90, 192–93

Friedmann, Harriet, 178, 179

Friends of the Earth (international environmental advocacy group), 32

"front groups," 127

Frost, Edmund, 45, 46

Gaines, Tianna, 147

Gates Foundation, corporate divestments, 141

GATT (Global Agreement on Tariffs and Trade), 178–79, 181–82, 187: and global expansion of free trade, 187–90. *See also* World Trade Organization (WTO)

gender: discrimination, 7, 104–6; and hunger in women of color, 147, 155; and international food sovereignty movements, 198–99; and restaurant workers, 112, 114, 115–16

immigrant workers *(continued)*
    pesticide exposure, 54–55; and Proposi-
    tion 170, 187; undocumented, 55, 106,
    170; and unionization, 108
Indigenous SeedKeepers Network, 43
industrial diets: and corporate alteration of
    what we eat, 1; defined, 121; and fast
    food expansion, 122; and food additives,
    123; health impacts of, 9, 121–22, 126,
    131, 138, 189; and health problems in
    Japan, 193; and the international food
    system, 192–93; and millennials, 128;
    and negative externalities, 122–23, 126;
    and plant based food alternatives, 128;
    and political will for change, 128
"inevitability narrative," 4–5, 86
insect die-off, 25
insecticidal toxins, 20
Institute for Agriculture and Trade Policy
    (IATP), 187
Intellectual Property Committee, 28
intellectual property (IP) rights: connec-
    tion with monopolies, 34, 35; cross-
    licensing agreements, 20–22; *Diamond
    v. Chakrabarty*, 27; in the EU, 27–28;
    impact on seed saving, 25, 27–28; and
    non-GE seeds (restrictions on use after
    purchase), 27; and open source/access
    licensing initiative, 40–41; and the
    Plant Patent Act of 1930, 27; Plant
    Variety Protection Act (PVPA) of 1970,
    27; and privatization of public
    resources, 9, 35, 39; public sector best
    practices statement on, 40; spread of US
    decisions to other countries, 27–28; and
    trade agreements, 28, 29
international capitalist food system: and
    agricultural chemical company domi-
    nance, 178; and the food industry's
    "stakeholder" status, 141; and free trade
    global politics, 176; and post-World War
    II overproduction, 177–78, 186; repeal
    of Corn Laws and early industrial
    development, 177; and state subordina-
    tion to private interests, 178–80. *See also*
    food system consolidation; *specific trade
    agreements*
"Invest an Acre" program (Monsanto), 151

Iowa Citizens for Community Improve-
    ment, 34
ISDS (investor-state dispute settlement)
    mechanism, 188–89
Ishii-Eiteman, Marcia, 9, 294
"Is Ronald McDonald the new Joe
    Camel?," 133

Japanese agriculture: and corporate inter-
    ests, 195; and farmer protests against the
    TPP, 196; and post-World War II
    decline, 192–93; restructuring for
    international trade (TPP and RCEP),
    194–95; and rice farmer wages, 193. *See
    also* Food Research Lab; Nouminren
Jayaraman, Saru, ix, 9, 106, 294
JBS and NAFTA, 187
Jefferson Elementary Federation of Teach-
    ers, 137
Joe Camel-Ronald McDonald juxtaposi-
    tion, 132–33
joint-ventures, in GE technologies, 20
junk food. *See* fast food
JWJ (Jobs with Justice) alliance, 165–66

Kegley, Susan, Dr., 63
Keidanren (Japanese business federation),
    195
Kellett, Gigi, 140, 141
Kinezuka, Ayumi, 10, 294–95
Kleeger, Sarah and Andrew Still, 43–44,
    45, 46
Kloppenburg, Jack, 4, 41
Korea Advanced Farmers Federation, 175
Korean Peasant Association, 175
Korean Peasant League, 175
Korten, David, 2, 6
Kraft, and SNAP program (food stamp
    sales), 153
Kroc, Ray, 126
Kroger, and food bank board composition,
    149
Kuzemchak, Sally, 133

labeling campaigns, corporate resistance to,
    21–22
labor: overview of in US economy, 101–2;
    and food industry consolidation, 18–19,

vertical integration, 2–3
La Vía Campesina, 175, 189, 191, 197, 199
Vollinger, Ellen, 153
"vote with our fork" narrative, 5–6, 205

wages: and the anti-hunger sector, 154–57; and corporate anti-hunger philanthropy, 150–51; and FRAC, 151; and tip theft, 104, 105*fig.*, 106, 110–12; and UFCW anti-hunger organizing strategies, 159–60; union and non-union in California, 161; and Walmart, 151; and working conditions of farmworkers, 108. *See also* minimum wages
Walmart: and anti-hunger philanthropy, 150–51; employee use of public assistance (low food security), 161–62; and food bank board composition, 149; opposition to $15 per hour minimum wage bill, 168; SNAP program beneficiary, 153
Warren, Elizabeth, 46–47
Water Defense, 87
Watts, Michael, 179
Wells Fargo, and food bank board composition, 149
Wells, Linda, 69
Western Growers Association, 61
Western Organization of Resource Councils, 36
Western States Council (UFCW), 161, 167, 168–69
When Corporations Rule the World (Korten), 2
WHO Framework Convention on Tobacco Control (Article 5.3), 141
wildlife refuges, 36

Winson, Anthony, 122
Wise, Timothy, 186
Witnesses to Hunger, 147–48
women of color, 147, 155. *See also* gender; race/ethnicity
workers' health and safety, 58, 99–101, 103–4
"World Food Board," 179
World Health Assembly (WHO), 140–41
World Trade Organization (WTO): and the comparative advantage myth (magical thinking), 180–82; and comparative advantage theory, 181–82; and country of origin labeling, 188; fallacious egalitarianism of comparative advantage (consumer benefits myth), 182–83; farmer resistance to, 175–77; historical overview of, 177–80; impact on Global South farmers, 175–76; and IP provisions in agricultural policy, 187–88; and ISDS (investor-state dispute settlement) mechanism, 188–89; and Japan, 194; and La Vía Campesina (LVC), 189–90; maintenance of superpower advantage, 183–85; Mexican opposition to, 175, 189, 191; and private global regulation, 178–79; reformist vs. populist responses to, 190–91; and state procurement policies, 188. *See also* GATT; NAFTA; TPP
"WTO! Kills. FARMERS," 175

"yogurt summit," 94
Yum! Brands (Taco Bell, KFC, Pizza Hut) and SNAP, 153

Zen master Dogen Zenji, 200–201

Founded in 1893,
UNIVERSITY OF CALIFORNIA PRESS
publishes bold, progressive books and journals
on topics in the arts, humanities, social sciences,
and natural sciences—with a focus on social
justice issues—that inspire thought and action
among readers worldwide.

The UC PRESS FOUNDATION
raises funds to uphold the press's vital role
as an independent, nonprofit publisher, and
receives philanthropic support from a wide
range of individuals and institutions—and from
committed readers like you. To learn more, visit
ucpress.edu/supportus.

lton Keynes UK
ram Content Group UK Ltd.
HW010117200124
347UK00005B/379